VOLUME EIGHTY THREE

ADVANCES IN PHARMACOLOGY

VOLUME EIGHTY THREE

ADVANCES IN PHARMACOLOGY

Pharmacogenetics

Edited by

KIM BRØSEN
Institute of Public Health, Clinical Pharmacology, Denmark

PER DAMKIER
Department of Clinical Biochemistry and Pharmacology, Odense University Hospital; Department of Clinical Research, University of Southern Denmark, Odense, Denmark

Serial Editor

S.J. ENNA
University of Kansas Medical Center, Kansas City, KS, United States

Managing Editor

LYNN LECOUNT
University of Kansas Medical Center, School of Medicine, Kansas City, KS, United States

ELSEVIER

ACADEMIC PRESS
An imprint of Elsevier

Academic Press is an imprint of Elsevier
50 Hampshire Street, 5th Floor, Cambridge, MA 02139, United States
525 B Street, Suite 1650, San Diego, CA 92101, United States
The Boulevard, Langford Lane, Kidlington, Oxford OX5 1GB, United Kingdom
125 London Wall, London, EC2Y 5AS, United Kingdom

First edition 2018

ISBN: 978-0-12-813381-1
ISSN: 1054-3589

Publisher: Zoe Kruze
Acquisition Editor: Zoe Kruze
Editorial Project Manager: Shellie Bryant
Production Project Manager: Vignesh Tamil
Cover Designer: Miles Hitchen

Typeset by SPi Global, India

CONTENTS

Contributors *xi*
Preface *xv*

Section I
Cytochrome P450

1. Cytochrome P450 in Pharmacogenetics: An Update **3**

Aleksi Tornio and Janne T. Backman

1. Introduction 4
2. Genetic Variability of CYP Enzymes 6
3. CYP1A Subfamily 7
4. CYP2A and CYP2B Subfamilies 8
5. CYP2C Subfamily 10
6. CYP2D6 18
7. CYP3A Subfamily 21
8. Conclusion 23

References 25

2. Epigenetics and MicroRNAs in Pharmacogenetics **33**

Ulrich M. Zanger, Kathrin Klein, Nicole Kugler, Tamara Petrikat, and Chang S. Ryu

1. Introduction 34
2. Epigenetics in Pharmacogenetics 36
3. miRNAs in Pharmacogenetics 40
4. Conclusion 56

Acknowledgments 57
References 57

3. Tamoxifen and CYP2D6: A Controversy in Pharmacogenetics **65**

Deirdre P. Cronin-Fenton and Per Damkier

1. Introduction 66
2. CYP2D6 and Tamoxifen Metabolism 69
3. Perspectives 79
4. Conclusion 83

Acknowledgments 83
References 83

Section II
Methods

4. Imaging in Pharmacogenetics **95**

Mikkel H. Vendelbo, Lars C. Gormsen, and Niels Jessen

1. Introduction 95
2. Imaging Modalities 96
3. Absorption 99
4. Distribution 100
5. Metabolism 102
6. Elimination 103
7. Conclusion 104

References 104

5. Pharmacoepidemiology in Pharmacogenetics **109**

Thomas P. Ahern

1. Introduction 109
2. Study Design 110
3. Bias and Validity 121
4. Conclusion 128

Further Reading 128

References 129

Section III
Special Themes

6. Population Diversity in Pharmacogenetics: A Latin American Perspective **133**

Guilherme Suarez-Kurtz and Esteban J. Parra

1. Introduction 134
2. Global Distribution of PGx Variants 139
3. Population Admixture in Latin America: Pharmacogenomic Implications 141
4. Pharmacogenetics of TAC: CYP3A5 Polymorphisms 145
5. Population Diversity and Warfarin Dosing Algorithms 147
6. Conclusion 150

Acknowledgments 151

References 151

7. Pharmacogenetics of Adverse Drug Reactions **155**
Orod Osanlou, Munir Pirmohamed, and Ann K. Daly
1. Introduction 156
2. Genetic Predisposition to Type A ADRs 161
3. Genetic Predisposition to Type B ADRs 165
4. Current Examples of Genetic Testing to Prevent ADRs 179
5. Future Prospects 180
6. Conclusion 181
References 182

8. Pharmacogenetics: Applications to Pediatric Patients **191**
Tiphaine Adam de Beaumais and Evelyne Jacqz-Aigrain
1. Introduction 192
2. Developmental Pharmacology and Pharmacogenetics 192
3. Clinical Applications 194
4. Conclusion 206
References 208

Section IV
Pharmacogenetics in Therapy

9. Implementation of Pharmacogenomics in Everyday Clinical Settings **219**
Paul C.D. Bank, Jesse J. Swen, and Henk-Jan Guchelaar
1. Introduction 220
2. Players in the Field 220
3. Challenges for Implementation of PGx 223
4. Conclusion 239
Acknowledgments 239
References 240

10. Pharmacogenetics in Pain Treatment **247**
Ana M. Peiró
1. Introduction 248
2. Pharmacogenetics Applied to the Treatment of Pain 253
3. Conclusion 267
Acknowledgments 268
References 268
Further Reading 272

11. The Pharmacogenetics of Immune-Modulating Therapy **275**
Ingolf Cascorbi
1. Introduction 276
2. Azathioprine/Mercaptopurine 277
3. Methotrexate 280
4. Mycophenolate 281
5. Calcineurin Inhibitors 283
6. Sirolimus 288
7. Conclusion 288
References 291

12. Pharmacogenetics in Psychiatry **297**
Filippo Corponi, Chiara Fabbri, and Alessandro Serretti
1. Introduction 299
2. Antidepressants 301
3. Mood Stabilizers 311
4. Antipsychotics 315
5. Conclusion 323
References 325

13. Pharmacogenetics in Cardiovascular Medicine **333**
Peter E. Weeke
1. Introduction 334
2. Cardiovascular-Specific Drug Responses 336
3. Drug-Induced Long QT Syndrome 346
4. Implementation Challenges 347
5. Conclusion 349
References 350
Further Reading 360

14. Pharmacogenetics of Antidiabetic Drugs **361**
Shylaja Srinivasan, Sook Wah Yee, and Kathleen M. Giacomini
1. Introduction 362
2. Discovery of Genetic Loci Related to Metformin Response Through Genome-Wide Approaches 362
3. Genome-Wide Screening to Elucidate Metformin Action Through in vitro Assays 369

4. Studies Related to Metformin Candidate Genes 371
5. Genetic Studies of Other Antidiabetic Drugs 375
6. Conclusion 381
Acknowledgment 382
References 382

CONTRIBUTORS

Thomas P. Ahern
Department of Surgery; Department of Biochemistry, The Robert Larner, M.D. College of Medicine, University of Vermont, Burlington, VT, United States

Janne T. Backman
Department of Clinical Pharmacology, University of Helsinki and Helsinki University Hospital, Helsinki, Finland

Paul C.D. Bank
Department of Clinical Pharmacy & Toxicology, Leiden University Medical Center, Leiden, The Netherlands

Ingolf Cascorbi
Institute of Experimental and Clinical Pharmacology, University Hospital Schleswig-Holstein, Kiel, Germany

Filippo Corponi
Department of Biomedical and Neuromotor Sciences, University of Bologna, Bologna, Italy

Deirdre P. Cronin-Fenton
Department of Clinical Epidemiology, Aarhus University, Aarhus, Denmark

Ann K. Daly
Institute of Cellular Medicine, Newcastle University, Medical School, Newcastle upon Tyne, United Kingdom

Per Damkier
Department of Clinical Biochemistry and Pharmacology, Odense University Hospital; Department of Clinical Research, University of Southern Denmark, Odense, Denmark

Tiphaine Adam de Beaumais
Department of Paediatric Pharmacology and Pharmacogenetics, Robert Debré Hospital, APHP, Paris, France

Chiara Fabbri
Department of Biomedical and Neuromotor Sciences, University of Bologna, Bologna, Italy

Kathleen M. Giacomini
Department of Bioengineering and Therapeutic Sciences, University of California, San Francisco, San Francisco, CA, United States

Lars C. Gormsen
Aarhus University Hospital, Aarhus, Denmark

Henk-Jan Guchelaar
Department of Clinical Pharmacy & Toxicology, Leiden University Medical Center, Leiden, The Netherlands

Evelyne Jacqz-Aigrain
Department of Paediatric Pharmacology and Pharmacogenetics, Robert Debré Hospital, APHP; University Paris Diderot Sorbonne Paris Cité; Clinical Investigation Center CIC1426, INSERM, Paris, France

Niels Jessen
Aarhus University Hospital; Aarhus University, Aarhus, Denmark

Kathrin Klein
Dr. Margarete Fischer-Bosch Institute of Clinical Pharmacology, Stuttgart, Germany

Nicole Kugler
Dr. Margarete Fischer-Bosch Institute of Clinical Pharmacology, Stuttgart, Germany

Orod Osanlou
Department of Molecular and Clinical Pharmacology, The University of Liverpool, Liverpool, United Kingdom

Esteban J. Parra
University of Toronto at Mississauga, Mississauga, ON, Canada

Ana M. Peiró
Clinical Pharmacology Unit, Department of Health of Alicante-General Hospital; Neuropharmacology on Pain (NED), Alicante Institute for Health and Biomedical Research (ISABIAL-FISABIO Foundation), Alicante, Spain

Tamara Petrikat
Dr. Margarete Fischer-Bosch Institute of Clinical Pharmacology, Stuttgart, Germany

Munir Pirmohamed
Department of Molecular and Clinical Pharmacology, The University of Liverpool, Liverpool, United Kingdom

Chang S. Ryu
Dr. Margarete Fischer-Bosch Institute of Clinical Pharmacology, Stuttgart, Germany

Alessandro Serretti
Department of Biomedical and Neuromotor Sciences, University of Bologna, Bologna, Italy

Shylaja Srinivasan
Department of Bioengineering and Therapeutic Sciences; Division of Pediatric Endocrinology and Diabetes, University of California, San Francisco, San Francisco, CA, United States

Guilherme Suarez-Kurtz
Instituto Nacional de Câncer and Rede Nacional de Farmacogenética, Rio de Janeiro, Brazil

Jesse J. Swen
Department of Clinical Pharmacy & Toxicology, Leiden University Medical Center, Leiden, The Netherlands

Aleksi Tornio
Department of Clinical Pharmacology, University of Helsinki and Helsinki University Hospital, Helsinki, Finland

Mikkel H. Vendelbo
Aarhus University Hospital; Aarhus University, Aarhus, Denmark

Peter E. Weeke
Department of Cardiology, Copenhagen University Hospital, Bispebjerg and Frederiksberg, Denmark

Sook Wah Yee
Department of Bioengineering and Therapeutic Sciences, University of California, San Francisco, San Francisco, CA, United States

Ulrich M. Zanger
Dr. Margarete Fischer-Bosch Institute of Clinical Pharmacology, Stuttgart; University Hospital Tübingen, Tübingen, Germany

PREFACE

The American geneticist Arno G. Motulsky published in 1957 the first review ever on certain genetic polymorphisms in enzymes predisposing to abnormal drug response. Two years later the German geneticist Friederich Vogel named this emerging science "pharmacogenetics," the study of genetic differences as underlying cause for individual variation in response to drug treatment. For the remainder of the 20th century pharmacogenetics was mainly devoted to the study of genetic polymorphism in drug-metabolizing enzymes, notably the *N*-acetyltransferase, cytochrome P4502D6 (CYP2D6), and CYP2C19. This relatively narrow focus changed dramatically in the beginning of the 21st century with the completion of the human genome project, in particular, because of the discovery that somatic mutations may play a pathophysiological role in disease and in particular cancer. Hence, the detection of such mutations can be used not only as a diagnostic tool but also as a means to develop new drugs and select the most appropriate treatment. However, the classical or germline pharmacogenetics is still an important component of what today is interchangeably referred to as personalized medicine, precision medicine, individualized therapy, or stratified medicine. Precision medicine and its aliases are the essence of modern medicine. Accordingly, patients should be divided into distinct groups and clinical decisions, practices, interventions, and products are personalized with respect to the underlying genetic, demographic, and pathophysiological characteristics to meet the needs of the individual patient. Until recently, it was implicit that the prediction and stratification of the individual patient's risk of disease or response to treatment could largely be deducted from genomic characteristics and testing. However, it is now increasingly recognized that environmental factors, epigenetic factors, as well as patient-specific host factors in most cases are equally important predictors of individual drug response.

This volume of *Advances in Pharmacology* aims at giving a broad update on germline pharmacogenetics. Chapters are written by internationally recognized authors (groups) within the specific subjects. The editors are clinical pharmacologists, and we are particularly interested in the application of pharmacogenetics in clinical medicine. Thus, there are chapters on pharmacogenetics in everyday clinical practice, cardiovascular disease, diabetes mellitus, immune-modulating therapy, psychiatry, pain and in children. Academic controversies within pharmacogenetics are not uncommon, as illustrated here with an overview of the highly contested issue of tamoxifen efficacy as related to CYP2D6 pharmacogenetics. There are also chapters on pharmacogenetics in adverse drug reactions and in ethnic differences and an update on cytochrome P450. Finally the exciting developments of epigenetics, imaging, and use of pharmacoepidemiology in germline pharmacogenetics are covered in separate chapters.

Kim Brøsen
Per Damkier

SECTION I

Cytochrome P450

CHAPTER ONE

Cytochrome P450 in Pharmacogenetics: An Update

Aleksi Tornio, Janne T. Backman[1]
Department of Clinical Pharmacology, University of Helsinki and Helsinki University Hospital, Helsinki, Finland
[1]Corresponding author: e-mail address: janne.backman@helsinki.fi

Contents

1. Introduction 4
2. Genetic Variability of CYP Enzymes 6
3. CYP1A Subfamily 7
   3.1 CYP1A2 7
4. CYP2A and CYP2B Subfamilies 8
   4.1 CYP2A6 8
   4.2 CYP2B6 9
5. CYP2C Subfamily 10
   5.1 CYP2C8 11
   5.2 CYP2C9 12
   5.3 CYP2C19 16
6. CYP2D6 18
7. CYP3A Subfamily 21
   7.1 CYP3A4 21
   7.2 CYP3A5 22
8. Conclusion 23
References 25

Abstract

Interindividual variability in drug disposition is a major cause of lack of efficacy and adverse effects of drug therapies. The majority of hepatically cleared drugs are metabolized by cytochrome P450 (CYP) enzymes, mainly in families CYP1, CYP2, and CYP3. Genes encoding these enzymes are highly variable with allele distribution showing considerable differences between populations. Genetic variability of especially *CYP2C9*, *CYP2C19*, *CYP2D6*, and *CYP3A5* is known to have clear clinical impact on drugs that are metabolized by these enzymes. *CYP1A2*, *CYP2A6*, *CYP2B6*, *CYP2C8*, and *CYP3A4* all show variability that affects pharmacokinetics of drugs as well, but so far the evidence regarding their clinical implications is not as conclusive. In this review, we provide an up-to-date summary of the pharmacogenetics of the major human drug-metabolizing CYP enzymes, focusing on clinically significant examples.

Advances in Pharmacology, Volume 83
ISSN 1054-3589
https://doi.org/10.1016/bs.apha.2018.04.007

ABBREVIATIONS

AhR	aryl hydrocarbon receptor
AS	activity score
CAR	constitutive androstane receptor
CNV	copy-number variant
CPIC	Clinical Pharmacogenetics Implementation Consortium
CYP	cytochrome P450
DPWG	Dutch Pharmacogenetics Working Group
GR	glucocorticoid receptor
IM	intermediate metabolizer
IWPC	International Warfarin Pharmacogenetics Consortium
MAF	minor allele frequency
NM	normal metabolizer
PM	poor metabolizer
PPI	proton pump inhibitor
PXR	pregnane X receptor
SNV	single-nucleotide variant
SSRI	selective serotonin reuptake inhibitor
TCA	tricyclic antidepressant
UM	ultrarapid metabolizer
VDR	vitamin D receptor
VKORC1	vitamin K epoxide reductase complex subunit 1

1. INTRODUCTION

The cytochrome P450 (CYP) enzymes are a superfamily of hemoproteins, which have crucial functions in the metabolism of both endogenous and xenobiotic compounds. In humans, 57 putatively functional genes and 58 pseudogenes have been described (Nelson et al., 2004). Most of the genes, which are divided into 18 families and 44 subfamilies based on their sequence similarity, have endogenous roles such as metabolism of bile acids, eicosanoids, and steroids (Nebert & Russell, 2002). Only about a dozen CYP enzymes belonging to families CYP1, CYP2, and CYP3 are important for drug metabolism (Table 1). However, the majority of clinically used drugs are metabolized by CYP enzymes (Zanger, Turpeinen, Klein, & Schwab, 2008), and many drugs are predominantly metabolized by a single CYP enzyme at clinically relevant concentrations in humans. Thus, intrinsic and extrinsic factors that influence CYP enzyme activity can have important effects on pharmacokinetics of drugs. For some drug-metabolizing CYP enzymes, in particular CYP2C9, CYP2C19, and CYP2D6, genetic variability explains a large proportion of variability in enzyme activity, whereas

Table 1 Drug-Metabolizing CYP Enzymes, Their Chromosomal Location, Clinical Significance of Their Genetic Variability, and Examples of Substrates

Enzyme/ Gene	Chromosome	Significance of Genetic Variability	Examples of Substrates
CYP1A2	15q24.1	±	Agomelatine, caffeine, clozapine, lidocaine, melatonin, tacrine, theophylline, tizanidine
CYP2A6	19q13.2	+	Cotinine, coumarin, letrozole, nicotine, tegafur
CYP2B6	19q13.2	+	Bupropion, efavirenz, cyclophosphamide
CYP2C8	10q23.33	+	Amodiaquine, cerivastatin, dasabuvir, imatinib, loperamide, montelukast, pioglitazone, paclitaxel, repaglinide, rosiglitazone
CYP2C9	10q23.33	++	Acenocoumarol, diclofenac, fluvastatin, glimepiride, glipizide, ibuprofen, losartan, **phenytoin, S-warfarin**
CYP2C19	10q23.33	++	**Amitriptyline** (**and other tertiary amine tricyclic antidepressants**), **clopidogrel**, (**es**)**citalopram**, omeprazole, pantoprazole, **sertraline, voriconazole**
CYP2D6	22q13.2	++	**Amitriptyline** (**and other tricyclic antidepressants**), aripiprazole, atomoxetine, **codeine**, dextromethorphan, **fluvoxamine**, metoprolol, mianserine, MDMA, **ondansetron, paroxetine**, propafenone, risperidone, **tamoxifen**, thioridazine, timolol, tramadol, **tropisetron**, venlafaxine
CYP2E1	10q26.3	±	Ethanol, halothane, paracetamol
CYP2J2	1p32.1	±	Amiodarone, arachidonic acid, astemizole, cyclosporine
CYP3A4	7q22.1	±	Alfentanil, alprazolam, atorvastatin, budesonide, buspirone, cyclosporine, dexamethasone, erythromycin, felodipine, gefitinib, ibrutinib, lovastatin, midazolam, nifedipine, quetiapine, saquinavir, sildenafil, simvastatin, tacrolimus, testosterone, triazolam, verapamil, vincristine
CYP3A5	7q22.1	++	Saquinavir, **tacrolimus**, verapamil, substrates overlap with CYP3A4

±, Minor or no clinical significance.
+, Moderate clinical significance.
++, Major clinical significance.
Substrates with an associated Clinical Pharmacogenetics Implementation (CPIC) guideline are given in *bold*.

for some other CYPs, such as CYP1A2 and CYP3A4, this proportion is much smaller (Zanger & Schwab, 2013). This review highlights the current knowledge on the pharmacogenetics of drug-metabolizing CYP enzymes, as well as its clinical relevance.

2. GENETIC VARIABILITY OF CYP ENZYMES

The drug-metabolizing CYP enzymes are genetically highly variable, in part due to low evolutionary constraint as many of them lack essential endogenous function. The variability is characterized by common and rare single-nucleotide variants (SNVs), as well as copy-number variants (CNVs), defined as duplications or deletions. The variants of *CYP* genes are defined by star (*) allele nomenclature for which the Human CYP Allele Nomenclature Database has served as a central repository for over 15 years. The database has recently been transitioned to be managed by the Pharmacogene Variation (PharmVar) Consortium available at www.PharmVar.org (Gaedigk et al., 2018). The functional status of the variant alleles can range from no function to increased function, and thus phenotypes ranging from poor metabolizer (PM) to ultrarapid metabolizer (UM) can be inferred from the genotype (Table 2). In order to standardize the terminology used to

Table 2 Assignment of Likely Phenotypes Based on Examples of Common Diplotypes

	Examples of Diplotypes			
Phenotype	**CYP2C9**	**CYP2C19**	**CYP2D6**	**CYP3A5**
Ultrarapid or rapid metabolizer	—	**17/*17*, **1/*17*	(**1/*1*)xN[a], (**1/*2*)xN, (**2/*2*)xN	—
Normal metabolizer	**1/*1*	**1/*1*	**1/*1*, **1/*2*, **2/*2*, **1/*9*, **1/*41*, **41/*41*, **1/*5*, **1/*4*	**1/*1*
Intermediate metabolizer	**1/*2*, **1/*3*	**1/*2*, **1/*3*, **2/*17*[b]	**4/*41*, **5/*9*, **4/*10*	**1/*3*
Poor metabolizer	**2/*2*, **2/*3*, **3/*3*	**2/*2*, **2/*3*, **3/*3*	**4/*4*, (**4/*4*)xN, **3/*4*, **5/*5*, **5/*6*	**3/*3*

[a]xN represents the number of CYP2D6 gene copies.
[b]Provisional classification.
Phenotype classification is based on consensus terms from the Clinical Pharmacogenetics Implementation Consortium (CPIC) (Caudle et al., 2017).

describe allele functional status and phenotype, a consensus paper was published by Clinical Pharmacogenetics Implementation Consortium (CPIC) (Caudle et al., 2017). To facilitate the transformation of pharmacogenetic knowledge into clinical practice and to provide evidence-based guidelines on how available genetic test results should be used to optimize drug therapy, several consortia have been established. Both CPIC and the Dutch Pharmacogenetics Working Group (DPWG) provide genotype-based dosing guidelines based on gene–drug pairs, with some differences in guideline development methods and the number of guidelines produced so far (Bank et al., 2018).

3. CYP1A SUBFAMILY

3.1 CYP1A2

CYP1A2 belongs to the CYP1 family and its gene is located on chromosome 15 along with *CYP1A1* and *CYP1B1*. Their expression is regulated by the aryl hydrocarbon receptor (AhR) pathway. CYP1A2 is abundantly expressed in the liver (Zhang et al., 2016), and it is involved in the metabolism of about 10% of clinically used drugs that are metabolized by CYP enzymes (Zhou, Wang, Yang, & Liu, 2010). In contrast, CYP1A1 and CYP1B1 are mostly extrahepatic, and are of lesser importance for drug metabolism. CYP1A2 is involved in the metabolism of, e.g., agomelatin, caffeine, clozapine, duloxetine, propranolol, tizanidine, and zolmitriptan, as well as some endogenous compounds, such as melatonin and estradiol. CYP1A2 activity is strongly affected by environmental factors. AhR-mediated induction by smoking or food components can markedly increase CYP1A2 activity. In contrast, oral contraceptives, fluoroquinolones, and fluvoxamine inhibit CYP1A2 to a clinically relevant degree.

Several SNVs have been identified that affect CYP1A2 function, but they only partially explain the variability in enzyme activity (Gunes & Dahl, 2008). The most common variants are located in the 5′ flanking region, including *CYP1A2*1F* (defining variant rs762551, c.-163C>A) which has a high frequency in many populations (Zhou, Ingelman-Sundberg, & Lauschke, 2017). On the other hand, nonsynonymous-coding variants (*CYP1A2*2* to **21*) are rare. Caffeine is frequently used to probe CYP1A2 activity, as caffeine N3-demethylation to paraxanthine is selectively catalyzed by CYP1A2 (Fuhr et al., 1996). *CYP1A2* and *AhR* loci have been identified in several genome-wide association studies to be linked with habitual coffee consumption (Amin et al., 2012; Coffee and Caffeine Genetics Consortium et al., 2015; Cornelis et al., 2011). *CYP1A2*1F* has been associated in many studies with increased inducibility of CYP1A2 by, e.g., smoking (Sachse, Brockmoller, Bauer, & Roots, 1999), but otherwise its functional consequence is less clear. In any case, genetic effects on CYP1A2 activity might be masked by environmental factors, in particular by smoking and oral contraceptive use (Matthaei et al., 2016), and the conclusions thus can depend on the population studied. Furthermore, earlier studies including only single variants might have missed more complex haplotypes including several variants. Taken together, the current available evidence does not support *CYP1A2* genotype-based dosing for any drug.

4. CYP2A AND CYP2B SUBFAMILIES

4.1 CYP2A6

CYP2A6 represents about 4% of total hepatic microsomal CYP enzyme content, and it is also expressed in some extrahepatic tissues, such as lungs and trachea (Di, Chow, Yang, & Zhou, 2009; Ding & Kaminsky, 2003; Zhang et al., 2016). In comparison to other CYP enzymes, CYP2A6 has a small active site (Yano, Hsu, Griffin, Stout, & Johnson, 2005). It has a major role in the metabolism of coumarin, letrozole, nicotine, and tegafur, and it contributes to the metabolism of other drugs, such as artemisinin, efavirenz, halothane, pilocarpine, and valproic acid.

CYP2A6 gene is highly variable, with over 40 star alleles described to date, along with additional suballeles (https://www.pharmvar.org/gene/CYP2A6, accessed 5 February 2018). The spectrum of *CYP2A6* variant alleles includes SNVs (e.g., *CYP2A6**2*, **6*), gene deletions (e.g., **4A-H*), a hybrid gene with CYP2A7 (e.g., **3*, **12A-C*), and gene conversions (e.g., **1B1-17*) (McDonagh et al., 2012). In principle, CYP2A6 phenotype, ranging from PM to UM, can be inferred from *CYP2A6* genotype. However, the effects of CYP2A6 variant alleles are known to be substrate specific (Fukami et al., 2005), and due to the high number of different variants and complex genetic architecture, variant allele carriers may be misclassified as, e.g., wild type due to limitations in genotyping methods used (Hoffman, Nelson, & Keeney, 2001). In addition, the distribution of variant alleles varies greatly between populations (Zhou et al., 2017). The decreased-function allele *CYP2A6**9* is common in all major populations (minor allele frequency (MAF) ranging from 8% in Africans to 23% in East Asians), whereas *CYP2A6**17*, *CYP2A6**23*, *CYP2A6**25*, and *CYP2A6**28* are only found in Africans, and *CYP2A6**7 and *CYP2A6**19* in East Asians. In Europeans, the most common variant alleles leading to decreased function are *CYP2A6**9* and *CYP2A6**35* with MAFs of 11% and 15%, respectively.

The metabolism of nicotine to cotinine is strongly related to CYP2A6 activity, and *CYP2A6* variants largely explain interindividual variability in the metabolism of nicotine to cotinine (Bloom et al., 2011; Hukkanen, Jacob, & Benowitz, 2005). *CYP2A6* variant alleles associated with reduced nicotine metabolism have been linked with lesser likelihood of becoming smoker, lower cigarette consumption, and better ability to quit than normal metabolizers (NMs) in many studies (McDonagh et al., 2012; Ray, Tyndale, & Lerman, 2009).

CYP2A6 is involved in the bioactivation of tegafur to 5-fluorouracil, and genetic variation of *CYP2A6* has been associated with altered tegafur metabolism, and also clinical outcomes in some studies (Kaida et al., 2008; Kong et al., 2009; Park et al., 2011). These results suggest that bioactivation of tegafur is impaired in CYP2A6 PMs, but the associations with clinical endpoints have not been replicated in all studies, and they may be dependent on the cancer type and combination treatment given (Tanner & Tyndale, 2017). In addition, decreased-function alleles of *CYP2A6* have been associated with increased plasma concentrations of another anticancer agent, letrozole (Desta et al., 2011; Tanii, Shitara, & Horie, 2011). It remains to be determined, however, whether the genotype has an impact on the efficacy and side effects of letrozole. In addition, *CYP2A6* variants have been reported to have an influence on the pharmacokinetics of efavirenz and valproic acid, even though also other enzymes contribute to the elimination of these drugs (Tanner & Tyndale, 2017).

4.2 CYP2B6

Similar to CYP2A6, the expression of CYP2B6 is highly variable, and it represents only a small percentage of the total hepatic microsomal CYP content (Wang & Tompkins, 2008; Zhang et al., 2016). *CYP2B6* and *CYP2A6* are located in close proximity to each other in chromosome 19, and their expression levels are correlated (Al Koudsi & Tyndale, 2010). In addition to the liver, CYP2B6 is also expressed in the brain (Miksys & Tyndale, 2004). It is involved in the metabolism of bupropion, cyclophosphamide, efavirenz, methadone, and nevirapine (Turpeinen & Zanger, 2012; Wang & Tompkins, 2008).

Currently, 38 *CYP2B6* variants with designated star alleles are described (https://www.pharmvar.org/gene/CYP2B6, accessed 5 February 2018).

The most widely studied allele is *CYP2B6*6*, (c.516G > T, c.785A > G) resulting in reduced expression, which is found with an MAF of 3% in Europeans, 6% in Africans, 3% in East Asians, 16% in South Asians, and 3% in admixed Americans (Zhou et al., 2017). The most common variant allele in all major populations is *CYP2B6*9* (c.516G > T), but its functional significance is less clear. Alleles with increased function have also been described (*CYP2B6*4* and *CYP2B6*22*), with an MAF of <2% in most major populations, with the exception of *CYP2B6*22* with an MAF of about 4% in Africans.

The nonnucleoside reverse transcriptase inhibitor efavirenz is metabolized predominantly by CYP2B6. Several studies have shown an association between *CYP2B6* genotype, in particular the reduced-function *CYP2B6*6* allele, and efavirenz-related adverse effects including central nervous system toxicity and hepatotoxicity (Vo & Varghese Gupta, 2016). On the other hand, the effect on clinical outcomes has not been as widely replicated. Genotype-based dose reduction of efavirenz in CYP2B6 PMs has been performed in some studies (Gatanaga et al., 2007). Interestingly, even though CYP2A6 is a minor metabolic pathway for efavirenz in general, *CYP2A6*9* has been associated with increased efavirenz plasma concentrations in CYP2B6 PMs (Haas et al., 2014). Efavirenz is a potential candidate for a genotype-based dosing guideline with emerging evidence.

*CYP2B6*6* has been associated with reduced metabolism of bupropion, a prodrug which is activated by CYP2B6. The effect of *CYP2B6*6* allele on the efficacy of bupropion in smoking cessation has been shown in some, but not all, studies (Chenoweth & Tyndale, 2017; Lee et al., 2007; Zhu et al., 2012). Pharmacokinetics of several other CYP2B6 substrates, such as cyclophosphamide, methadone, and nevirapine, have been reported to be influenced by *CYP2B6* genotype, but evidence regarding them is not yet conclusive (Zanger & Klein, 2013).

5. CYP2C SUBFAMILY

The CYP2C subfamily consists of four highly homologous genes *CYP2C18–CYP2C19–CYP2C9–CYP2C8*, which are located in this order from centromere to telomere on chromosome 10q23.33. Even though CYP2C18 mRNA is highly expressed in the liver, it does not get efficiently translated into protein (Läpple et al., 2003). The other CYP2C enzymes are expressed in the liver in the order CYP2C9 > CYP2C8 > CYP2C19, and, to a lesser extent, in the small intestine (Zhang et al., 2016). CYP2C enzyme activities can be markedly altered by environmental factors. A variety of xenobiotics such as rifampicin and hyperforin can induce the transcriptional expression of CYP2C genes in hepatocytes and thereby increase the metabolism of CYP2C substrates. Several drug-activated nuclear receptors including CAR, PXR, VDR, and GR have been implicated in this induction (Chen & Goldstein, 2009). Many drugs can also act as reversible or time-dependent inhibitors of CYP2C enzymes, such as clopidogrel and gemfibrozil for CYP2C8, fluconazole and miconazole for CYP2C9, and fluvoxamine and omeprazole for CYP2C19.

5.1 CYP2C8

CYP2C8 has been established as one of the key drug-metabolizing CYP enzymes during the last 15 years (Backman, Filppula, Niemi, & Neuvonen, 2016). CYP2C8 metabolizes a variety of xenobiotics and drugs, including amodiaquine, dasabuvir, imatinib, paclitaxel, loperamide, montelukast, pioglitazone, repaglinide, and rosiglitazone, for example.

There are tens of SNVs, short deletions, and essential splice site variants that have been found in the *CYP2C8* gene. Fourteen *CYP2C8* alleles have a designated star allele (https://www.pharmvar.org/gene/CYP2C8, accessed 31 Jan 2018). The alleles *CYP2C8**2*, **3*, and **4* account for the majority of nonsynonymous variability of *CYP2C8* in humans (Zhou et al., 2017). *CYP2C8**2** (c.805A > T, p.Ile269Phe; rs11572103) occurs with an allele frequency ranging from about 10% to 37% in individuals with a Sub-Saharan African ancestry. However, this allele is rare or absent in most Asian, European, and admixed American populations. The *CYP2C8**3** allele consists of two nonsynonymous variants (c.416G > A, p.Arg139Lys; rs11572080, and c.1196A > G, p.Lys399Arg; rs10509681) that are in complete or nearly complete linkage. *CYP2C8**3** is also in linkage disequilibrium with the *CYP2C9**2** allele (Yasar et al., 2002). In individuals with a European ancestry, the allele frequency of *CYP2C8**3** approximates 11% (Zhou et al., 2017). In South Asian and admixed American populations the frequency of the allele is about 4% and 7%, respectively, while in Sub-Saharan African populations the frequency is generally very low, albeit highly variable. Like *CYP2C8**3**, the *CYP2C8**4** allele (c.792C.G, p.Ile264Met; rs1058930) is more common in European than in other populations. In most populations, its frequency is lower (by a factor of about two) than that of *CYP2C8**3**.

The clinical significance of CYP2C8 pharmacogenetics seems to be limited (Backman et al., 2016). Most in vitro studies have suggested that the *CYP2C8**2*, **3*, and **4* alleles result in moderately decreased CYP2C8 function. However, also opposite findings have been reported regarding the

**3* and **4* alleles, for example, with respect to the metabolism of cerivastatin (Kaspera et al., 2010). Many clinical studies have suggested an increased CYP2C8 activity for carriers of the **3* allele. Individuals with the *CYP2C8*1/*3* genotype have had an approximately 40%–50% lower repaglinide AUC than individuals with the *CYP2C8*1/*1* genotype (Backman et al., 2016). In addition, the AUCs of rosiglitazone or pioglitazone have been about 20%–40% lower in *CYP2C8*3* carriers than in noncarriers, with an apparent gene-dose effect. In accordance with the pharmacokinetic findings, *CYP2C8*3* has been associated with reduced glycemic response to rosiglitazone treatment in two studies in patients with type 2 diabetes mellitus (Dawed et al., 2016; Stage, Christensen, Feddersen, Beck-Nielsen, & Brøsen, 2013). Furthermore, in a recent study, *CYP2C8*3* carriers ($n = 34$) had a slightly higher imatinib metabolic ratio than did *CYP2C8*1/*1* ($n = 147$) patients (Barratt et al., 2017).

In contrast to the clinical findings with repaglinide and thiazolidinediones, the *CYP2C8*3* allele has been associated with a slightly impaired clearance of paclitaxel (Bergmann et al., 2011; Henningsson et al., 2005) and an increased risk for paclitaxel-induced neurotoxicity or myelosuppression (Backman et al., 2016; Boora et al., 2016; Lam et al., 2016). Thus, it seems that the influence of *CYP2C8*3* on drug metabolism may be substrate dependent and is usually only modest. Based on limited evidence, *CYP2C8*2* and **4* alleles appear to have some, but limited, effect on the pharmacokinetics of CYP2C8 substrates. Inactive *CYP2C8* alleles, such as **5*, **7*, and **11*, are rare (Zhou et al., 2017), but as case reports have shown, such alleles can drastically increase the risk of adverse reactions (Backman et al., 2016). At present, there are no genotype-based consensus guidelines for CYP2C8.

5.2 CYP2C9

CYP2C9 is one of the most important CYP enzymes in terms of the number of substrates; it has been estimated to contribute to the metabolism of approximately 15% of all drugs that are metabolized by CYP enzymes (Daly, Rettie, Fowler, & Miners, 2018; Kirchheiner & Brockmöller, 2005). Important CYP2C9 substrates include warfarin (S-isomer), acenocoumarol, phenytoin, losartan, fluvastatin, bosentan, most sulfonylureas, and several nonsteroidal antiinflammatory agents.

Two nonsynonymous polymorphisms, rs1799853 (c.430C>T, p.Arg144Cys) and rs1057910 (c.1075A>C, p.Ile359Leu), define the

*CYP2C9*2* and *CYP2C9*3* alleles, respectively (https://www.pharmvar.org/gene/CYP2C9, accessed 31 Jan 2018). They are the best-studied alleles largely because they are functionally detrimental and globally the most common *CYP2C9* variants. Altogether, there are 60 *CYP2C9* variants with a star allele name and tens of other SNVs in the regulatory and coding regions of the *CYP2C9* gene. Apart from *CYP2C9*2* and *CYP2C9*3*, some of the alleles are also relatively common and at least *CYP2C9*5*, *CYP2C9*6*, *CYP2C9*11*, *CYP2C9*12*, and *CYP2C9*13* can produce an enzyme with markedly reduced activity (Daly et al., 2018).

The allele frequencies of *CYP2C9*2* and *CYP2C9*3* are around 12% and 6% in European subjects (Zhou et al., 2017). *CYP2C9*2* is also relatively common in admixed Americans (7%), South Asians (5%), and Africans (2%) but very rare in East Asians, while *CYP2C9*3* is remarkably common in South Asians (11%) and fairly common in East Asians and Americans (3%–4%). *CYP2C9*3* is generally associated with a more than 80% reduction in CYP2C9-mediated intrinsic clearance, while the effect of *CYP2C9*2* is generally slightly smaller and varies considerably, depending on the substrate (Daly et al., 2018). Interestingly, *CYP2C9*8* and *CYP2C9*9* are more common (6% and 8%) than the **2* and **3* alleles in Africans, but extremely rare in Europeans (Zhou et al., 2017). In addition, also *CYP2C9*5*, *CYP2C9*6*, and *CYP2C9*11* are much more common among Africans than among Europeans and *CYP2C9*14* is fairly common in South Asians. All other star alleles are rare in major populations. Based on genotypes, individuals can be classified as normal (**1/*1*), intermediate (IM, carrier of one decreased-function allele), or poor (carrier of two decreased-function alleles) metabolizers (Table 2). About 30% of Europeans are IMs and 4% are PMs, and the frequencies of these phenotypes are somewhat lower in other populations (Table 3).

One of the most sensitive drugs to genetic variability in CYP2C9 activity is warfarin, since its S-isomer is metabolized almost exclusively by CYP2C9 (Baker & Johnson, 2016; Rettie et al., 1992). Consequently, the oral clearance of S-warfarin is reduced by 70%–85% in CYP2C9 PMs and about 40% in IMs, leading to a longer S-warfarin half-life, longer delay in reaching a stable INR, lower warfarin dose requirement, and increased risk of bleeding during warfarin treatment, particularly in PMs (Jorgensen, FitzGerald, Oyee, Pirmohamed, & Williamson, 2012). Apart from *CYP2C9* variants (explaining about 6%–19% of variability in dose requirement), a number of other factors contribute to warfarin dose requirement, including vitamin K epoxide reductase complex subunit 1 (*VKORC1*) and *CYP4F2* genotypes, patient age, body size, smoking status, and certain concomitant medications. Various algorithms have been developed to guide warfarin dosing on the basis of these factors. The first algorithm developed on a sufficient patient population was published 10 years ago by Gage et al. (2008) and is currently in use as a modified and updated web-based calculator (www.warfarindosing.org). A large worldwide project, International Warfarin Pharmacogenetics Consortium (IWPC), also developed a definitive warfarin-dosing algorithm using clinical and genetic data on about 5000 patients treated with warfarin, including different ethnicities (International Warfarin Pharmacogenetics Consortium et al., 2009).

Three large randomized controlled trials, termed CoumaGen-II, EU-PACT, and GIFT, comparing the above warfarin-dosing algorithms to various conventional nongenetic approaches suggested that genotype-based dosing can be beneficial when warfarin treatment is initiated (Anderson et al., 2012; Gage et al., 2017; Pirmohamed et al., 2013). However, in the fourth randomized study, COAG, the time within therapeutic range in the first 4 weeks of warfarin treatment was not improved by genotype-based dosing, and the outcome was worse in the genotyped African-Americans than in the respective controls (Kimmel et al., 2013). The poor result of the COAG study may be partly explained by that *CYP2C9* genotyping included only the **2* and **3* alleles, but not the common African alleles. Accordingly, more comprehensive algorithms have been developed, and the warfarindosing.org website now contains both the Gage algorithm and the IWPC algorithm and enables adjustments for *CYP4F2*, *CYP2C9*5* and **6*. The CPIC guideline for pharmacogenetics-guided warfarin dosing and its annotations (https://cpicpgx.org/guidelines/guideline-for-warfarin-and-cyp2c9-and-vkorc1/) provide detailed instructions on how to use pharmacogenetic algorithms for warfarin dosing (Johnson et al., 2017). Apart from warfarin, CYP2C9 genotype influences to some degree also the pharmacokinetics of the other coumarins acenocoumarol and phenprocoumon.

In addition to anticoagulants, *CYP2C9*2* and **3* alleles can markedly reduce the clearances of sulfonylureas, particularly tolbutamide and glipizide (Kirchheiner & Brockmöller, 2005). Clinical studies and case reports have suggested that *CYP2C9* variant allele carriers are more sensitive to the hypoglycemic effect of sulfonylureas and may be at risk of hypoglycemia (Daly et al., 2018). In addition, *CYP2C9* variant alleles markedly affect the pharmacokinetics of a number of nonsteroidal antiinflammatory drugs, including celecoxib, ibuprofen, and flurbiprofen. There are also several studies suggesting that *CYP2C9* variant carriers are at an increased risk of NSAID-associated gastrointestinal bleeding (Figueiras et al., 2016).

Table 3 Population Frequencies of CYP2C9, CYP2C19, and CYP2D6 Phenotypes in Major Populations

Enzyme	Poor Metabolizer	Intermediate Metabolizer	Normal Metabolizer	Ultrarapid Metabolizer[a]	Unknown/ Indeterminate[b]
CYP2C9					
Africans	1.8%	23%	75%	—	—
Europeans	4.0%	32%	64%	—	—
East Asians	0.1%	6.6%	93%	—	—
South Asians	4.5%	33%	62%	—	—
Americans	1.2%	20%	79%	—	—
CYPC19					
Africans	4.8%	24%	17%	16%	38%
Europeans	2.5%	27%	39%	32%	0.0%
East Asians	14%	47%	37%	1.7%	0.2%
South Asians	12%	46%	23%	19%	0.0%
Americans	2.3%	26%	47%	24%	0.0%
CYP2D6					
Africans	1.9%	13%	72%	4.5%	9.2%
Europeans	6.1%	7.2%	75%	3.3%	8.5%
East Asians	0.9%	8.7%	86%	1.2%	3.7%
South Asians	1.3%	6.3%	89%	2.8%	0.4%
Americans	3.7%	4.5%	81%	4.8%	5.8%

[a]For CYP2C19, rapid (*CYP2C19**1/*17*) and ultrarapid (*CYP2C19**17/*17*) metabolizers are combined.

[b]For CYP2C9, phenotypes are based on genotyping for defining SNVs of the decreased-function alleles *CYP2C9**2*, **3*, **5*, **6*, **8*, and **11*, and all alleles that are negative for these SNVs are defaulted to *CYP2C9**1*. For CYP2C19 and CYP2D6, alleles whose functional status is indeterminate are included in the calculations.

Based on phenotype frequencies provided by PharmGKB and CPIC in Gene-specific Information Tables (https://www.pharmgkb.org/page/cyp2c9RefMaterials, https://www.pharmgkb.org/page/cyp2c19RefMaterials, https://www.pharmgkb.org/page/cyp2d6RefMaterials; accessed 6 February 2018).

The antiepileptic drug phenytoin has a narrow therapeutic index and complex pharmacokinetic characteristics, including saturable metabolism and dependence on CYP2C9 activity (Caudle et al., 2014). Both *CYP2C9*2* and *CYP2C9*3* are associated with impaired clearance of phenytoin. Consequently, it has been reported that phenytoin maintenance doses are about 30% lower in heterozygous carriers of these *CYP2C9* alleles and 30%–50% lower in homozygous carriers than in noncarriers. Furthermore, case reports suggest that CYP2C9 PMs are at increased risk for dose-related phenytoin toxicity. Accordingly, the respective CPIC guideline recommends a 25%–50% reduction of phenytoin starting maintenance dose in decreased-function *CYP2C9* allele carriers, with subsequent maintenance doses adjusted based on therapeutic drug monitoring or response (Caudle et al., 2014).

5.3 CYP2C19

CYP2C19 participates in the metabolism of many clinically relevant drugs such as benzodiazepines, proton pump inhibitors (PPIs), selective serotonin reuptake inhibitors (SSRIs), tricyclic antidepressants (TCAs), and voriconazole, and it is important for the metabolic activation of the prodrug clopidogrel.

CYP2C19 is highly variable with 35 defined haplotypes with a designated star allele so far (https://www.pharmvar.org/gene/CYP2C19, accessed 14 Jan 2018). The most common no-function allele is *CYP2C19*2* (c.681G > A; rs4244285), occurring with an allele frequency of 18% in Africans and Europeans, and over 30% in Asian populations (Zhou et al., 2017). Other decreased or no-function alleles (**3*–**8*) are typically rare, with the exception of *CYP2C19*3* (c.636G > A; rs4986893) in East Asians with an MAF of about 7%. On the other hand, the increased-function *CYP2C19*17* allele (c.-806C > T; rs12248560) results in enhanced transcription probably due to the modulation of GATA4 binding (Mwinyi et al., 2010). It is common in Europeans and Africans (MAF about 23%), less common in admixed Americans and South Asians (12%–14%), and almost absent in East Asians. Thus, CYP2C19 phenotype ranges from PM to UM (Table 3).

The clinical significance of CYP2C19 pharmacogenetics is well established. For example, clopidogrel is a prodrug, which is activated in two sequential oxidative steps involving several CYP enzymes, including CYP2C19 (Kazui et al., 2010). Many studies have indicated that the bioactivation of clopidogrel is impaired in CYP2C19 PMs and that these PMs have lower levels of clopidogrel active metabolite than NMs (Scott et al., 2013). Moreover, there is substantial evidence linking *CYP2C19* genotype with clinical outcomes, especially in patients with acute coronary syndrome who have undergone percutaneous coronary intervention (Mao et al., 2013; Mega et al., 2010). More recently, a meta-analysis of clopidogrel-treated patients with stroke or transient ischemic attack suggested a similar level of CYP2C19 genotype-related risk for vascular events than that reported for patients with coronary artery disease (Pan, Chen, et al., 2017), and the risk seems to be more pronounced in stroke patients treated with clopidogrel monotherapy (Sun et al., 2015; Tornio et al., 2018). On the other hand, the increased-function *CYP2C19*17* allele has been associated with increased risk of bleeding in some studies (Sibbing et al., 2010). Based on the current available evidence, alternative antiplatelet therapy is recommended for CYP2C19 IMs and PMs in the CPIC guideline (Scott et al., 2013).

There is also strong evidence on the influence of *CYP2C19* genotype on TCAs and SSRIs that are metabolized by CYP2C19 (Hicks et al., 2017). Tertiary amine TCAs, namely, amitriptyline, clomipramine, doxepin, imipramine, and trimipramine, are demethylated by CYPC19 to corresponding pharmacologically active secondary amines (e.g., amitriptyline to nortriptyline), and both the tertiary amines and secondary amines are metabolized by CYP2D6 to less active hydroxy metabolites. Tertiary amines have a stronger serotonergic effect, whereas secondary amines have a more pronounced noradrenergic effect, and thus changes in CYP2C19 activity can have an impact on clinical response or adverse effects of tertiary amines (Gillman, 2007). Both CYP2C19 poor and ultrarapid/rapid metabolizers are at risk of suboptimal response to tertiary amines, and other TCAs not metabolized by CYP2C19 are recommended for these individuals in the CPIC guideline (Hicks et al., 2017). Furthermore, the SSRIs citalopram, escitalopram, and sertraline are metabolized by CYP2C19, and especially for citalopram and escitalopram, CYP2C19 UMs are at risk of therapeutic failure and PMs at increased risk of side effects if normal recommended doses are used (Hicks et al., 2015; Jukic, Haslemo, Molden, & Ingelman-Sundberg, 2018).

Most PPIs are metabolized by CYP2C19 and their pharmacokinetics are affected by CYP2C19 phenotype (Furuta et al., 1998). Both CYP2C19 IMs and PMs have higher PPI plasma concentrations compared to NMs, and consequently, the success rate of *Helicobacter pylori* eradication therapy depends on *CYP2C19* genotype (Zhao et al., 2008). In contrast, CYP2C19 UMs are at risk of treatment failure, and consequently dose escalation is recommended for esomeprazole, lansoprazole, omeprazole, and pantoprazole in *H. pylori* eradication in the UM patients according to the DPWG guideline (Swen et al., 2011). Also the triazole antifungal voriconazole is metabolized by CYP2C19, and choosing an alternative antifungal agent not metabolized by CYP2C19 is recommended for rapid metabolizers and UMs due to risk of subtherapeutic concentrations and for PMs due to risk of adverse effects (Moriyama et al., 2017).

6. CYP2D6

Although the protein abundancy of CYP2D6 in the liver is only about 5% of the total hepatic CYP amount (Zhou et al., 2017), CYP2D6 contributes significantly to the metabolism of roughly 25% of all drugs in clinical use (He, Chen, Zhou, & Zhou, 2015). CYP2D6 substrates include TCAs, SSRIs (paroxetine, fluoxetine, fluvoxamine), other psychiatric drugs (venlafaxine, aripiprazole, risperidone), atomoxetine, opioids (codeine, tramadol, oxycodone), antiemetics (ondansetron, tropisetron), primaquine, tamoxifen, and cardiovascular drugs (metoprolol, timolol, propafenone). CYP2D6 is inhibited strongly by various drugs, including fluoxetine, paroxetine, terbinafine, and moclobemide. Moreover, although it has been thought that CYP2D6 is not inducible, accumulating data indicate that transcriptional regulation of CYP2D6 may account for part of CYP2D6 variability (Pan, Ning, & Jeong, 2017).

The *CYP2D6* gene is located on Chr22q13.1 in close proximity to the nonfunctional pseudogenes, *CYP2D7* and *CYP2D8*. There are more than 100 variants with a designated star allele in the highly polymorphic *CYP2D6* locus, including CNVs (https://www.pharmvar.org/gene/CYP2D6, accessed 31 Jan 2018). Overall, the different variations confer no, decreased, normal, or increased function, leading to huge variability in enzyme activity between individuals and populations, ranging from PMs (individuals with two nonfunctional alleles) to UMs (usually carriers of more than two functional *CYP2D6* alleles due to gene duplication) (Table 3). The *CYP2D6* diplotypes can be translated into predicted more definitive phenotypes using the activity score (AS) system (Gaedigk, Sangkuhl, Whirl-Carrillo, Klein, & Leeder, 2017; Gaedigk et al., 2008). To calculate the AS, alleles are grouped according to their crude functionality, and a value is assigned to each allele to calculate the AS of each diplotype: no-function (0) alleles (**3, *4, *4xN,*5, *6, *7, *8, *11, *12, *36, *40, *42, *56*), decreased-function (0.5) alleles (**9, *10, *17, *29, *41, *44, *49*), normal-function (1) alleles (**2, *35, *43, *45*), and increased-function (2) alleles (**1xN, *2xN*). Accordingly, the CYP2D6 phenotype can thus be inferred as poor

(AS 0), intermediate (0.5), normal (1–2), or ultrarapid (>2) metabolizer. There is lack of consensus concerning whether patients with an AS of 1.0 should be assigned a normal or intermediate phenotype, and in some reports, they have been classified as normal–slow metabolizers, and individuals with an AS of 1.5–2 as normal–fast metabolizers (Gaedigk et al., 2017, 2008).

CYP2D6 allele frequencies vary substantially between populations. The *CYP2D6*2* allele, conferring normal CYP2D6 function, and the variant defining *CYP2D6*4* (rs3892097), causing a splicing defect and an inactive CYP2D6 gene product, are frequent in European, African, South Asian, and admixed American populations, with allele frequencies of 27%–36% and 12%–16%, respectively (Zhou et al., 2017). On the other hand, the inactive alleles *CYP2D6*3* (4%) and *CYP2D6*6* (2%) are only found in individuals of European ancestry, while the decreased-function allele *CYP2D6*10* is almost exclusively found in African, South Asian, and particularly in East Asian populations, where it is the most common *CYP2D6* allele (59%). *CYP2D6*14* is only found in East Asian populations (2%), while *CYP2D6*17* (20%), *CYP2D6*29* (9%), and *CYP2D6*43* (2%) are African haplotypes. The duplicated increased-function alleles *CYP2D6*1xN* and *CYP2D6*2xN* occur with frequencies of 1%–2% in whites and Asians but are much more common in certain African populations, in which their frequency can be up to 29%, and can be enriched in some smaller populations, such as the Finns (7%) (Pietarinen, Tornio, & Niemi, 2016). The frequencies of deletions (*CYP2D6*5*) vary from 1% to 7% (Gaedigk et al., 2017).

Codeine is a weak opioid analgesic, whose opioid effect is dependent on morphine formed by CYP2D6 (Crews et al., 2014). Accordingly, the rate of bioactivation and analgesic efficacy of codeine is markedly decreased in CYP2D6 PMs and increased in UMs, even though clinical evidence from pain studies regarding the effect of CYP2D6 genotype is still lacking (Somogyi, Coller, & Barratt, 2015). There are several case reports of severe or life-threatening adverse effects following standard codeine doses in CYP2D6 UMs. Consequently, the CPIC guideline recommends using alternative analgesics in PMs and UMs, and codeine is contraindicated by the medicines agencies in known CYP2D6 UMs. In addition to codeine, also other opioids, including tramadol, hydrocodone, and oxycodone, are *O*-demethylated by CYP2D6. As *O*-desmethyltramadol is mainly responsible for the opioid effects of tramadol, similar to codeine, CYP2D6 PMs and UMs can be susceptible to treatment failure when tramadol is used (Orliaguet et al., 2015). However, the effect of genetic variability in

CYP2D6 on the analgesic efficacy and risk of toxicity with oxycodone and hydromorphone seems to be smaller due to the variable significance of parent drug and metabolites to the opioid effects.

All TCAs are metabolized to less active hydroxylated metabolites almost exclusively by CYP2D6 (Hicks et al., 2017). Therefore, there is huge *CYP2D6* genotype-dependent variability in their metabolic clearance. Accordingly, clinical studies have shown particularly for amitriptyline and nortriptyline that standard doses of TCAs can fail to produce sufficient drug concentrations in the systemic circulation in UMs, while the concentrations of TCAs may reach supratherapeutic levels in PMs, resulting in risk of therapeutic failure or intolerable adverse effects, respectively. The CPIC guideline therefore recommends avoiding TCAs in CYP2D6 UMs and PMs.

Of the SSRIs, fluoxetine, and particularly fluvoxamine and paroxetine are metabolized by CYP2D6 (Hicks et al., 2015). CYP2D6 UMs have been shown to be at risk of low or undetectable plasma paroxetine concentrations, which may be associated with an increased likelihood of therapeutic failure. Therefore, it is advisable to select an alternative antidepressant in UMs. CYP2D6 PMs, on the other hand, have greater drug exposure to fluvoxamine and paroxetine, compared to NMs, and therefore it is recommended that their doses should be reduced by 30%–50% in PMs, if alternative antidepressants cannot be selected. Fluoxetine itself is pharmacologically active, and it is converted to a major active metabolite, R-norfluoxetine by CYP2D6. Therefore, CYP2D6 PMs have high fluoxetine levels and low norfluoxetine levels, and their total sum may not vary to a clinically significant degree between CYP2D6 genotypes.

The 5-hydroxytryptamine receptor antagonists ondansetron and tropisetron, that are used as antiemetics, are metabolized to inactive metabolites to a significant degree by CYP2D6 (Bell et al., 2017). Based on some pharmacokinetic data, the metabolism and clearance of tropisetron are highly dependent on CYP2D6 phenotype, while the effect on ondansetron pharmacokinetics is only moderate. More importantly, there is clinical evidence showing that CYP2D6 UMs are at risk of reduced antiemetic response to ondansetron and tropisetron. Accordingly, the CPIC guideline gives a moderate recommendation to select an alternative antiemetic approach in CYP2D6 UMs.

Tamoxifen is an antiestrogenic agent that is used in treatment of breast cancer. It is bioactivated to 4-hydroxytamoxifen and endoxifen by CYP2D6 (Goetz et al., 2018). Compared to NMs, CYP2D6 PMs exhibit lower endoxifen concentrations and a higher risk of cancer recurrence when tamoxifen is used as an adjuvant in early breast cancer. The CPIC guideline for tamoxifen therefore recommends the use of alternative hormonal therapy for CYP2D6 PMs. For CYP2D6 IMs and NMs with an AS of 1, the recommendation is to consider alternative hormonal therapy, or if aromatase inhibitor use is contraindicated, to consider a higher but approved tamoxifen dose. For PMs, higher dose tamoxifen (40 mg/day) can be considered if there are contraindications to aromatase inhibitor therapy.

7. CYP3A SUBFAMILY

The CYP3A subfamily consists of four genes, namely, *CYP3A4*, *CYP3A5*, *CYP3A7*, *CYP3A43* located on chromosome 7q22.1. CYP3A4 and CYP3A5 are abundantly expressed in the adult liver (Zhang et al., 2016), while the expression of the other two isoforms is much lower. However, CYP3A7 is highly expressed in fetal liver, contributing to about 50% of the total microsomal CYP protein content. CYP3A4 is important for the metabolism of about 50% of clinically used drugs including wide range of drugs and drug classes: benzodiazepines, calcium channel blockers, cyclosporine, macrolide antibiotics, opioids, several statins, and it also contributes to the metabolism of steroid hormones (Zhou, 2008). CYP3A4 is inhibited by a wide range of xenobiotics, such as erythromycin, grapefruit juice, ketoconazole, and HIV protease inhibitors. CYP3A4 is also highly inducible by PXR and CAR ligands. CYP3A5 is structurally very similar to CYP3A4, resulting in an overlapping substrate selectivity.

7.1 CYP3A4

CYP3A4 activity is highly variable, but genetic variants in the *CYP3A4* gene have explained only a minor portion of this variability (Werk & Cascorbi, 2014). So far, the most relevant *CYP3A4* variant to explain CYP3A4 activity appears to be the intronic *CYP3A4*22* (rs35599367 C > T) variant, which occurs with an MAF of 5% in Europeans, and about 3% in admixed Americans, but is rare in many other populations (Zhou et al., 2017). In 2011 it was shown to be associated with reduced CYP3A4 mRNA expression in liver samples, and with lower statin dose requirement for lipid control (Wang, Guo, Wrighton, Cooke, & Sadee, 2011). These findings have been subsequently replicated in several studies (Werk & Cascorbi, 2014). On the other hand, another widely studied variant, *CYP3A4*1B*, appears to have no or very limited functional impact on CYP3A4 (García-Martín et al., 2002), in contrast to some initial reports which may have been influenced by its linkage disequilibrium with *CYP3A5*1*. In addition to several nonsynonymous exonic variants, two total loss-of-function variants have been described (*CYP3A4**20* and **26*), both initially discovered based on single individuals with abnormal pharmacokinetics (Werk et al., 2014; Westlind-Johnsson et al., 2006). The frequency of these alleles is generally very low, but, for example, *CYP3A4**20* is present in the Spanish population with an allele frequency of 1.2% (Apellaniz-Ruiz et al., 2015).

The association of *CYP3A4**22* with reduced metabolic activity for several CYP3A4 substrates such as cyclosporine, erythromycin, sunitinib, tamoxifen, and quetiapine is well established (Werk & Cascorbi, 2014). Few studies have reported effects on pharmacodynamic endpoints for, e.g., fluticasone in asthma and CYP3A4-metabolized statins in lipid control. However, no genotype-based dosing guidelines have been published for CYP3A4.

7.2 CYP3A5

CYP3A5 substrate selectivity overlaps with that of CYP3A4, and CYP3A5 contributes significantly to the CYP3A metabolic activity in individuals who express fully functional CYP3A5, i.e., in carriers of at least one *CYP3A5**1* allele (Kuehl et al., 2001). The most common and well-studied nonfunctional variant allele is the *CYP3A5**3* (Lamba, Hebert, Schuetz, Klein, & Altman, 2012). This allele is very common in admixed Americans, Europeans, East Asians, and South Asians, constituting the major allele with a frequency of 80%, 94%, 71%, and 67%, respectively (Zhou et al., 2017). The allele frequency has been reported to correlate with the distance from the equator (Thompson et al., 2004), and it is considerably rarer in Africans (allele frequency 17%) than in other superpopulations. Other nonfunctional alleles are generally rare, but *CYP3A5**6* and *7 occur in African populations with allele frequencies of 15% and 10% (Zhou et al., 2017).

The strongest evidence for clinical implications of *CYP3A5* variation is available for tacrolimus, which is one of the most widely used immunosuppressive medications in solid organ transplantation. Blood concentrations of tacrolimus have been associated with *CYP3A5* genotype in numerous studies, and CYP3A5 expressors have a higher tacrolimus clearance than nonexpressors (Birdwell et al., 2015). Therapeutic drug monitoring is employed with tacrolimus therapy, and studies have shown that *CYP3A5* genotyping is helpful for achieving target trough whole blood concentrations when treatment is initiated. Less evidence is available on its effect on clinical outcomes. Furthermore, in liver transplant patients, both the genotype of the recipient and that of the donor liver can influence tacrolimus clearance, since CYP3A5 is expressed in both the intestine and the liver. However, the evidence is inconclusive at the moment regarding the relative significance of donor's and recipient's genotypes in liver transplants where the genotype is different between the two.

The evidence regarding *CYP3A5* genotype and statins metabolized by CYP3A enzymes is somewhat controversial, as some studies have shown poorer LDL response to statin therapy in CYP3A5 expressors than in nonexpressors (Kivistö et al., 2004), whereas other studies have implicated reduced response in CYP3A5 nonexpressors (Willrich et al., 2008). Furthermore, there is limited evidence that *CYP3A5*3* is associated with statin-induced myopathy. In one study, atorvastatin-associated myalgia cases with the *CYP3A5*3/*3* genotype had higher creatine kinase levels than those with the *CYP3A5*1/*3* genotype (Wilke, Moore, & Burmester, 2005). In addition, an association with the *CYP3A5* genotype and treatment-related toxicity has been reported for the anticancer agents sunitinib and vincristine, which are both metabolized by CYP3A enzymes (Egbelakin et al., 2011; Garcia-Donas et al., 2011). However, due to limited evidence, no other genotype-based dosing guidelines than those for tacrolimus have been published for CYP3A5 to date.

8. CONCLUSION

Due to substantial research efforts, there has been tremendous progress in understanding the genetic variability of drug-metabolizing CYP enzymes, their genotype–phenotype relationships, as well as their clinical significance. During the last decade, important advances have included:

- the discovery and characterization of the clinical relevance of certain fairly common functionally relevant CYP alleles (particularly *CYP2C19*17* and *CYP3A4*22*),
- recognition of the significance of CYP alleles common in individuals of non-European ancestry (e.g., certain decreased-function *CYP2C9* alleles),
- understanding of the significance of rare loss-of-function CYP variants,
- realization that in all populations, the proportion that possesses an "actionable pharmacogene" (i.e., a pharmacogenetic variant which is associated with actionable prescribing decision for a specific drug) is very high,

- detailed characterization of the clinical usefulness of pharmacogenetic approaches related to specific drugs (even prospective, randomized controlled clinical trials of pharmacogenetics vs conventional approaches have been conducted with warfarin),
- and perhaps most importantly the systematic production of drug-specific evidence-based pharmacogenetic guidelines.

At the same time with increased understanding of the pharmacogenetics of CYP enzymes, there has been a rapid movement from traditional genotyping toward an era of large-scale exome and genome sequencing. This has already now increased the number of reported rare nonsynonymous CYP variants to thousands (Fujikura, Ingelman-Sundberg, & Lauschke, 2015). Such variants of uncertain significance will pose a special challenge to pharmacogenetics, since they may have a very large impact on drug pharmacokinetics when they are present as a diplotype together with a common loss-of-function variant. Improvement of various computational approaches and large-scale functional assays will be needed to make significant progress in understanding the significance of such a multitude of rare variants, since there will be no possibility to investigate each of them clinically.

Despite all the scientific advances, the incorporation of pharmacogenetic information to clinical routine has been slow. So far, only few hospitals worldwide have adapted large-scale preemptive genotyping in clinical use. The reasons for the slow progress include organizational, ethical, legal, and financial issues, in addition to medical issues. Sometimes, a main reason has been that alternative drugs with a perceived or known more reliable clinical effect have become preferred, in order to avoid pharmacogenetic complexities (Azmoon & Angiolillo, 2013).

In the future, the discovery and characterization of pharmacogenes and their variants will continue at a considerable rate, and work will be continued to compose and update pharmacogenetics consensus guidelines. In addition, research efforts will be needed to characterize the clinical utility and practicality of CYP genotyping in properly designed clinical trials. Moreover, incorporation of the pharmacogenetics guidelines to health care routines will require development of computational approaches, as well as electronic medical records and their interfaces, so that the use of pharmacogenetics information to support medical decisions is smooth and effective; a key challenge will be the provision of clear, unambiguous guidance to health care providers. At the same time, it should be kept in mind that in addition to genetic variability, CYP phenotypes are altered by multiple other individual factors, such as disease states and drug interactions.

CONFLICT OF INTEREST

The authors declare no conflict of interest.

REFERENCES

Al Koudsi, N., & Tyndale, R. F. (2010). Hepatic CYP2B6 is altered by genetic, physiologic, and environmental factors but plays little role in nicotine metabolism. *Xenobiotica*, *40*(6), 381–392. https://doi.org/10.3109/00498251003713958.

Amin, N., Byrne, E., Johnson, J., Chenevix-Trench, G., Walter, S., Nolte, I. M., et al. (2012). Genome-wide association analysis of coffee drinking suggests association with CYP1A1/CYP1A2 and NRCAM. *Molecular Psychiatry*, *17*(11), 1116–1129. https://doi.org/10.1038/mp.2011.101.

Anderson, J. L., Horne, B. D., Stevens, S. M., Woller, S. C., Samuelson, K. M., Mansfield, J. W., et al. (2012). A randomized and clinical effectiveness trial comparing two pharmacogenetic algorithms and standard care for individualizing warfarin dosing (CoumaGen-II). *Circulation*, *125*(16), 1997–2005. https://doi.org/10.1161/CIRCULATIONAHA.111.070920.

Apellaniz-Ruiz, M., Inglada-Perez, L., Naranjo, M. E., Sanchez, L., Mancikova, V., Curras-Freixes, M., et al. (2015). High frequency and founder effect of the CYP3A4*20 loss-of-function allele in the Spanish population classifies CYP3A4 as a polymorphic enzyme. *The Pharmacogenomics Journal*, *15*(3), 288–292. https://doi.org/10.1038/tpj.2014.67.

Azmoon, S., & Angiolillo, D. J. (2013). Switching antiplatelet regimens: Alternatives to clopidogrel in patients with acute coronary syndrome undergoing PCI: A review of the literature and practical considerations for the interventional cardiologist. *Catheterization and Cardiovascular Interventions*, *81*(2), 232–242. https://doi.org/10.1002/ccd.24480.

Backman, J. T., Filppula, A. M., Niemi, M., & Neuvonen, P. J. (2016). Role of cytochrome P450 2C8 in drug metabolism and interactions. *Pharmacological Reviews*, *68*(1), 168–241. https://doi.org/10.1124/pr.115.011411. 68/1/168 [pii].

Baker, W. L., & Johnson, S. G. (2016). Pharmacogenetics and oral antithrombotic drugs. *Current Opinion in Pharmacology*, *27*, 38–42. https://doi.org/10.1016/j.coph.2016.01.008.

Bank, P. C., Caudle, K. E., Swen, J. J., Gammal, R. S., Whirl-Carrillo, M., Klein, T. E., et al. (2018). Comparison of the guidelines of the Clinical Pharmacogenetics Implementation Consortium and the Dutch Pharmacogenetics Working Group. *Clinical Pharmacology and Therapeutics*, *103*, 599–618. https://doi.org/10.1002/cpt.762.

Barratt, D. T., Cox, H. K., Menelaou, A., Yeung, D. T., White, D. L., Hughes, T. P., et al. (2017). CYP2C8 genotype significantly alters imatinib metabolism in chronic myeloid leukaemia patients. *Clinical Pharmacokinetics*, *56*(8), 977–985. https://doi.org/10.1007/s40262-016-0494-0.

Bell, G. C., Caudle, K. E., Whirl-Carrillo, M., Gordon, R. J., Hikino, K., Prows, C. A., et al. (2017). Clinical Pharmacogenetics Implementation Consortium (CPIC) guideline for CYP2D6 genotype and use of ondansetron and tropisetron. *Clinical Pharmacology and Therapeutics*, *102*(2), 213–218. https://doi.org/10.1002/cpt.598.

Bergmann, T. K., Brasch-Andersen, C., Green, H., Mirza, M., Pedersen, R. S., Nielsen, F., et al. (2011). Impact of CYP2C8*3 on paclitaxel clearance: A population pharmacokinetic and pharmacogenomic study in 93 patients with ovarian cancer. *The Pharmacogenomics Journal*, *11*(2), 113–120. https://doi.org/10.1038/tpj.2010.19.

Birdwell, K. A., Decker, B., Barbarino, J. M., Peterson, J. F., Stein, C. M., Sadee, W., et al. (2015). Clinical Pharmacogenetics Implementation Consortium (CPIC) guidelines for CYP3A5 genotype and tacrolimus dosing. *Clinical Pharmacology and Therapeutics*, *98*(1), 19–24. https://doi.org/10.1002/cpt.113.

Bloom, J., Hinrichs, A. L., Wang, J. C., von Weymarn, L. B., Kharasch, E. D., Bierut, L. J., et al. (2011). The contribution of common CYP2A6 alleles to variation in nicotine metabolism among European-Americans. *Pharmacogenetics and Genomics, 21*(7), 403–416. https://doi.org/10.1097/FPC.0b013e328346e8c0.

Boora, G. K., Kanwar, R., Kulkarni, A. A., Abyzov, A., Sloan, J., Ruddy, K. J., et al. (2016). Testing of candidate single nucleotide variants associated with paclitaxel neuropathy in the trial NCCTG N08C1 (Alliance). *Cancer Medicine, 5*(4), 631–639. https://doi.org/10.1002/cam4.625.

Caudle, K. E., Dunnenberger, H. M., Freimuth, R. R., Peterson, J. F., Burlison, J. D., Whirl-Carrillo, M., et al. (2017). Standardizing terms for clinical pharmacogenetic test results: Consensus terms from the Clinical Pharmacogenetics Implementation Consortium (CPIC). *Genetics in Medicine, 19*(2), 215–223. https://doi.org/10.1038/gim.2016.87.

Caudle, K. E., Rettie, A. E., Whirl-Carrillo, M., Smith, L. H., Mintzer, S., Lee, M. T., et al. (2014). Clinical pharmacogenetics implementation consortium guidelines for CYP2C9 and HLA-B genotypes and phenytoin dosing. *Clinical Pharmacology and Therapeutics, 96*(5), 542–548. https://doi.org/10.1038/clpt.2014.159.

Chen, Y., & Goldstein, J. A. (2009). The transcriptional regulation of the human CYP2C genes. *Current Drug Metabolism, 10*(6), 567–578.

Chenoweth, M. J., & Tyndale, R. F. (2017). Pharmacogenetic optimization of smoking cessation treatment. *Trends in Pharmacological Sciences, 38*(1), 55–66. https://doi.org/10.1016/j.tips.2016.09.006.

Coffee and Caffeine Genetics Consortium, Cornelis, M. C., Byrne, E. M., Esko, T., Nalls, M. A., Ganna, A., et al. (2015). Genome-wide meta-analysis identifies six novel loci associated with habitual coffee consumption. *Molecular Psychiatry, 20*(5), 647–656. https://doi.org/10.1038/mp.2014.107.

Cornelis, M. C., Monda, K. L., Yu, K., Paynter, N., Azzato, E. M., Bennett, S. N., et al. (2011). Genome-wide meta-analysis identifies regions on 7p21 (AHR) and 15q24 (CYP1A2) as determinants of habitual caffeine consumption. *PLoS Genetics,* 7(4), e1002033. https://doi.org/10.1371/journal.pgen.1002033.

Crews, K. R., Gaedigk, A., Dunnenberger, H. M., Leeder, J. S., Klein, T. E., Caudle, K. E., et al. (2014). Clinical Pharmacogenetics Implementation Consortium guidelines for cytochrome P450 2D6 genotype and codeine therapy: 2014 Update. *Clinical Pharmacology and Therapeutics, 95*(4), 376–382. https://doi.org/10.1038/clpt.2013.254.

Daly, A. K., Rettie, A. E., Fowler, D. M., & Miners, J. O. (2018). Pharmacogenomics of CYP2C9: Functional and clinical considerations. *Journal of Personalized Medicine, 8*(1). https://doi.org/10.3390/jpm8010001.

Dawed, A. Y., Donnelly, L., Tavendale, R., Carr, F., Leese, G., Palmer, C. N., et al. (2016). CYP2C8 and SLCO1B1 variants and therapeutic response to thiazolidinediones in patients with type 2 diabetes. *Diabetes Care, 39*(11), 1902–1908. https://doi.org/10.2337/dc15-2464.

Desta, Z., Kreutz, Y., Nguyen, A. T., Li, L., Skaar, T., Kamdem, L. K., et al. (2011). Plasma letrozole concentrations in postmenopausal women with breast cancer are associated with CYP2A6 genetic variants, body mass index, and age. *Clinical Pharmacology and Therapeutics, 90*(5), 693–700. https://doi.org/10.1038/clpt.2011.174.

Di, Y. M., Chow, V. D., Yang, L. P., & Zhou, S. F. (2009). Structure, function, regulation and polymorphism of human cytochrome P450 2A6. *Current Drug Metabolism, 10*(7), 754–780.

Ding, X., & Kaminsky, L. S. (2003). Human extrahepatic cytochromes P450: Function in xenobiotic metabolism and tissue-selective chemical toxicity in the respiratory and gastrointestinal tracts. *Annual Review of Pharmacology and Toxicology, 43*, 149–173. https://doi.org/10.1146/annurev.pharmtox.43.100901.140251.

Egbelakin, A., Ferguson, M. J., MacGill, E. A., Lehmann, A. S., Topletz, A. R., Quinney, S. K., et al. (2011). Increased risk of vincristine neurotoxicity associated with low CYP3A5 expression genotype in children with acute lymphoblastic leukemia. *Pediatric Blood & Cancer*, *56*(3), 361–367. https://doi.org/10.1002/pbc.22845.

Figueiras, A., Estany-Gestal, A., Aguirre, C., Ruiz, B., Vidal, X., Carvajal, A., et al. (2016). CYP2C9 variants as a risk modifier of NSAID-related gastrointestinal bleeding: A case-control study. *Pharmacogenetics and Genomics*, *26*(2), 66–73. https://doi.org/10.1097/FPC.0000000000000186.

Fuhr, U., Rost, K. L., Engelhardt, R., Sachs, M., Liermann, D., Belloc, C., et al. (1996). Evaluation of caffeine as a test drug for CYP1A2, NAT2 and CYP2E1 phenotyping in man by in vivo versus in vitro correlations. *Pharmacogenetics*, *6*(2), 159–176.

Fujikura, K., Ingelman-Sundberg, M., & Lauschke, V. M. (2015). Genetic variation in the human cytochrome P450 supergene family. *Pharmacogenetics and Genomics*, *25*(12), 584–594. https://doi.org/10.1097/FPC.0000000000000172.

Fukami, T., Nakajima, M., Higashi, E., Yamanaka, H., Sakai, H., McLeod, H. L., et al. (2005). Characterization of novel CYP2A6 polymorphic alleles (CYP2A6*18 and CYP2A6*19) that affect enzymatic activity. *Drug Metabolism and Disposition*, *33*(8), 1202–1210. https://doi.org/10.1124/dmd.105.004994.

Furuta, T., Ohashi, K., Kamata, T., Takashima, M., Kosuge, K., Kawasaki, T., et al. (1998). Effect of genetic differences in omeprazole metabolism on cure rates for Helicobacter pylori infection and peptic ulcer. *Annals of Internal Medicine*, *129*(12), 1027–1030.

Gaedigk, A., Ingelman-Sundberg, M., Miller, N. A., Leeder, J. S., Whirl-Carrillo, M., Klein, T. E., et al. (2018). The Pharmacogene Variation (PharmVar) Consortium: Incorporation of the human cytochrome P450 (CYP) allele nomenclature database. *Clinical Pharmacology and Therapeutics*, *103*, 399–401. https://doi.org/10.1002/cpt.910.

Gaedigk, A., Sangkuhl, K., Whirl-Carrillo, M., Klein, T., & Leeder, J. S. (2017). Prediction of CYP2D6 phenotype from genotype across world populations. *Genetics in Medicine*, *19*(1), 69–76. https://doi.org/10.1038/gim.2016.80.

Gaedigk, A., Simon, S. D., Pearce, R. E., Bradford, L. D., Kennedy, M. J., & Leeder, J. S. (2008). The CYP2D6 activity score: Translating genotype information into a qualitative measure of phenotype. *Clinical Pharmacology and Therapeutics*, *83*(2), 234–242. https://doi.org/10.1038/sj.clpt.6100406.

Gage, B. F., Bass, A. R., Lin, H., Woller, S. C., Stevens, S. M., Al-Hammadi, N., et al. (2017). Effect of genotype-guided warfarin dosing on clinical events and anticoagulation control among patients undergoing hip or knee arthroplasty: The GIFT randomized clinical trial. *JAMA*, *318*(12), 1115–1124. https://doi.org/10.1001/jama.2017.11469.

Gage, B. F., Eby, C., Johnson, J. A., Deych, E., Rieder, M. J., Ridker, P. M., et al. (2008). Use of pharmacogenetic and clinical factors to predict the therapeutic dose of warfarin. *Clinical Pharmacology and Therapeutics*, *84*(3), 326–331. https://doi.org/10.1038/clpt.2008.10.

Garcia-Donas, J., Esteban, E., Leandro-Garcia, L. J., Castellano, D. E., del Alba, A. G., Climent, M. A., et al. (2011). Single nucleotide polymorphism associations with response and toxic effects in patients with advanced renal-cell carcinoma treated with first-line sunitinib: A multicentre, observational, prospective study. *The Lancet Oncology*, *12*(12), 1143–1150. https://doi.org/10.1016/S1470-2045(11)70266-2.

García-Martín, E., Martínez, C., Pizarro, R. M., Garcia-Gamito, F. J., Gullsten, H., Raunio, H., et al. (2002). CYP3A4 variant alleles in white individuals with low CYP3A4 enzyme activity. *Clinical Pharmacology and Therapeutics*, *71*(3), 196–204. https://doi.org/10.1067/mcp.2002.121371.

Gatanaga, H., Hayashida, T., Tsuchiya, K., Yoshino, M., Kuwahara, T., Tsukada, H., et al. (2007). Successful efavirenz dose reduction in HIV type 1-infected individuals with cytochrome P450 2B6 *6 and *26. *Clinical Infectious Diseases*, *45*(9), 1230–1237. https://doi.org/10.1086/522175.

Gillman, P. K. (2007). Tricyclic antidepressant pharmacology and therapeutic drug interactions updated. *British Journal of Pharmacology*, *151*(6), 737–748. https://doi.org/10.1038/sj.bjp.0707253.

Goetz, M. P., Sangkuhl, K., Guchelaar, H. J., Schwab, M., Province, M., Whirl-Carrillo, M., et al. (2018). Clinical pharmacogenetics implementation consortium (CPIC) guideline for CYP2D6 and tamoxifen therapy. *Clinical Pharmacology and Therapeutics*, *103*, 770–777. https://doi.org/10.1002/cpt.1007.

Gunes, A., & Dahl, M. L. (2008). Variation in CYP1A2 activity and its clinical implications: Influence of environmental factors and genetic polymorphisms. *Pharmacogenomics*, *9*(5), 625–637. https://doi.org/10.2217/14622416.9.5.625.

Haas, D. W., Kwara, A., Richardson, D. M., Baker, P., Papageorgiou, I., Acosta, E. P., et al. (2014). Secondary metabolism pathway polymorphisms and plasma efavirenz concentrations in HIV-infected adults with CYP2B6 slow metabolizer genotypes. *The Journal of Antimicrobial Chemotherapy*, *69*(8), 2175–2182. https://doi.org/10.1093/jac/dku110.

He, Z. X., Chen, X. W., Zhou, Z. W., & Zhou, S. F. (2015). Impact of physiological, pathological and environmental factors on the expression and activity of human cytochrome P450 2D6 and implications in precision medicine. *Drug Metabolism Reviews*, *47*(4), 470–519. https://doi.org/10.3109/03602532.2015.1101131.

Henningsson, A., Marsh, S., Loos, W. J., Karlsson, M. O., Garsa, A., Mross, K., et al. (2005). Association of CYP2C8, CYP3A4, CYP3A5, and ABCB1 polymorphisms with the pharmacokinetics of paclitaxel. *Clinical Cancer Research*, *11*(22), 8097–8104. https://doi.org/10.1158/1078-0432.CCR-05-1152.

Hicks, J. K., Bishop, J. R., Sangkuhl, K., Müller, D. J., Ji, Y., Leckband, S. G., et al. (2015). Clinical Pharmacogenetics Implementation Consortium (CPIC) guideline for CYP2D6 and CYP2C19 genotypes and dosing of selective serotonin reuptake inhibitors. *Clinical Pharmacology and Therapeutics*, *98*(2), 127–134. https://doi.org/10.1002/cpt.147.

Hicks, J. K., Sangkuhl, K., Swen, J. J., Ellingrod, V. L., Muller, D. J., Shimoda, K., et al. (2017). Clinical pharmacogenetics implementation consortium guideline (CPIC) for CYP2D6 and CYP2C19 genotypes and dosing of tricyclic antidepressants: 2016 Update. *Clinical Pharmacology and Therapeutics*, *102*(1), 37–44. https://doi.org/10.1002/cpt.597.

Hoffman, S. M., Nelson, D. R., & Keeney, D. S. (2001). Organization, structure and evolution of the CYP2 gene cluster on human chromosome 19. *Pharmacogenetics*, *11*(8), 687–698.

Hukkanen, J., Jacob, P., 3rd, & Benowitz, N. L. (2005). Metabolism and disposition kinetics of nicotine. *Pharmacological Reviews*, *57*(1), 79–115. https://doi.org/10.1124/pr.57.1.3.

International Warfarin Pharmacogenetics Consortium, Klein, T. E., Altman, R. B., Eriksson, N., Gage, B. F., Kimmel, S. E., et al. (2009). Estimation of the warfarin dose with clinical and pharmacogenetic data. *The New England Journal of Medicine*, *360*(8), 753–764. https://doi.org/10.1056/NEJMoa0809329.

Johnson, J. A., Caudle, K. E., Gong, L., Whirl-Carrillo, M., Stein, C. M., Scott, S. A., et al. (2017). Clinical Pharmacogenetics Implementation Consortium (CPIC) guideline for pharmacogenetics-guided warfarin dosing: 2017 Update. *Clinical Pharmacology and Therapeutics*, *102*(3), 397–404. https://doi.org/10.1002/cpt.668.

Jorgensen, A. L., FitzGerald, R. J., Oyee, J., Pirmohamed, M., & Williamson, P. R. (2012). Influence of CYP2C9 and VKORC1 on patient response to warfarin: A systematic review and meta-analysis. *PLoS One*, 7(8), e44064. https://doi.org/10.1371/journal.pone.0044064.

Jukic, M. M., Haslemo, T., Molden, E., & Ingelman-Sundberg, M. (2018). Impact of CYP2C19 genotype on escitalopram exposure and therapeutic failure: A retrospective study based on 2,087 patients. *The American Journal of Psychiatry*, *175*(5), 463–470. https://doi.org/10.1176/appi.ajp.2017.17050550. appiajp201717050550.

Kaida, Y., Inui, N., Suda, T., Nakamura, H., Watanabe, H., & Chida, K. (2008). The CYP2A6*4 allele is determinant of S-1 pharmacokinetics in Japanese patients with non-small-cell lung cancer. *Clinical Pharmacology and Therapeutics*, *83*(4), 589–594. https://doi.org/10.1038/sj.clpt.6100484.

Kaspera, R., Naraharisetti, S. B., Tamraz, B., Sahele, T., Cheesman, M. J., Kwok, P. Y., et al. (2010). Cerivastatin in vitro metabolism by CYP2C8 variants found in patients experiencing rhabdomyolysis. *Pharmacogenetics and Genomics*, *20*(10), 619–629. https://doi.org/10.1097/FPC.0b013e32833ecace.

Kazui, M., Nishiya, Y., Ishizuka, T., Hagihara, K., Farid, N. A., Okazaki, O., et al. (2010). Identification of the human cytochrome P450 enzymes involved in the two oxidative steps in the bioactivation of clopidogrel to its pharmacologically active metabolite. *Drug Metabolism and Disposition*, *38*(1), 92–99. https://doi.org/10.1124/dmd.109.029132.

Kimmel, S. E., French, B., Kasner, S. E., Johnson, J. A., Anderson, J. L., Gage, B. F., et al. (2013). A pharmacogenetic versus a clinical algorithm for warfarin dosing. *The New England Journal of Medicine*, *369*(24), 2283–2293. https://doi.org/10.1056/NEJMoa1310669.

Kirchheiner, J., & Brockmöller, J. (2005). Clinical consequences of cytochrome P450 2C9 polymorphisms. *Clinical Pharmacology and Therapeutics*, 77(1), 1–16. https://doi.org/10.1016/j.clpt.2004.08.009.

Kivistö, K. T., Niemi, M., Schaeffeler, E., Pitkälä, K., Tilvis, R., Fromm, M. F., et al. (2004). Lipid-lowering response to statins is affected by CYP3A5 polymorphism. *Pharmacogenetics*, *14*(8), 523–525.

Kong, S. Y., Lim, H. S., Nam, B. H., Kook, M. C., Kim, Y. W., Ryu, K. W., et al. (2009). Association of CYP2A6 polymorphisms with S-1 plus docetaxel therapy outcomes in metastatic gastric cancer. *Pharmacogenomics*, *10*(7), 1147–1155. https://doi.org/10.2217/pgs.09.48.

Kuehl, P., Zhang, J., Lin, Y., Lamba, J., Assem, M., Schuetz, J., et al. (2001). Sequence diversity in CYP3A promoters and characterization of the genetic basis of polymorphic CYP3A5 expression. *Nature Genetics*, *27*(4), 383–391. https://doi.org/10.1038/86882.

Lam, S. W., Frederiks, C. N., van der Straaten, T., Honkoop, A. H., Guchelaar, H. J., & Boven, E. (2016). Genotypes of CYP2C8 and FGD4 and their association with peripheral neuropathy or early dose reduction in paclitaxel-treated breast cancer patients. *British Journal of Cancer*, *115*(11), 1335–1342. https://doi.org/10.1038/bjc.2016.326.

Lamba, J., Hebert, J. M., Schuetz, E. G., Klein, T. E., & Altman, R. B. (2012). PharmGKB summary: Very important pharmacogene information for CYP3A5. *Pharmacogenetics and Genomics*, *22*(7), 555–558. https://doi.org/10.1097/FPC.0b013e328351d47f.

Läpple, F., von Richter, O., Fromm, M. F., Richter, T., Thon, K. P., Wisser, H., et al. (2003). Differential expression and function of CYP2C isoforms in human intestine and liver. *Pharmacogenetics*, *13*(9), 565–575. https://doi.org/10.1097/01.fpc.0000054122.14659.1e.

Lee, A. M., Jepson, C., Hoffmann, E., Epstein, L., Hawk, L. W., Lerman, C., et al. (2007). CYP2B6 genotype alters abstinence rates in a bupropion smoking cessation trial. *Biological Psychiatry*, *62*(6), 635–641. https://doi.org/10.1016/j.biopsych.2006.10.005.

Mao, L., Jian, C., Changzhi, L., Dan, H., Suihua, H., Wenyi, T., et al. (2013). Cytochrome CYP2C19 polymorphism and risk of adverse clinical events in clopidogrel-treated patients: A meta-analysis based on 23,035 subjects. *Archives of Cardiovascular Diseases*, *106*(10), 517–527. https://doi.org/10.1016/j.acvd.2013.06.055.

Matthaei, J., Tzvetkov, M. V., Strube, J., Sehrt, D., Sachse-Seeboth, C., Hjelmborg, J. B., et al. (2016). Heritability of caffeine metabolism: Environmental effects masking genetic effects on CYP1A2 activity but not on NAT2. *Clinical Pharmacology and Therapeutics*, *100*(6), 606–616. https://doi.org/10.1002/cpt.444.

McDonagh, E. M., Wassenaar, C., David, S. P., Tyndale, R. F., Altman, R. B., Whirl-Carrillo, M., et al. (2012). PharmGKB summary: Very important pharmacogene information for cytochrome P-450, family 2, subfamily A, polypeptide 6. *Pharmacogenetics and Genomics*, *22*(9), 695–708. https://doi.org/10.1097/FPC.0b013e3283540217.

Mega, J. L., Simon, T., Collet, J. P., Anderson, J. L., Antman, E. M., Bliden, K., et al. (2010). Reduced-function CYP2C19 genotype and risk of adverse clinical outcomes among patients treated with clopidogrel predominantly for PCI: A meta-analysis. *JAMA*, *304*(16), 1821–1830. https://doi.org/10.1001/jama.2010.1543.

Miksys, S., & Tyndale, R. F. (2004). The unique regulation of brain cytochrome P450 2 (CYP2) family enzymes by drugs and genetics. *Drug Metabolism Reviews*, *36*(2), 313–333. https://doi.org/10.1081/DMR-120034149.

Moriyama, B., Obeng, A. O., Barbarino, J., Penzak, S. R., Henning, S. A., Scott, S. A., et al. (2017). Clinical Pharmacogenetics Implementation Consortium (CPIC) guidelines for CYP2C19 and voriconazole therapy. *Clinical Pharmacology and Therapeutics*, *102*(1), 45–51. https://doi.org/10.1002/cpt.583.

Mwinyi, J., Hofmann, Y., Pedersen, R. S., Nekvindova, J., Cavaco, I., Mkrtchian, S., et al. (2010). The transcription factor GATA-4 regulates cytochrome P4502C19 gene expression. *Life Sciences*, *86*(19–20), 699–706. https://doi.org/10.1016/j.lfs.2010.02.021.

Nebert, D. W., & Russell, D. W. (2002). Clinical importance of the cytochromes P450. *Lancet*, *360*(9340), 1155–1162. https://doi.org/10.1016/S0140-6736(02)11203-7.

Nelson, D. R., Zeldin, D. C., Hoffman, S. M., Maltais, L. J., Wain, H. M., & Nebert, D. W. (2004). Comparison of cytochrome P450 (CYP) genes from the mouse and human genomes, including nomenclature recommendations for genes, pseudogenes and alternative-splice variants. *Pharmacogenetics*, *14*(1), 1–18.

Orliaguet, G., Hamza, J., Couloigner, V., Denoyelle, F., Loriot, M. A., Broly, F., et al. (2015). A case of respiratory depression in a child with ultrarapid CYP2D6 metabolism after tramadol. *Pediatrics*, *135*(3), e753–755. https://doi.org/10.1542/peds.2014-2673.

Pan, Y., Chen, W., Xu, Y., Yi, X., Han, Y., Yang, Q., et al. (2017). Genetic polymorphisms and clopidogrel efficacy for acute ischemic stroke or transient ischemic attack: A systematic review and meta-analysis. *Circulation*, *135*(1), 21–33. https://doi.org/10.1161/CIRCULATIONAHA.116.024913.

Pan, X., Ning, M., & Jeong, H. (2017). Transcriptional regulation of CYP2D6 expression. *Drug Metabolism and Disposition*, *45*(1), 42–48. https://doi.org/10.1124/dmd.116.072249.

Park, S. R., Kong, S. Y., Nam, B. H., Choi, I. J., Kim, C. G., Lee, J. Y., et al. (2011). CYP2A6 and ERCC1 polymorphisms correlate with efficacy of S-1 plus cisplatin in metastatic gastric cancer patients. *British Journal of Cancer*, *104*(7), 1126–1134. https://doi.org/10.1038/bjc.2011.24.

Pietarinen, P., Tornio, A., & Niemi, M. (2016). High frequency of CYP2D6 ultrarapid metabolizer genotype in the Finnish population. *Basic & Clinical Pharmacology & Toxicology*, *119*(3), 291–296. https://doi.org/10.1111/bcpt.12590.

Pirmohamed, M., Burnside, G., Eriksson, N., Jorgensen, A. L., Toh, C. H., Nicholson, T., et al. (2013). A randomized trial of genotype-guided dosing of warfarin. *The New England Journal of Medicine*, *369*(24), 2294–2303. https://doi.org/10.1056/NEJMoa1311386.

Ray, R., Tyndale, R. F., & Lerman, C. (2009). Nicotine dependence pharmacogenetics: Role of genetic variation in nicotine-metabolizing enzymes. *Journal of Neurogenetics*, *23*(3), 252–261. https://doi.org/10.1080/01677060802572887.

Rettie, A. E., Korzekwa, K. R., Kunze, K. L., Lawrence, R. F., Eddy, A. C., Aoyama, T., et al. (1992). Hydroxylation of warfarin by human cDNA-expressed cytochrome P-450: A role for P-4502C9 in the etiology of (S)-warfarin-drug interactions. *Chemical Research in Toxicology*, *5*(1), 54–59.

Sachse, C., Brockmoller, J., Bauer, S., & Roots, I. (1999). Functional significance of a C→A polymorphism in intron 1 of the cytochrome P450 CYP1A2 gene tested with caffeine. *British Journal of Clinical Pharmacology*, *47*(4), 445–449.

Scott, S. A., Sangkuhl, K., Stein, C. M., Hulot, J. S., Mega, J. L., Roden, D. M., et al. (2013). Clinical Pharmacogenetics Implementation Consortium guidelines for CYP2C19 genotype and clopidogrel therapy: 2013 Update. *Clinical Pharmacology and Therapeutics*, *94*(3), 317–323. https://doi.org/10.1038/clpt.2013.105. clpt2013105 [pii].

Sibbing, D., Koch, W., Gebhard, D., Schuster, T., Braun, S., Stegherr, J., et al. (2010). Cytochrome 2C19*17 allelic variant, platelet aggregation, bleeding events, and stent thrombosis in clopidogrel-treated patients with coronary stent placement. *Circulation*, *121*(4), 512–518. https://doi.org/10.1161/CIRCULATIONAHA.109.885194.

Somogyi, A. A., Coller, J. K., & Barratt, D. T. (2015). Pharmacogenetics of opioid response. *Clinical Pharmacology and Therapeutics*, *97*(2), 125–127. https://doi.org/10.1002/cpt.23.

Stage, T. B., Christensen, M. M., Feddersen, S., Beck-Nielsen, H., & Brøsen, K. (2013). The role of genetic variants in CYP2C8, LPIN1, PPARGC1A and PPARgamma on the trough steady-state plasma concentrations of rosiglitazone and on glycosylated haemoglobin A1c in type 2 diabetes. *Pharmacogenetics and Genomics*, *23*(4), 219–227. https://doi.org/10.1097/FPC.0b013e32835f91fc.

Sun, W., Li, Y., Li, J., Zhang, Z., Zhu, W., Liu, W., et al. (2015). Variant recurrent risk among stroke patients with different CYP2C19 phenotypes and treated with clopidogrel. *Platelets*, *26*(6), 558–562. https://doi.org/10.3109/09537104.2014.953044.

Swen, J. J., Nijenhuis, M., de Boer, A., Grandia, L., Maitland-van der Zee, A. H., Mulder, H., et al. (2011). Pharmacogenetics: From bench to byte—An update of guidelines. *Clinical Pharmacology and Therapeutics*, *89*(5), 662–673. https://doi.org/10.1038/clpt.2011.34.

Tanii, H., Shitara, Y., & Horie, T. (2011). Population pharmacokinetic analysis of letrozole in Japanese postmenopausal women. *European Journal of Clinical Pharmacology*, *67*(10), 1017–1025. https://doi.org/10.1007/s00228-011-1042-3.

Tanner, J. A., & Tyndale, R. F. (2017). Variation in CYP2A6 activity and personalized medicine. *Journal of Personalized Medicine*, 7(4). https://doi.org/10.3390/jpm7040018.

Thompson, E. E., Kuttab-Boulos, H., Witonsky, D., Yang, L., Roe, B. A., & Di Rienzo, A. (2004). CYP3A variation and the evolution of salt-sensitivity variants. *American Journal of Human Genetics*, *75*(6), 1059–1069. https://doi.org/10.1086/426406.

Tornio, A., Flynn, R., Morant, S., Velten, E., Palmer, C. N. A., MacDonald, T. M., et al. (2018). Investigating real-world clopidogrel pharmacogenetics in stroke using a bioresource linked to electronic medical records. *Clinical Pharmacology and Therapeutics*, *103*(2), 281–286. https://doi.org/10.1002/cpt.780.

Turpeinen, M., & Zanger, U. M. (2012). Cytochrome P450 2B6: Function, genetics, and clinical relevance. *Drug Metabolism and Drug Interactions*, *27*(4), 185–197. https://doi.org/10.1515/dmdi-2012-0027.

Vo, T. T., & Varghese Gupta, S. (2016). Role of cytochrome P450 2B6 pharmacogenomics in determining efavirenz-mediated central nervous system toxicity, treatment outcomes, and dosage adjustments in patients with human immunodeficiency virus infection. *Pharmacotherapy*, *36*(12), 1245–1254. https://doi.org/10.1002/phar.1852.

Wang, D., Guo, Y., Wrighton, S. A., Cooke, G. E., & Sadee, W. (2011). Intronic polymorphism in CYP3A4 affects hepatic expression and response to statin drugs. *The Pharmacogenomics Journal*, *11*(4), 274–286. https://doi.org/10.1038/tpj.2010.28.

Wang, H., & Tompkins, L. M. (2008). CYP2B6: New insights into a historically overlooked cytochrome P450 isozyme. *Current Drug Metabolism*, *9*(7), 598–610.

Werk, A. N., & Cascorbi, I. (2014). Functional gene variants of CYP3A4. *Clinical Pharmacology and Therapeutics*, *96*(3), 340–348. https://doi.org/10.1038/clpt.2014.129.

Werk, A. N., Lefeldt, S., Bruckmueller, H., Hemmrich-Stanisak, G., Franke, A., Roos, M., et al. (2014). Identification and characterization of a defective CYP3A4 genotype in a kidney transplant patient with severely diminished tacrolimus clearance. *Clinical Pharmacology and Therapeutics*, *95*(4), 416–422. https://doi.org/10.1038/clpt.2013.210.

Westlind-Johnsson, A., Hermann, R., Huennemeyer, A., Hauns, B., Lahu, G., Nassr, N., et al. (2006). Identification and characterization of CYP3A4*20, a novel rare CYP3A4 allele without functional activity. *Clinical Pharmacology and Therapeutics*, *79*(4), 339–349. https://doi.org/10.1016/j.clpt.2005.11.015.

Wilke, R. A., Moore, J. H., & Burmester, J. K. (2005). Relative impact of CYP3A genotype and concomitant medication on the severity of atorvastatin-induced muscle damage. *Pharmacogenetics and Genomics*, *15*(6), 415–421.

Willrich, M. A., Hirata, M. H., Genvigir, F. D., Arazi, S. S., Rebecchi, I. M., Rodrigues, A. C., et al. (2008). CYP3A53A allele is associated with reduced lowering-lipid response to atorvastatin in individuals with hypercholesterolemia. *Clinica Chimica Acta*, *398*(1–2), 15–20. https://doi.org/10.1016/j.cca.2008.07.032.

Yano, J. K., Hsu, M. H., Griffin, K. J., Stout, C. D., & Johnson, E. F. (2005). Structures of human microsomal cytochrome P450 2A6 complexed with coumarin and methoxsalen. *Nature Structural & Molecular Biology*, *12*(9), 822–823. https://doi.org/10.1038/nsmb971.

Yasar, U., Lundgren, S., Eliasson, E., Bennet, A., Wiman, B., de Faire, U., et al. (2002). Linkage between the CYP2C8 and CYP2C9 genetic polymorphisms. *Biochemical and Biophysical Research Communications*, *299*(1), 25–28.

Zanger, U. M., & Klein, K. (2013). Pharmacogenetics of cytochrome P450 2B6 (CYP2B6): Advances on polymorphisms, mechanisms, and clinical relevance. *Frontiers in Genetics 4* , 24. https://doi.org/10.3389/fgene.2013.00024.

Zanger, U. M., & Schwab, M. (2013). Cytochrome P450 enzymes in drug metabolism: Regulation of gene expression, enzyme activities, and impact of genetic variation. *Pharmacology & Therapeutics*, *138*(1), 103–141. https://doi.org/10.1016/j.pharmthera.2012.12.007.

Zanger, U. M., Turpeinen, M., Klein, K., & Schwab, M. (2008). Functional pharmacogenetics/genomics of human cytochromes P450 involved in drug biotransformation. *Analytical and Bioanalytical Chemistry*, *392*(6), 1093–1108. https://doi.org/10.1007/s00216-008-2291-6.

Zhang, H. F., Wang, H. H., Gao, N., Wei, J. Y., Tian, X., Zhao, Y., et al. (2016). Physiological content and intrinsic activities of 10 cytochrome P450 isoforms in human normal liver microsomes. *The Journal of Pharmacology and Experimental Therapeutics*, *358*(1), 83–93. https://doi.org/10.1124/jpet.116.233635.

Zhao, F., Wang, J., Yang, Y., Wang, X., Shi, R., Xu, Z., et al. (2008). Effect of CYP2C19 genetic polymorphisms on the efficacy of proton pump inhibitor-based triple therapy for Helicobacter pylori eradication: A meta-analysis. *Helicobacter*, *13*(6), 532–541. https://doi.org/10.1111/j.1523-5378.2008.00643.x.

Zhou, S. F. (2008). Drugs behave as substrates, inhibitors and inducers of human cytochrome P450 3A4. *Current Drug Metabolism*, *9*(4), 310–322.

Zhou, Y., Ingelman-Sundberg, M., & Lauschke, V. M. (2017). Worldwide distribution of cytochrome P450 alleles: A meta-analysis of population-scale sequencing projects. *Clinical Pharmacology and Therapeutics*, *102*(4), 688–700. https://doi.org/10.1002/cpt.690.

Zhou, S. F., Wang, B., Yang, L. P., & Liu, J. P. (2010). Structure, function, regulation and polymorphism and the clinical significance of human cytochrome P450 1A2. *Drug Metabolism Reviews*, *42*(2), 268–354. https://doi.org/10.3109/03602530903286476.

Zhu, A. Z., Cox, L. S., Nollen, N., Faseru, B., Okuyemi, K. S., Ahluwalia, J. S., et al. (2012). CYP2B6 and bupropion's smoking-cessation pharmacology: The role of hydroxybupropion. *Clinical Pharmacology and Therapeutics*, *92*(6), 771–777. https://doi.org/10.1038/clpt.2012.186.

CHAPTER TWO

Epigenetics and MicroRNAs in Pharmacogenetics

Ulrich M. Zanger*,†,1, Kathrin Klein*, Nicole Kugler*, Tamara Petrikat*, Chang S. Ryu*

*Dr. Margarete Fischer-Bosch Institute of Clinical Pharmacology, Stuttgart, Germany
†University Hospital Tübingen, Tübingen, Germany
[1]Corresponding author: e-mail address: uli.zanger@ikp-stuttgart.de

Contents

1. Introduction 34
2. Epigenetics in Pharmacogenetics 36
   2.1 Polymorphisms Interacting With DMET Gene Methylation 36
   2.2 Polymorphisms Affecting Methylation Machinery 39
3. miRNAs in Pharmacogenetics 40
   3.1 miR-SNPs Affecting Enzymes 41
   3.2 miR-SNPs Affecting Transporters 54
   3.3 miR-SNPs Affecting Regulators and miRNA Machinery 55
4. Conclusion 56
Acknowledgments 57
References 57

Abstract

Germline pharmacogenetics has so far mainly studied common variants in "pharmacogenes," i.e., genes encoding drug metabolizing enzymes and transporters (DMET genes), certain auxiliary and regulatory genes, and drug target genes. Despite remarkable progress in understanding genetically determined differences in pharmacokinetics and pharmacodynamics of drugs, currently known common variants even in important pharmacogenes explain genetic variability only partially. This suggests "missing heritability" that may in part be due to rare variants in the classical pharmacogenes, but current evidence suggests that largely unexplored resources with potential for pharmacogenetics exist, both within already known pharmacogenes and in entirely new areas. In particular, recent studies suggest that epigenetic processes and noncoding RNAs, including mostly microRNAs (miRNAs), represent important and largely unexplored layers of DMET gene regulation that may fill some of the gaps in understanding interindividual variability and lead to new biomarkers. In this chapter we summarize recent advances in the understanding of genetic variability in epigenetic and miRNA-mediated processes with focus on their significance for DMET regulation and pharmacokinetic or pharmacological endpoints.

Advances in Pharmacology, Volume 83
ISSN 1054-3589
https://doi.org/10.1016/bs.apha.2018.02.003

ABBREVIATIONS

5-FU	5-fluorouracil
ABC	ATP-binding cassette
AGO-CLIP	Argonaute cross-linking immunoprecipitation
ALDH	aldehyde dehydrogenase
CNV	copy number variation
CpG	5′—C—phosphate—G—3′
CYP	cytochrome P450
DHFR	dihydrofolate reductase
DMET	drug metabolizing enzymes and transporters
DNMT	DNA methyltransferase
DPYD, DPD	dihydropyrimidine dehydrogenase
eQTL	expression quantitative trait loci
HIF	hypoxia-inducible factor
HNF	hepatic nuclear factor
LD	linkage disequilibrium
LPL	lipoprotein lipase
MAF	minor allele frequency
MDR	multidrug resistance protein, p-glycoprotein
MGMT	O-6-methylguanine-DNA methyltransferase
miR, miRNA	microRNA
MTHFR	methylenetetrahydrofolate reductase
OR	odds ratio
PD	pharmacodynamics
PK	pharmacokinetics
PXR	pregnane X receptor
RAN	Ras-related nuclear protein
RISC	RNA-induced silencing complex
SLC	solute carrier family
SNP	single-nucleotide polymorphism
SULT	sulfotransferase
TYMS	thymidylate synthase
UGT	UDP-glucuronosyltransferase
UTR	untranslated region
VKORC1	vitamin K epoxide reductase complex subunit 1
XPO	exportin

1. INTRODUCTION

Previous decades of research on germline pharmacogenetics have focused on the impact of common variants in "pharmacogenes," i.e., genes encoding drug metabolizing enzymes and transporters (DMET genes), some auxiliary and regulatory genes (e.g., nuclear receptors), and drug target genes on drug pharmacokinetics (PK) and pharmacodynamics (PD) (Zhang & Nebert, 2017; Zanger & Schwab, 2013). Despite remarkable progress in understanding heritable differences in drug disposition, currently known common variants even in important pharmacogenes such as CYP2D6, CYP2C9, or the transporter OATP1B1 contribute only to a minor extent to the total genetic variability as estimated in twin studies (Matthaei et al., 2015). This suggests "missing heritability" that may in part be due to rare variants in these genes, although advanced prediction tools will have to be developed for them to become meaningful (Lauschke & Ingelman-Sundberg, 2016; Zanger et al., 2014). Recent research has demonstrated that epigenetic processes and microRNAs (miRNAs) constitute important and largely unexplored layers of DMET gene regulation that may fill some of the gaps in understanding interindividual variability and lead to new biomarkers.

"Epigenetics" refers to heritable changes or differences in gene expression that are not due to DNA sequence differences in the encoding gene but due to heritable changes in DNA methylation or chromatin architecture and their consequences. Epigenetic mechanisms may affect gene expression in a short term, for example, through induction/repression of noncoding RNA transcription, but also over years (and transmitted through cell divisions within a tissue) or even generations (transmitted through the germline) by mechanisms involving DNA methylation or histone modifications (Baer-Dubowska, Majchrzak-Celińska, & Cichocki, 2011; Fisel, Schaeffeler, & Schwab, 2016; Ivanov, Kacevska, & Ingelman-Sundberg, 2012). However, unlike genetic information, epigenetic information stored in the germ lineage can be modified with every generation, so that epigenetically modified phenotypes may not always be transgenerationally stable. Today's molecular concepts about epigenetics hold that the genetic information stored in DNA can exist in different "on" (euchromatin) or "off" (heterochromatin) functional states that are maintained by epigenetic mechanisms involving covalent modifications on histones such as acetylation, methylation, and phosphorylation, as well as methylation, hydroxymethylation, and other modifications at DNA CpG sites (Allis & Jenuwein, 2016; Lauschke, Barragan, & Ingelman-Sundberg, 2018). These processes involve numerous enzymes classified as "writers" or "readers" depending on whether they introduce or delete such modifications on their substrate (e.g., histone acetylases and deacetylases, DNA methyltransferases, and demethylases), or whether they recognize them leading to a change in outcome (e.g., DNA methylation-sensitive transcription factors).

miRNAs represent so far the most extensively studied subclass of non-coding RNAs. The wide influence of miRNAs on the expression and function of DMET genes has been summarized in several excellent reviews (Dluzen & Lazarus, 2015; Yokoi & Nakajima, 2013; Yu, Tian, Tu, Ho, & Jilek, 2016). It is thus an interesting question, how genetic polymorphisms in the miRNA machinery, the miRNA genes, or in their corresponding target sequences modulate the interactions between miRNAs and their targets, and how this may affect today's pharmacogenetic concepts and predictions. The focus of this chapter is therefore not the epigenetic or miRNA-mediated regulation of drug metabolism and response itself, nor is it the development or use of epigenetic or miRNA-based drugs (both of which have been summarized in the above-mentioned references), but on *interactions* between epigenetics/miRNAs and defined genetic polymorphisms that influence the metabolism and/or the response to pharmacological agents.

2. EPIGENETICS IN PHARMACOGENETICS

Polymorphisms relating to both epigenetics and pharmacogenetics may reside in any gene of the epigenetic enzymatic machinery, i.e., methylating/demethylating or acetylating/deacetylating enzymes, effector genes that recognize epigenetic modifications, or in the target genes themselves, e.g., in CpG islands of DMET or other genes related to drug response and subject to epigenetic modification (Table 1). While the former variants would be classified as *trans*-acting, the latter ones would be classical *cis*-acting variants. Generally, genetic variants acting in *cis* are expected to be of higher impact and more specific, while *trans*-acting variants have often been found to be of lower impact and difficult to reproduce (e.g., Glubb, Dholakia, & Innocenti, 2012). In the following section, studies with implications for PK/PD or DMET gene regulation are presented (Table 1).

2.1 Polymorphisms Interacting With DMET Gene Methylation

Aldehyde dehydrogenase 2 (ALDH2) is the primary enzyme for the metabolism of acetaldehyde derived from oxidation of ethanol by alcohol dehydrogenases and CYP2E1. The toxic effects of acetaldehyde are mainly responsible for the acute adverse effects following excessive ethanol consumption like nausea and headache, but also influence diverse long-term health risks. Carriers of a polymorphism (rs671) common in Asia that leads to acetaldehyde consumption are particularly sensitive to the adverse effects of ethanol, but

Table 1 Epigenetic SNPs

SNP	Gene	Location	Position (HGVS) (ref > var)	MAF (Allele)[a]	Effect	References
rs1128503	ABCB1	Exonic	c.1236T > C (G412)	0.41 (T)	Methylation	Gupta et al. (2017)
rs2032582	ABCB1	Exonic	c.2677T > G,A (S893T)	0.46 (T)	Methylation	Gupta et al. (2017)
rs886205	ALDH2	Promoter	c.–360A > G	0.17 (G)	Methylation	Pathak et al. (2017) and Haschemi Nassab et al. (2016)
rs2228612	DNMT1	Exonic	c.979A > G (I327F)	0.07 (G)	Expression	Li, Liu, Sun, and Yuan (2017)
rs377577594	DNMT3A	Exonic	c.2188C > A,G,T (R882H/C/S)	0.0004 (A)	Unknown	Zhang et al. (2017)
rs2424909	DNMT3B	Promoter	c.-149C > T	0.63 (T)	Unknown	Zhang et al. (2017)
rs910083	DNMT3B	Intronic	c.688–717 A > C,G	0.42 (C)	Unknown	Hancock et al. (2017)
rs2424913	DNMT3B	Promoter	c.-149C > T	0.41 (T)	Expression	Lai et al. (2017)
rs16906252	MGMT	Exonic	c.66C > T (R22)	0.06 (T)	Methylation	Rapkins et al. (2015)
rs1801133	MTHFR	Exonic	c.665C > T *"677C > T"* (A222V)	0.36 (T)	Reduced MTHFR activity	Lin et al. (2016), Spellicy, Kosten, Hamon, Harding, and Nielsen (2012), and Aarabi et al. (2015)

[a]Minor allele frequency for EUR population as given in dbSNP, minor allele is noted in brackets.

risk factors in other ethnicities have been less well studied (Quertemont, 2004). *ALDH2* transcriptional regulation involves several nonsteroidal nuclear receptors and is inducible by ethanol. The rs886205 polymorphism in the *ALDH2* promoter, originally identified as a risk marker for alcohol-associated upper digestive tract cancers in non-Asian populations, is associated with decreased promoter activity. The mechanism involves methylation at CpG sites located in negative and positive regulatory regions of the promoter (Pathak et al., 2017). Interestingly, the A-allele is more readily methylated during the first 24 h of alcohol withdrawal leading to an almost 50% decrease in ALDH2 protein within 1 week, while G-allele carriers show retarded epigenetic adaptation and no change in protein levels (Haschemi Nassab et al., 2016). These studies support the emerging evidence that alcohol and other drugs can have a permanent influence on gene expression via epigenetic processes and show furthermore that allele-specific genetic–epigenetic interactions modulate the effects of classical pharmacogenetics markers.

The *ABCB1 gene encoding the P-glycoprotein transporter,* also called multidrug resistance protein 1 (MDR1), is one of the most important drug transporters acting to export drugs and other xenobiotics as well as endogenous toxic substances from tissues. The *ABCB1* gene is highly polymorphic, and several common variants have been associated with altered drug exposure in various tissues, drug resistance, and/or altered susceptibility to a range of different diseases including malaria (Chinn & Kroetz, 2007; Kerb et al., 2009). Earlier studies in breast cancer cells have suggested that changes in *ABCB1* promoter methylation can regulate *ABCB1* transcription and be temporally and causally related to the acquisition of drug resistance toward paclitaxel that moreover appeared to be even allele-specifically determined (Reed, Hembruff, Sprowl, & Parissenti, 2010). Hypothesizing that epigenetic changes may be causally related to the distinction between complicated (severe) and uncomplicated (less severe) malaria, a recent study investigated *ABCB1* promoter methylation in malaria patients and related them to transcript and protein levels as well as three important polymorphisms (Gupta et al., 2017). They found differences in methylation levels between patients and healthy controls and that two of the three analyzed polymorphisms correlated with methylation as well as with ABCB1 protein levels in the complicated malaria group (Table 1). These data suggest that genetic–epigenetic interactions may be involved in the etiology of malaria susceptibility as well as prognosis and drug response.

2.2 Polymorphisms Affecting Methylation Machinery

Most work in this area has been done in regard to the DNA methylation machinery, which plays critical roles for chromatin structure and gene expression and comprises DNA methyltransferases (DNMTs), demethylating enzymes such as the ten-eleven translocation (TET) family of 5mC dioxygenases, which together regulate levels and patterns of DNA methylation, while the effects are mediated by and DNA "reader" proteins. Variants in these genes have been identified mainly in cancer and developmental disorders (Hamidi, Singh, & Chen, 2015). In addition, enzymes involved in DNA repair mechanisms (MGMT) or required for supply of methyl groups (MTHFR) may also be considered as components of the epigenetic machinery (see below). Although to our knowledge variants in the DNMT/TET genes have not been shown to directly affect DMET gene expression or pharmacokinetics of drugs, a few examples related to xenobiotic exposure and/or cancer risk are mentioned in Table 1.

Promoter methylation of *O-6-methylguanine-DNA methyltransferase (MGMT)*, an enzyme involved in repair of DNA lesions caused by temozolomide and other alkylating agents, is an established predictive biomarker associated with lower MGMT expression and greater benefit of treatment with a significant increase of survival (Hegi et al., 2005). However, since methylation status alone did not seem to explain all data satisfactorily, MacDonald and colleagues hypothesized that a combination of single-nucleotide polymorphisms (SNPs) and differential *MGMT* promoter methylation determines sensitivity to alkylating agents (Rapkins et al., 2015). The SNP rs16906252 (Table 1), which is located within a *cis*-acting enhancer element within the *MGMT* coding region, was shown by allelic bisulfite sequencing to be a key determinant for acquisition of *MGMT* promoter methylation. Interestingly, however, the SNP was associated with better survival in temozolomide-treated patients irrespective of tumor *MGMT* methylation status. This finding, obtained in two independent temozolomide-treated glioblastoma cohorts, one Australian and one American, may be useful to more precisely define patients who profit from the treatment.

Methylenetetrahydrofolate reductase (MTHFR) is a key enzyme for the supply of methyl groups for protein and DNA methylation as it catalyzes the conversion of 5,10-methyltetrahydrofolate to 5-methyltetrahydrofolate in the remethylation cycle. MTHFR can thus be regarded as a primary suspect to explain interindividual differences in methylation epigenetics. The common MTHFR variant rs1801133 (A222V) codes for a more thermolabile enzyme with lower activity (Table 1) and has been investigated thoroughly in relation to folate status in a variety of metabolic and disease contexts (Hiraoka & Kagawa, 2017). The significance of *MTHFR* polymorphisms for global methylation has been investigated in several studies. For example, since folate is considered to be essential for spermatogenesis, one study investigated methylation levels across different regions of the sperm genome by bisulfate pyrosequencing in men with idiopathic infertility under high-dose folic acid supplementation (Aarabi et al., 2015). Surprisingly they did not find improved sperm parameters as expected, but a marked loss of DNA methylation across the genome including promoter regions of genes involved in cancer and neurological diseases. This loss was exacerbated in carriers of the T-allele, showing an interaction between a well-known genetic polymorphism and DNA methylation, and the authors suggest a personalized approach to high-dose folic acid supplementation in male infertility, taking genetic background in consideration. In another study DNA methylation in the context of atherosclerosis was studied, and long interspersed nuclear element (LINE-1) methylation was determined in relation to the MTHFR A222V polymorphism in coronary atherosclerosis patients and controls (Lin et al., 2012). The T-allele was associated with increased risk of atherosclerosis and with lower LINE-1 methylation levels, further suggesting that the *MTHFR* gene polymorphism affects global DNA methylation, thereby possibly influencing atherosclerosis morbidity. However, not all studies confirmed an influence of the common MTHFR variant A222V on global methylation (Wang, Shangguan et al., 2016).

3. MIRNAS IN PHARMACOGENETICS

The effect a miRNA has on its target can be influenced by genetic variants in different locations and mechanisms: variants in genes of the miRNA biogenesis machinery may influence miRNA processing and maturation; variants in pre-miRNAs could alter stem–loop structures and also influence maturation; variants in mature miRNAs, especially within seed regions, and in their cognate target gene-binding sites, could modulate miRNA–mRNA interaction by creating or destroying miRNA-binding sites or by altering mRNA secondary structures that may affect mRNA recognition and cleavage by the RNA-induced silencing complex (RISC). Since a single miRNA can affect many genes, a single SNP in the seed-sequence of the miRNA gene may affect many target genes, in contrast to an SNP in the miRNA-binding sequence. We will refer to all these types of SNPs as miR-SNPs. Table 2 presents some useful publically available databases for miR-SNPs.

A number of studies explored polymorphisms that may affect interactions between miRNAs and pharmacogenes on a more general basis. In an in silico study different algorithms and databases were used to predict miRNAs that regulate the 12 most important drug metabolizing CYPs, and within the predicted target sites 38 SNPs that potentially interfere with miRNA binding were identified (Ramamoorthy & Skaar, 2011). In a systematic sequence analysis of genetic variation within 3′-UTRs of four CYPs (1A2, 2B6, 2D6, 3A4), the nuclear pregnane X receptor (PXR, NR1I2), and UGT2B7 in black South Africans, several variants were found (Swart & Dandara, 2014). The PolymiRTS database was used to predict whether they alter the targeting of more than 200 miRNAs; however, no functional association data have been provided in that study. Using publically available expression quantitative trait loci (eQTL) datasets generated from HAPMAP lymphoblastoid cell lines and human liver and brain tissues, another study identified 308 significant eQTL signals associated with mRNA expression of 101 xenobiotic enzymes and transporter genes and identified 26 SNPs in the 3′-UTRs of 14 of these genes that were strongly correlated with these traits and that were predicted to affect miRNA target sites (Wei et al., 2012). However, only 12 of these correlations were found in liver (the others in brain) and to our knowledge, only those in CYP2E1 have so far been confirmed (see below). A similar, more integrative study identified miRNA-binding site polymorphisms associated with eQTLs and used Argonaute cross-linking immunoprecipitation (AGO-CLIP) datasets to predict interference with miRNA response elements on a global scale (Võsa, Esko, Kasela, & Annilo, 2015).

In the following section, we discuss distinct genetic variants according to their affected target genes phase I enzymes, phase II enzymes, phase 0/III transporters, pharmacogene effectors and regulators, and various miRNA machinery genes (Fig. 1; Table 3).

3.1 miR-SNPs Affecting Enzymes

Cytochrome P450 (CYP) 2B6 (CYP2B6) is one of the minor CYPs in human liver. Expression is highly variable due to extensive genetic polymorphism and inducibility. Drugs metabolized by CYP2B6 include artemisinin,

Table 2 Selected Databases for Analysis of Epigenetic Variants

Title	Description	URL	References
Databases miRNA + SNP			
lncRNASNP2	SNPs in human/mouse lncRNAs, functional SNP selection for genetic association studies	http://bioinfo.life.hust.edu.cn/lncRNASNP2#!/	Miao, Liu, Zhang, and Guo (2017)
Mir2Drug	Genetic variations in miRNA target sites and their potential function in drug response	http://bioinfo.njmu.edu.cn/Mir2Drug/	Wang et al. (2017)
miRdSNP	Disease-associated SNPs and microRNA target sites on 3′-UTRs of human genes, manually curated	http://mirdsnp.ccr.buffalo.edu/	Bruno et al. (2012)
miRNA SNiPer	Variations within different regions of miRNA	http://www.integratomics-time.com/miRNA-SNiPer/	Zorc, Obsteter, Dovc, and Kunej (2015)
miRNASNP	SNPs in miRNAs and genes that may impact miRNA biogenesis and/or miRNA target binding	http://bioinfo.life.hust.edu.cn/miRNASNP2/	Gong et al. (2015)
MirSNP	Putative human miRNA-related SNPs from GWAS and eQTLs researches	http://bioinfo.bjmu.edu.cn/mirsnp/search/	Liu et al. (2012)
Mirsnpscore	SNPs effects associated with diseases on microRNA targeting computer-based predictions	http://www.bigr.medisin.ntnu.no/mirsnpscore/	Thomas, Saito, and Sætrom (2011)
PolymiRTS	Functional impact of SNPs in miRNA seed regions and miRNA target sites	http://compbio.uthsc.edu/miRSNP/	Bhattacharya, Ziebarth, and Cui (2014)
General genotype–phenotype databases			
NHGRI GWAS catalog	The NHGRI-EBI Catalog of published genome-wide association studies	http://www.ebi.ac.uk/gwas/	Welter et al. (2014)
PheGenI	Phenotype–genotype integrator	https://www.ncbi.nlm.nih.gov/gap/phegeni	Ramos et al. (2014)

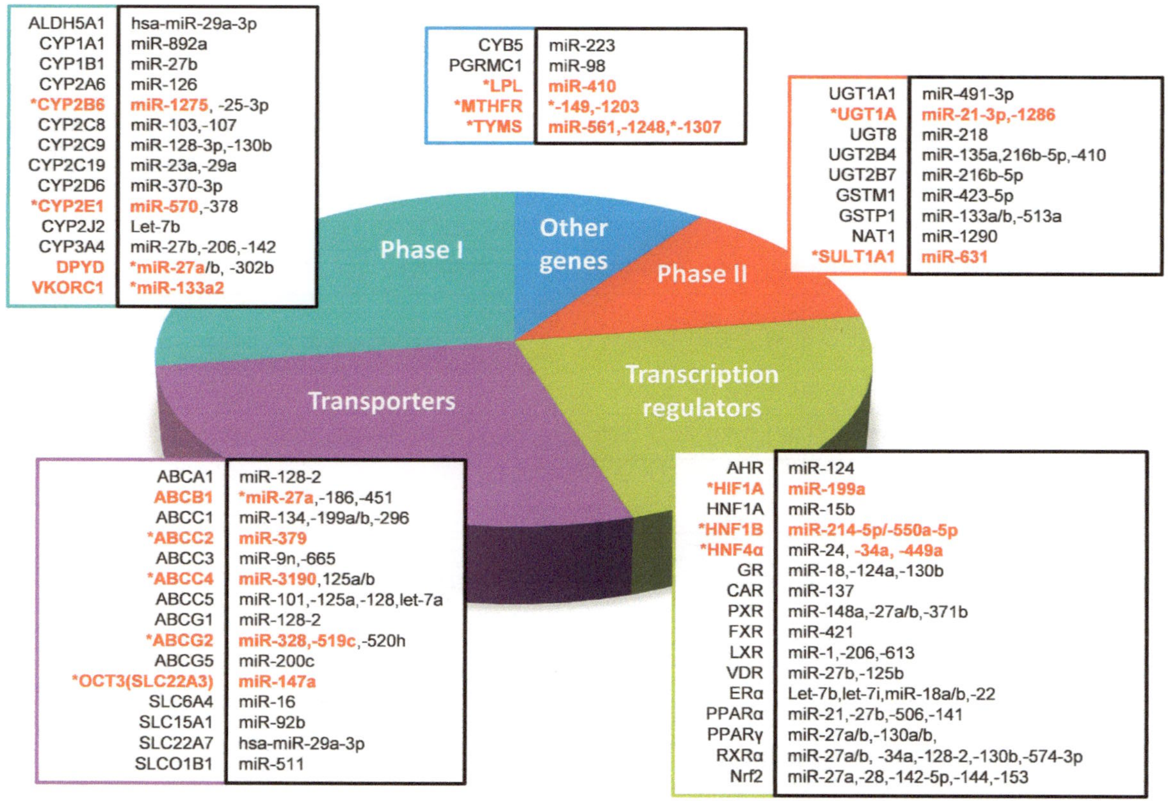

Fig. 1 Interactions between pharmacogenes and miRNAs. The figure depicts miRNAs that have been shown to directly interact with pharmacogenes comprising phase I and phase II enzymes, drug transporters, transcription regulators, and other genes. Polymorphisms in either the target gene or the interacting miRNA are indicated by an asterisk and mutual influence is marked additionally by red color text.

Table 3 Polymorphisms Affecting miRNA-Mediated Regulation

SNP	Gene	Location	Position (HGVS) ref > var	MAF (Allele)[a]	Effect	References
Enzyme SNPs affecting miRNA binding						
rs12979270 and rs12979898 (combined rs70950385)	CYP2B6	3′-UTR	c.*1399A > C c.*1400G > A (combined: AG > CA)	0.21 (C) 0.21 (A)	miR-1275 target site generated	Burgess et al. (2017)
rs2480256	CYP2E1	3′-UTR	c.*46A > G (=1561A > G)	0.28 (A)	miR-570 binding	Liao et al. (2011) and Nakano et al. (2015)
rs2480257	CYP2E1	3′-UTR	c.*41T > A(=1556T > A)	0.28 (T)	miR-570 binding	Liao et al. (2011) and Nakano et al. (2015)
rs13702	LPL	3′-UTR	c.*1671T > C	0.32 (C)	miR-410 target site	Richardson et al. (2013) and Corella et al. (2014)
rs868014	MTHFR	3′-UTR	c.*1290T > C	0.24[b] (T)	miR-1203 binding	He et al. (2017)
rs1042157	SULT1A1	3′-UTR	c.*85C > G,T	0.33 (T)	miR-631 binds to T-allele	Yu et al. (2010)
rs2790	TYMS	3′-UTR	c.*89A > G	0.21 (G)	miR-1248 binding verified	Xu et al. (2014), Shen et al. (2015), and Guan et al. (2015)
rs11280056	TYMS	3′-UTR	c.*450_*455delAAGTTA	0.33 (del)	miR-561 (predicted)	Shen et al. (2015) and Guan et al. (2015)
rs1059394	TYMS	3′-UTR/ intron	c.805–68C > T	0.33 (T)	miR-892a (predicted)	Shen et al. (2015) and Guan et al. (2015)
rs10929303	UGT1A	3′-UTR	c.*211T > C	0.22 (T)	miR-21-3p binds preferentially to the variant allele	Papageorgiou and Court (2017a) and Mehboob et al. (2017)
rs8330	UGT1A	3′-UTR	c.*440G > C	0.24 (G)	miR-1286 binds to ref allele	Papageorgiou and Court (2017a) and Mehboob et al. (2017)

Transporter SNPs affecting miRNA binding						
rs3740066	ABCC2	3′-UTR	c.3972C > T (linked to rs717620 c.-24C > T)	0.37 (T)	miR-379	Werk, Bruckmueller, Haenisch, and Cascorbi (2014)
rs3742106	ABCC4	3′-UTR	c.*38T > G	0.47 (G)	miR-3190-5p	Chen, Meng, et al. (2017)
rs2231142	ABCG2	Exonic	c.421C > A (Q141K)	0.094 (A)	miR-519c and miR-328	Ripperger and Benndorf (2016)
rs3088442	SLC22A3 (OCT3)	3′-UTR	c.*564G > A (2282G > A)	0.35 (A)	G-allele suppress binding of miR-147a	Wang, Chen, et al. (2016)
MicroRNA SNPs						
rs895819	miR-27a	3′ Flanking	n.182 A > C,T,G hairpin loop of pre-miRNA	0.32 (G)	Elevated expression of miR-27a; reduced DPD activity; 5-FU toxicity risk	Offer et al. (2014), Falvella, Caporale, et al. (2015), Amstutz et al. (2015), and Meulendijks et al. (2016)
rs45547937 (and linked SNPs)	miR-133a-2	Near 5′	n.-102 G > A	0.21 (A)	VKORC1 expression; warfarin dosage	Ciccacci et al. (2015)
rs2292832	Pre-miR-149	3′ Arm	n.86 T > C	0.28 (T)	Expression of miR-149 and its target MTHFR increased	An, Yang, and An (2017)
rs7911488	Pre-miR-1307	Terminal loop	n.70 T > C	0.35 (C)	Lower miR-1307 and elevated TYMS expression	Chen, Mao, et al. (2017)
rs56292801	Pri-miR-5189	5′ Arm	n.16 G > A	0.27 (A)	MTX plasma levels associated (SLC46A1, SLC19A1, SLCO1A2)	Iparraguirre et al. (2016)

Continued

Table 3 Polymorphisms Affecting miRNA-Mediated Regulation—cont'd

SNP	Gene	Location	Position (HGVS) ref > var	MAF (Allele)	Effect	References
rs4909237	Pri-miR-595	5′ Arm	n.3 G > T,A	0.18 (A)	MTX plasma levels associated (SLC46A1, SLC19A1, SLCO1A2)	Iparraguirre et al. (2016)
rs78790512	Pri-miR-6083	5′ Arm	n.42 G > A	0.18 (A)	MTX plasma levels associated (SLC46A1, SLC19A1, SLCO1A2)	Iparraguirre et al. (2016)
SNPs in regulators and miRNA processing machinery						
rs2057482	HIF1A	3′-UTR	c.*45T > C	0.14 (T)	miR-199a-binding site impaired by C	Wang, Ren, et al. (2016)
rs11574744	HNF4A	3′-UTR	c.*167T > A	0.04 (A)[b]	miR-34a/miR-449a	Ramamoorthy et al. (2012)
rs2229295	HNF1B	3′-UTR	c.*99C > A	0.2 (A)	miR-214-5p/miR-550a-5p binding increased	Goda, Murase, Kasezawa, Goda, and Yamakawa-Kobayashi (2015)
rs11077	XPO5	3′-UTR	c.*659A > C	0.43 (C)	Expression	Geng et al. (2016) and Lund, Güttinger, Calado, Dahlberg, and Kutay (2004)

[a]Minor allele frequency for EUR population as given in dbSNP, minor allele is noted in brackets.
[b]Allele does not occur in EUR, minor allele frequency for AFR population as given in dbSNP.

bupropion, cyclophosphamide, efavirenz, ketamine, methadone, and others (Zanger & Klein, 2013). In a study among 187 healthy volunteers pharmacokinetically characterized for CYP2B6 activity with the non-nucleoside reverse transcriptase inhibitor efavirenz (8-hydroxylation) and genotyped for the most important CYP2B6 polymorphic alleles **6* and **18* revealed 25 variants within the 3′-UTR, five of which showed association with either increased or decreased efavirenz metabolism, sometimes depending on *CYP2B6* genotype (Burgess et al., 2017). One variant, the dinucleotide polymorphism rs70950385 (AG > CA; Table 3), was associated with decreased efavirenz and bupropion hydroxylation activity in microsomes of genotyped pediatric and adult human liver specimens. The authors showed in further in vitro studies that CA on the variant allele created a functional binding site for miR-1275 causing an 11% decrease in activity compared to the AG-allele (Burgess et al., 2017). The other 3′-UTR SNPs that are associated with activity changes could so far not be related to miRNA targeting events through the PolymiRTS database. It would be interesting whether any of these *CYP2B6* 3′-UTR variants can be independently confirmed as robust predictor of CYP2B6 functional variation. An expanded analysis of 30 SNPs, including the 3′-UTR, in South African HIV-infected patients receiving efavirenz-containing highly active antiretroviral therapy treatment came however to the conclusion that *CYP2B6* c.516G > T and c.983T > C SNPs remain the most powerful predictors of efavirenz plasma concentration (Swart et al., 2016).

CYP2E1 is one of the major CYP enzymes of human liver with several characteristic features among the drug metabolizing CYPs, including a unique substrate specificity comprising ethanol and other small molecules, several of which act also as inducers, and is of particular toxicological relevance. Many studies on the regulation of *CYP2E1* gene expression indicate that posttranscriptional regulation of both constitutive and inducible expression (e.g., induction by ethanol) is of greater importance for CYP2E1 as compared to other CYPs, while genetic variation has comparably little influence (Zanger & Schwab, 2013).

Following an initial report of a *CYP2E1* 3′-UTR variant that is linked to decreased mRNA levels in peripheral blood mononuclear cells (Liao et al., 2011; see below), the group of Nakajima investigated the mechanism of this association (Nakano et al., 2015). Two adjacent variants in complete linkage disequilibrium (LD) (rs2480256/7; Table 3) form two haplotypes (TA and AG), one of which (the wild-type TA) was shown by luciferase assay to harbor a target site for miR-570. The group had previously identified a functional miR-378-binding site located closely downstream of the miR-570 site that had been found to regulate *CYP2E1* posttranscriptionally (Mohri et al., 2010). Further experiments in human embryonic kidney 293 (HEK293) cell lines stably expressing the two 3′-UTR variants of human *CYP2E1* showed that while miR-378 regulates *CYP2E1* independent of the 3′-UTR haplotype at the mRNA and protein level, miR-570 downregulates only the wild-type haplotype on the protein level by 60% of control (Nakano et al., 2015). Interestingly, when miRNA levels were determined in human livers, both were found to be significantly inversely correlated to CYP2E1 protein levels but not to mRNA levels. In summary, these data show that human *CYP2E1* is posttranscriptionally regulated by at least two miRNAs, miR-378 and miR-570, by the latter one in a genotype-dependent manner. According to the initial report, the polymorphic miR-570 site could be of clinical value as it was found to be associated with systemic lupus erythematosus in a Chinese population (Liao et al., 2011).

Dihydrofolate reductase (DHFR) was the first gene reported to harbor a functional miR-SNP located in the 3′-UTR (rs34764978, *DHFR* 829C > T) that decreased binding of miR-24 to its target site resulting in methotrexate resistance in mutant cells (Mishra et al., 2007). However, a reinvestigation study was unable to confirm its existence as a natural polymorphism and suggested that its detection was in fact a genotyping artifact caused by a homologous SNP in the *DHFRP1* pseudogene (Hayashi et al., 2012). To our knowledge, no confirmative studies or follow-up studies on the effect or use of this polymorphism as biomarker of methotrexate response was published.

Dihydropyrimidine dehydrogenase (DPYD) is a ubiquitous and rate-limiting enzyme of the uracil catabolic pathway, and as such also a major enzyme for the degradation of 5-fluorouracil (5-FU), a chemotherapeutic drug of the antimetabolite class that has been in wide use since the 1950s. The cellular level of DPD is therefore a determinant of drug response as well as toxicity. While high levels of DPD tend to be associated with poor response, low levels can cause severe toxicity. *DPYD* polymorphisms have been widely studied as possible predictors of 5-FU toxicity (Campbell et al., 2016; Meulendijks et al., 2015). The search for epigenetic markers and miRNAs that influence 5-FU toxicity and response is motivated by the fact that currently prediction of severe toxicity as well as drug response is unsatisfactory (Deng, Wang, Lei, Lei, & Xiong, 2017).

The *DPYD* 3′-UTR (1230 nt) has been shown by luciferase assays to be directly targeted by miRNAs miR-27a, miR-27b, miR-134, miR-582-5p

(Hirota et al., 2012), miR-494 (Chai et al., 2015), and in the coding sequence by hsa-miR-302b-3p (Cai, He, Chang, Tong, & Huang, 2015). The highly conserved and homologous miR-27a and miR-27b species can both bind to two target sites close to the *DPYD* stop codon, and down-regulate endogenous DPD expression by 31% and 51%, respectively, in colorectal carcinoma cells transduced with lentiviral particles encoding miR-27a and miR-27b (Offer et al., 2014). Mechanistically, cells that overexpress miR-27a and miR-27b were shown to accumulate AGO proteins, catalytic components of RISC, on *DPYD* mRNA, leading to RISC-mediated repression of *DPYD* and higher sensitivity to 5-FU. In this study the authors also showed that a common variant (rs895819), that had been associated with colorectal cancer (Liu et al., 2016), stabilizes the hairpin loop region of hsa-miR-27a leading to higher miR-27a levels and reduced DPD activity in a cohort of 40 healthy volunteers, suggesting rs895819 as a potential marker of 5-FU toxicity (Offer et al., 2014).

The clinical relevance of the miR-27a polymorphism was so far evaluated in three later studies on patients treated with fluoropyrimidines. Amstutz and colleagues sequenced miR-27a in 514 cancer patients genetically characterized for *DPYD* risk alleles (Amstutz et al., 2015). In carriers of such risk alleles, the miR-27a polymorphism was associated with increased early-onset toxicity (odds ratio, OR 7.6), and while in patients without DPYD risk alleles, it was moderately protective (OR 0.62). In a follow-up meta-analysis including a total of 1592 patients, the predictive value of the rs895819 and an additional miR-27a related but rarer polymorphism, rs11671784 C>T, was tested in multivariable logistic regression models (Meulendijks et al., 2016). The interaction of the miR-27a polymorphism with *DPYD* risk variants was confirmed, i.e., in patients carrying *DPYD* risk alleles, the miR-27a variant allele was associated with significantly increased risk of grade 3 or 4 toxicity, while the beneficial effect of the miR-27a wild-type allele was not confirmed in the multivariable models. The rare rs11671784 variant was also not associated with fluoropyrimidine toxicity in this meta-analysis. In a considerably smaller study, the miR-27a variant was associated with increased toxicity in the univariate, but not in the multivariate analysis, but this may have been due to the small number of patients studied ($n = 64$; Falvella, Cheli, et al., 2015). Thus, all three patient studies provided evidence that the miR-27a polymorphism rs895819 may have predictive value to assess the risk of severe toxicity from fluoropyrimidines.

Lipoprotein lipase (LPL) is an important enzyme in the triglyceride homeostasis, and its deficiency is associated with hypertriglyceridemia.

miR-410 targets and downregulates LPL, and a 3′-UTR polymorphism rs13702 T>C modulates lipid phenotypes in response to dietary fatty acids through disruption of the miR-410 seed sequence (Richardson et al., 2013). For example, in a study with >7000 participants the C-allele was associated with lower triglycerides, and this association was modulated by fat intake. The variant was also associated with stroke incidence, depending on diet (Corella et al., 2014).

MTHFR (see Section 2.2) contains several 3′-UTR polymorphisms that have been partially investigated in the context of various conditions including ischemic stroke. The rs868014 (T>C) SNP was shown in vitro to enhance or create a miR-1203-binding site that leads to downregulation of MTHFR and increased plasma homocysteine formation in C-allele carriers and poor ischemic stroke outcome (He et al., 2017). The variant is however strongly linked to the tightly linked nonsynonymous MTHFR variants A222V (Table 1) and E429A that are known to result in decreased enzyme activity, and mechanistically, the contribution of each variant to *MTHFR* regulation has still to be clarified. Another miRNA that interacts with MTHFR is miR-149, which harbors a polymorphism rs2292832 C>T (Table 3). In a study on effects of fatty acids on MTHFR, hepatocytes genotyped TT upregulated miR-149, while MTHFR was downregulated by about 40% following treatment with long-chain fatty acids. No changes occurred in CC hepatocytes. The effects could be reproduced using miR-149 mimics and inhibitors, and regulation of *MTHFR* by miR-149 was confirmed by luciferase assays (An et al., 2017). The authors further discussed the roles of miR-149 and MTHFR in the context of nonalcoholic fatty liver disease.

Sulfotransferase 1A1 (SULT1A1) is the most highly expressed sulfotransferase in human liver and catalyzes the sulfation of a wide variety of endogenous and exogenous substances including phenolic steroids, acetaminophen, 4-hydroxytamoxifen, many benzylic alcohols, aromatic amines, hydroxylamines, and many more (Glatt & Meinl, 2004). *SULT1A1* is genetically highly variable and displays in addition to SNPs also highly frequent copy number variations (CNVs) which affect expression and function (Tremmel et al., 2017). Several common, tightly linked SNPs in the 3′ area including rs1042157 C>G,T were found to be associated with hepatic mRNA and enzyme activity independent of copy number (Yu et al., 2010). Functional characterization using luciferase constructs as well as breast cell lines with homozygous WT, heterozygous and homozygous variant alleles showed that miR-631 binds preferentially to the rs1042157 variant T-allele resulting in downregulation of *SULT1A1*. It should however be noted that these SNPs are also absolutely linked to the nonsynonymous *SULT1A1*2*. It remains to be shown which of the variants are causative. A recent study has shown that **2* has much less predictive effects on *SULT1A1* mRNA and protein levels as compared to the CNVs (Tremmel et al., 2017).

Thymidylate synthase (TYMS) catalyzes the conversion of deoxyuridine-5′-monophosphate (dUMP) to deoxythymidine-5′-monophosphate (dTMP), the essential precursor of DNA synthesis and is therefore a key enzyme for DNA synthesis and repair and involved in tumorigenesis, cell senescence, and apoptosis (Lima, Azevedo, Sousa, Seabra, & Medeiros, 2013). Impairment of TYMS is therefore associated with chromosomal and DNA damage. TYMS is an important target for a variety of fluoropyrimidine-based chemotherapeutic drugs, and its expression level predicts response to 5-FU-based chemotherapy. *TYMS* polymorphisms, in particular a 28-bp variable number of tandem repeats (VNTR) polymorphism in the 5′-UTR of *TYMS*, and the 6 bp deletion/insertion polymorphism rs11280056 (former rs16430) in the 3′-UTR, have been widely studied in the context of 5-FU toxicity and response (Lee et al., 2015; Lima et al., 2013; Schwab et al., 2008).

In addition to the above-mentioned rs11280056 within a predicted binding site for miR-561, two further 3′-UTR SNPs which are quite common (minor allele frequency, MAF > 0.05) in Caucasians have been described and are located within predicted miR-binding sites, namely, rs1059394 C > T (predicted binding site miR-892a), which is tightly linked to rs11280056, and rs2790 A > G (Table 3). For the latter variant rs2790 A > G it has been shown that miR-1248 binds specifically to the G-allele and suppresses its expression in vitro by approximately 70% (Xu et al., 2014).

The *TYMS* 3′-UTR variants have been mainly studied in the context of risk assessment of various cancers (Guan et al., 2015; Shen et al., 2015); however, in some studies there seemed to be an influence also on chemotherapy outcome. Thus, in a study on gastric cancer patients the minor alleles of the three aforementioned SNPs were associated with increased gastric cancer risk, and homozygous carriers of the rs11280056 and rs1059394 minor alleles were also associated with poor survival in gastric cancer patients receiving chemotherapy (Shen et al., 2015). The rs2790 A > G SNP influenced overall survival of nonsmall cell lung cancer patients on platinum-based chemotherapy (Xu et al., 2014). To our knowledge, an association between these common 3′-UTR variants and toxicity has so far not been described. In fact, the TYMS-3′-UTR 6-bp deletion/insertion polymorphism was not associated with severe 5-FU toxicity in a prospective study (Schwab et al., 2008). Further 3′-UTR SNPs with unclear relation to miRNAs but related to capecitabine toxicity have been identified by Pellicer et al. (2017).

TYMS is also a direct target of pre-miR-1307, which harbors the rs7911488 T>C polymorphism found to be associated with the efficacy of capecitabine chemotherapy in colon cancer patients (Chen, Mao, et al., 2017). The authors of this study pointed out that in patients carrying the C-allele, miR-1307-3p is downregulated, causing upregulation of TYMS, which in turn leads to insensitivity of cancer cells to capecitabine chemotherapy. Cancer cells with rs7911488 C-allele were furthermore found to be resistant to 5-FU treatment in vitro and in vivo.

UDP-glucuronosyltransferases (UGTs) are conjugation enzymes that detoxify a wide variety of both endogenous and exogenous substrates by glucuronidation of free alcohol and phenol groups. In humans there are 19 functional enzymes classified into three subfamilies, UGT1A, UGT2A, and UGT2B, with considerable and clinically relevant genetic variation (Guillemette, Lévesque, & Rouleau, 2014). A number of recent studies have identified miRNAs that interact with various UGTs (Dluzen et al., 2016; Margaillan, Lévesque, & Guillemette, 2016; Papageorgiou & Court, 2017a, 2017b; Wijayakumara, Mackenzie, McKinnon, Hu, & Meech, 2017). Some of them appear to be susceptible to target gene polymorphisms. Papageorgiou and Court have recently performed a systematic analysis of posttranscriptional repression of UDP-glucuronosyltransferase UGT1A and UGT2B subfamily expression by miRNAs (Papageorgiou & Court, 2017a, 2017b). All UGT1A enzymes share a common, polymorphic 3′-UTR containing three linked SNPs (rs10929303, rs1042640, and rs8330; Table 3) that may influence miRNA binding. A common SNP is also present within the 3′-UTR of *UGT2B15*, one of seven functional enzymes of the UGT2B subfamily. Using luciferase reporter constructs that contain reference or variant 3′-UTR Papageorgiou and Court screened a 2048 human miRNA library for inhibitory miRNAs and for miRNAs that show differential effects on reference and variant 3′-UTRs (Papageorgiou & Court, 2017a, 2017b). They identified a total of 24 novel miRNAs that repressed either UGT1A or UGT2B 3′-UTRs, with several of them selectively repressing either the reference or the variant UGT1A (Table 1). In particular, miR-1286 was found to bind in an allele-specific way to the more common reference 3′-UTR, while miR-21-3p showed allele-selective binding preferentially to the rarer variant sequence. The rs3100 in *UGT2B15* did not seem to have an impact on binding of the identified miRNAs. With additional experiments these authors further characterized miRNA-binding sites and the abundance of miRNAs.

While miR-21-3p is known to be rather highly expressed in hepatocytes, miR-1286 is apparently expressed at low levels and its potential functional impact in liver remains to be shown. Interestingly, in previous work by the same authors rs8330 had been associated with higher acetaminophen glucuronidation activity in liver samples and decreased risk of unintentional acetaminophen-induced liver failure, but also a changed splice variant ratio (Court et al., 2013). Together these studies open up a variety of interesting pharmacogenetic possibilities on polymorphic regulation of glucuronidation pathways through miR-SNPs.

Vitamin K epoxide reductase (VKORC1), a 163 residue microsomal membrane protein, converts vitamin K epoxide to vitamin K and thus is a key enzyme for the physiological recycling of vitamin K, which is required by several coagulation proteins as a cofactor (Owen, Gong, Sagreiya, Klein, & Altman, 2010). Therapeutically VKORC1 is of significance because it contributes to the high and clinically relevant variability in coumarin anticoagulant dose requirement. *VKORC1* polymorphisms have been extensively studied along with *CYP2C9* and *CYP2F3* polymorphisms as predictors of warfarin response (Johnson et al., 2011). The *VKORC1* 3′-UTR contains conserved binding sites for miR-133a and miR-137 at 145 and 254 bp downstream of the stop codon, respectively. A functional binding site that mediates downregulation of *VKORC1* mRNA and protein by up to 50% and 30%, respectively, could be shown for miR-133a, which is also constitutively expressed in hepatocytes (Pérez-Andreu et al., 2012). Since this binding site could also bind other miR-133 family members, Ciccacci and colleagues investigated miRNA polymorphisms in the corresponding miRNA genes *MIR133A1*, *MIR133A2*, and *MIR133B* (Ciccacci et al., 2015). Direct sequencing of the genes in a sample of patients treated with warfarin revealed four SNPs in the *MIR133A2* gene of which three were in complete LD with a MAF of 0.2. When variant rs45547937 G>A at −102 bp in the 5′-flanking sequence (Table 3) was taken as a tag SNP for this LD block, a trend correlation with warfarin dose requirement was found (Ciccacci et al., 2015). Interestingly, when patients were stratified according to the *VKORC1* promoter polymorphism, GG homozygous wild types, who need a higher warfarin dose compared to variant A-allele carriers, had an even higher dose requirement when they carried one or two *MIR133A2* variant alleles. The *MIR133A2* polymorphism had no significant effect on *VKORC1* variant carriers, but this was probably due to the small number of patients with AA genotype. To our knowledge, unfortunately no larger studies have yet been presented to confirm these interesting data.

3.2 miR-SNPs Affecting Transporters

The *ATP-binding cassette subfamily C member 2 (ABCC2)* encodes the membrane transporter multidrug resistance-associated protein 2 (MRP2) that is expressed at many compartment barriers and functions as an efflux pump for various conjugated and unconjugated substances. Regulation of ABCC2 expression includes transcriptional inducibility by PXR ligands such as rifampicin as well as various genetic polymorphisms and several miRNAs. Induction of ABCC2 was shown in HepG2 cells to lead to increased mRNA but decreased protein, and this was explained by the concomitant induction of miR-379 (Haenisch et al., 2011). In a subsequent study the influence of a triple haplotype involving c.-24C>T, c.1249G>A (V417I), and the silent c.3972C>T SNPs (Table 3) on regulation by miR-379 was investigated (Werk et al., 2014). It was shown that the CGC wild-type haplotype was only modestly affected, whereas the variant haplotypes CGT and TGT lead to more substantial ABCC2 downregulation. The authors hypothesized that haplotype-dependent differences in mRNA secondary structures lead to changes in mRNA accessibility and consequently differential regulation by the miRNA.

ABCC4 is also expressed at compartment barriers and is involved in the export of fluoropyrimidine drugs, among others, and may thus be an important factor for drug response and resistance. A polymorphism rs3742106 T>G (Table 3) in the ABCC4 3′-UTR disrupts or weakens a binding site for miR-3190-5p which was shown to inhibit *ABCC4* expression in cultured cells by approximately 40%, thereby leading to increased intracellular 5-FU concentration and enhanced cellular sensitivity to 5-FU (Chen, Meng, et al., 2017). In a cohort of colorectal cancer patients it was found that homozygous carriers of the G-allele responded less well to 5-FU/capecitabine-based chemotherapy, which may be consequently be explained by lower intracellular 5-FU concentrations due to higher ABCC4 expression.

ABCG2, also known as BCRP/MXR, is another important and widely expressed transporter for numerous xenobiotic and endogenous drugs, including uric acid. A nonsynonymous polymorphism c.421C>A (Q141K) is known to reduce ABCG2 protein levels and to be associated with gout (Table 3). A recent study showed that the downregulation of protein but not mRNA expression by the SNP was markedly enhanced by the presence of the 3′-UTR in an expression plasmid, suggesting translational repression of the mutant transcript (Ripperger & Benndorf, 2016). A role of miRNAs in mediating the 3′-UTR-dependent downregulation was indicated by experimental interference with miRNA biogenesis by DICER knockdown as well as mutagenesis of putative miRNA-binding sites in the 3′-UTR. The authors suggested miR-519c and miR-328 as potential candidates supported by respective antagomirs which partially reversed the effect of the mutation. The authors conclude that the mutation decreases ABCG2 expression not only by affecting cellular protein stability but also via miRNA-mediated translational inhibition, although the exact mechanism remains to be elucidated.

3.3 miR-SNPs Affecting Regulators and miRNA Machinery

Hepatic nuclear receptors and other liver-enriched transcription factors are the most important regulators of constitutive and inducible expression of most DMET genes. Polymorphisms in nuclear receptor genes like PXR, hepatic nuclear factors (HNFs), and others would be expected to influence a range of target genes simultaneously. However, it has been difficult to identify common germline polymorphisms in such regulators that show reproducible effects with predictive value for pharmacogenetics (Zanger & Schwab, 2013). A reason for this may be, as already mentioned, that *trans* effects on downstream genes are generally more difficult to assess and reproduce (Glubb et al., 2012). A few examples of variants in *trans*-regulators are discussed later. An early investigation of the 3′-UTR of human PXR identified 12 SNPs in five major haplotypes, one of which was associated with increased midazolam clearance reflecting higher CYP3A4 expression in African-American carriers (Oleson, von Moltke, Greenblatt, & Court, 2010). However, using luciferase constructs, no evidence for the direct involvement of miRNAs in the mechanism by which this haplotype affects CYP3A4 was obtained. A later study screened the PXR 3′-UTR in Indian breast cancer patients and identified rs3732360, rs1054190, and rs1054191 as being located in binding sites for miR-500a-3p, miR-532-3p, and miR-374a-3p, respectively, by in silico prediction (Revathidevi et al., 2016). To our knowledge these polymorphisms still lack any direct evidences for impact on gene regulation.

HNF4α, a nuclear receptor considered to be a master regulator for hepatic gene expression, is regulated by several miRNAs, including miR-34a and miR-449a, which were found to downregulate the expression of HNF4α and the target gene PXR by blocking translation. This regulation was less effective for a variant (rs11574744 T>A) found exclusively in African-Americans (Ramamoorthy et al., 2012).

HNF1B, a liver-enriched homeodomain-containing transcription factor that is linked to maturity-onset diabetes of the young type (MODY5), was shown to harbor a 3′-UTR SNP rs2229295 C>A (Table 3) that enhanced binding of miR-214-5p and miR-550a-5p (Goda et al., 2015). Whether this influences HNF1B protein levels is not known, but the authors found an association of the variant with type 2 diabetes.

Hypoxia-inducible factor-1 alpha (HIF-1α) is a hypoxically inducible subunit of HIF-1 and overexpressed in many cancers and correlated with poor prognosis. A 3′-UTR variant (rs2057482 T>C; Table 3) was found to be associated with increased risk for pancreatic ductal adenocarcinoma risk and worse clinical outcome (Wang, Ren, et al., 2016). The SNP is located close to miR-199a seed sequence and was shown to affect miR-199a binding in that the T-allele is more repressed than the C-allele, leading to increased expression of HIF-1α protein and mRNA in pancreatic tissues.

Numerous polymorphisms in the miRNA machinery have been investigated in the context of cancer and other diseases, but little evidence is so far available as to whether such variants influence drug pharmacokinetics or response. One example included in Table 3 concerns the nuclear envelope transporter exportin-5 (XPO-5), that is, responsible for the export of pre-miRNAs from the nucleus to the cytoplasm. Although no mechanism for the 3′-UTR SNP rs11077 A>C (Table 3) was so far reported, a variant in the 3′-UTR rs11077 A>C (Table 3) was associated with better prognosis and chemotherapy response in nonsmall cell lung cancer patients (Geng et al., 2016). The authors speculated that XPO5 expression changes may affect global miRNA expression levels, thereby modulating tumor development and chemotherapy response. However, no mechanistic explanation has been provided so far.

4. CONCLUSION

In this chapter we discussed polymorphisms that impact genes and gene products related to drug metabolism, transport and response, and/or clinical endpoints through interactions with epigenetic and miRNA-mediated processes. It appears that quite a large number of such polymorphisms may exist and that some of them can have profound influence on the expression and function of DMET genes, thereby broadening the repertoire of pharmacogenetic tools and approaches. This contributes to our understanding of the origin of interindividual variability in drug disposition and may help to develop predictive tests for clinical practice.

Yet most of the studies are still in a very initial phase, having shown only a mechanism or an influence on gene expression, in some cases also an influence on clinical outcome. In most cases this was only shown in a single study or in one cohort without independent confirmation. Nevertheless some studies involving interactions of epigenetic and genetic factors point already at exact clinical settings in which these new polymorphisms may have a role for better prediction. These clinical implications should be motivation for future studies, especially with respect to confirmation of effect, determination of effect size, and relationship to already known polymorphisms and other existing biomarkers and variability factors. In this regard these new avenues should be useful to improve translation of pharmacogenetics into clinical practice.

Finally we are aware of some important omissions. Numerous additional studies on interactions between epigenetics, noncoding RNAs, and genetics describing many more mutations and polymorphisms in the genes of the epigenetic machinery have been identified and investigated particularly with respect to their significance for cancer and a variety of other disorders. Due to the limited scope of this chapter we could not discuss these areas, although many of these studies bear principal pharmacogenetic relevance.

ACKNOWLEDGMENTS

This work was supported by the Robert Bosch Foundation, Stuttgart, Germany.

CONFLICT OF INTEREST

The authors have no conflicts of interest to declare.

REFERENCES

Aarabi, M., San Gabriel, M. C., Chan, D., Behan, N. A., Caron, M., Pastinen, T., et al. (2015). High-dose folic acid supplementation alters the human sperm methylome and is influenced by the MTHFR C677T polymorphism. *Human Molecular Genetics*, *24*(22), 6301–6313.

Allis, C. D., & Jenuwein, T. (2016). The molecular hallmarks of epigenetic control. *Nature Reviews Genetics*, *17*(8), 487.

Amstutz, U., Offer, S. M., Sistonen, J., Joerger, M., Diasio, R. B., & Largiadèr, C. R. (2015). Polymorphisms in MIR27A associated with early-onset toxicity in fluoropyrimidine-based chemotherapy. *Clinical Cancer Research*, *21*(9), 2038–2044.

An, X., Yang, Z., & An, Z. (2017). MiR-149 compromises the reactions of liver cells to fatty acid via its polymorphism and increases non-alcoholic fatty liver disease (NAFLD) risk by targeting methylene tetrahydrofolate reductase (MTHFR). *Medical Science Monitor: International Medical Journal of Experimental and Clinical Research*, *23*, 2299–2307.

Baer-Dubowska, W., Majchrzak-Celińska, A., & Cichocki, M. (2011). Pharmocoepigenetics: A new approach to predicting individual drug responses and targeting new drugs. *Pharmacological Reports: PR*, *63*(2), 293–304.

Bhattacharya, A., Ziebarth, J. D., & Cui, Y. (2014). PolymiRTS database 3.0: Linking polymorphisms in microRNAs and their target sites with human diseases and biological pathways. *Nucleic Acids Research*, *42*(Database issue), D86–D91.

Bruno, A. E., Li, L., Kalabus, J. L., Pan, Y., Yu, A., & Hu, Z. (2012). miRdSNP: A database of disease-associated SNPs and microRNA target sites on 3'UTRs of human genes. *BMC Genomics*, *13*, 44.

Burgess, K. S., Ipe, J., Swart, M., Metzger, I. F., Lu, J., Gufford, B. T., et al. (2017). Variants in the CYP2B6 3'UTR alter in vitro and in vivo CYP2B6 activity: Potential role of microRNAs. *Clinical Pharmacology and Therapeutics*. https://doi.org/10.1002/cpt.892.

Cai, D., He, K., Chang, S., Tong, D., & Huang, C. (2015). MicroRNA-302b enhances the sensitivity of hepatocellular carcinoma cell lines to 5-FU via targeting Mcl-1 and DPYD. *International Journal of Molecular Sciences*, *16*(10), 23668–23682.

Campbell, J. M., Bateman, E., Peters, M. D., Bowen, J. M., Keefe, D. M., & Stephenson, M. D. (2016). Fluoropyrimidine and platinum toxicity pharmacogenetics: An umbrella review of systematic reviews and meta-analyses. *Pharmacogenomics*, *17*(4), 435–451.

Chai, J., Dong, W., Xie, C., Wang, L., Han, D.-L., Wang, S., et al. (2015). MicroRNA-494 sensitizes colon cancer cells to fluorouracil through regulation of DPYD. *IUBMB Life*, *67*(3), 191–201.

Chen, Q., Mao, Y., Meng, F., Wang, L., Zhang, H., Wang, W., et al. (2017). Rs7911488 modified the efficacy of capecitabine-based therapy in colon cancer through altering miR-1307-3p and TYMS expression. *Oncotarget*, *8*(43), 74312–74319.

Chen, Q., Meng, F., Wang, L., Mao, Y., Zhou, H., Hua, D., et al. (2017). A polymorphism in ABCC4 is related to efficacy of 5-FU/capecitabine-based chemotherapy in colorectal cancer patients. *Scientific Reports*, 7(1), 7059.

Chinn, L. W., & Kroetz, D. L. (2007). ABCB1 pharmacogenetics: Progress, pitfalls, and promise. *Clinical Pharmacology and Therapeutics*, *81*(2), 265–269.

Ciccacci, C., Rufini, S., Politi, C., Novelli, G., Forte, V., & Borgiani, P. (2015). Could MicroRNA polymorphisms influence warfarin dosing? A pharmacogenetics study on mir133 genes. *Thrombosis Research*, *136*(2), 367–370.

Corella, D., Sorlí, J. V., Estruch, R., Coltell, O., Ortega-Azorín, C., Portolés, O., et al. (2014). MicroRNA-410 regulated lipoprotein lipase variant rs13702 is associated with stroke incidence and modulated by diet in the randomized controlled PREDIMED trial. *The American Journal of Clinical Nutrition*, *100*(2), 719–731.

Court, M. H., Freytsis, M., Wang, X., Peter, I., Guillemette, C., Hazarika, S., et al. (2013). The UDP-glucuronosyltransferase (UGT) 1A polymorphism c.2042C>G (rs8330) is associated with increased human liver acetaminophen glucuronidation, increased UGT1A exon 5a/5b splice variant mRNA ratio, and decreased risk of unintentional acetaminophen-induced acute liver failure. *Journal of Pharmacology and Experimental Therapeutics*, *345*(2), 297–307.

Deng, J., Wang, Y., Lei, J., Lei, W., & Xiong, J. P. (2017). Insights into the involvement of noncoding RNAs in 5-fluorouracil drug resistance. *Tumor Biology*, *39*(4), 1010428317697553.

Dluzen, D. F., & Lazarus, P. (2015). MicroRNA regulation of the major drug-metabolizing enzymes and related transcription factors. *Drug Metabolism Reviews*, *47*(3), 320–334.

Dluzen, D. F., Sutliff, A. K., Chen, G., Watson, C. J. W., Ishmael, F. T., & Lazarus, P. (2016). Regulation of UGT2B expression and activity by miR-216b-5p in liver cancer cell lines. *Journal of Pharmacology and Experimental Therapeutics*, *359*(1), 182–193.

Falvella, F. S., Caporale, M., Cheli, S., Martinetti, A., Berenato, R., Maggi, C., et al. (2015). Undetected toxicity risk in pharmacogenetic testing for dihydropyrimidine dehydrogenase. *International Journal of Molecular Sciences*, *16*(4), 8884–8895.

Falvella, F. S., Cheli, S., Martinetti, A., Mazzali, C., Iacovelli, R., Maggi, C., et al. (2015). DPD and UGT1A1 deficiency in colorectal cancer patients receiving triplet chemotherapy with fluoropyrimidines, oxaliplatin and irinotecan. *British Journal of Clinical Pharmacology*, *80*(3), 581–588.

Fisel, P., Schaeffeler, E., & Schwab, M. (2016). DNA methylation of ADME genes. *Clinical Pharmacology & Therapeutics*, *99*(5), 512–527.

Geng, J.-Q., Wang, X.-C., Li, L.-F., Zhao, J., Wu, S., Yu, G.-P., et al. (2016). MicroRNA-related single-nucleotide polymorphism of XPO5 is strongly correlated with the prognosis and chemotherapy response in advanced non-small-cell lung cancer patients. *Tumour Biology: The Journal of the International Society for Oncodevelopmental Biology and Medicine*, *37*(2), 2257–2265.

Glatt, H., & Meinl, W. (2004). Pharmacogenetics of soluble sulfotransferases (SULTs). *Naunyn-Schmiedeberg's Archives of Pharmacology*, *369*(1), 55–68.

Glubb, D. M., Dholakia, N., & Innocenti, F. (2012). Liver expression quantitative trait loci: A foundation for pharmacogenomic research. *Frontiers in Genetics*, *3*, 153.

Goda, N., Murase, H., Kasezawa, N., Goda, T., & Yamakawa-Kobayashi, K. (2015). Polymorphism in microRNA-binding site in HNF1B influences the susceptibility of type 2 diabetes mellitus: A population based case-control study. *BMC Medical Genetics*, *16*, 75.

Gong, J., Liu, C., Liu, W., Wu, Y., Ma, Z., Chen, H., et al. (2015). An update of miRNASNP database for better SNP selection by GWAS data, miRNA expression and online tools. *Database: The Journal of Biological Databases and Curation*, *2015* . bav029.

Guan, X., Liu, H., Ju, J., Li, Y., Li, P., Wang, L.-E., et al. (2015). Genetic variant rs16430 6bp > 0bp at the microRNA-binding site in TYMS and risk of sporadic breast cancer risk in non-Hispanic white women aged ≤55 years. *Molecular Carcinogenesis*, *54*(4), 281–290.

Guillemette, C., Lévesque, É., & Rouleau, M. (2014). Pharmacogenomics of human uridine diphospho-glucuronosyltransferases and clinical implications. *Clinical Pharmacology and Therapeutics*, *96*(3), 324–339.

Gupta, H., Chaudhari, S., Rai, A., Bhat, S., Sahu, P. K., Hande, M. H., et al. (2017). Genetic and epigenetic changes in host ABCB1 influences malaria susceptibility to Plasmodium falciparum. *PLoS One*, *12*(4), e0175702.

Haenisch, S., Laechelt, S., Bruckmueller, H., Werk, A., Noack, A., Bruhn, O., et al. (2011). Down-regulation of ATP-binding cassette C2 protein expression in HepG2 cells after rifampicin treatment is mediated by microRNA-379. *Molecular Pharmacology*, *80*(2), 314–320.

Hamidi, T., Singh, A. K., & Chen, T. (2015). Genetic alterations of DNA methylation machinery in human diseases. *Epigenomics*, 7(2), 247–265.

Hancock, D. B., Guo, Y., Reginsson, G. W., Gaddis, N. C., Lutz, S. M., Sherva, R., et al. (2017). Genome-wide association study across European and African American ancestries identifies a SNP in *DNMT3B* contributing to nicotine dependence. *Molecular Psychiatry*. https://doi.org/10.1038/mp.2017.193.

Haschemi Nassab, M., Rhein, M., Hagemeier, L., Kaeser, M., Muschler, M., Glahn, A., et al. (2016). Impaired regulation of ALDH2 protein expression revealing a yet unknown epigenetic impact of rs886205 on specific methylation of a negative regulatory promoter region in alcohol-dependent patients. *European Addiction Research*, *22*(2), 59–69.

Hayashi, H., Tazoe, Y., Horino, M., Fujimaki-Katoh, C., Tsuboi, S., Matsuyama, T., et al. (2012). An artifact derived from a pseudogene led to the discovery of microRNA binding site polymorphism in the 3′-untranslated region of the human dihydrofolate reductase gene. *Drug Metabolism and Pharmacokinetics*, *27*(2), 263–267.

He, W., Lu, M., Li, G., Sun, Z., Gu, L., & Liu, D. (2017). Methylene tetrahydrofolate reductase (MTHFR) rs868014 polymorphism regulated by miR-1203 associates with risk and short term outcome of ischemic stroke. *Cellular Physiology and Biochemistry*, *41*(2), 701–710.

Hegi, M. E., Diserens, A.-C., Gorlia, T., Hamou, M.-F., de Tribolet, N., Weller, M., et al. (2005). MGMT gene silencing and benefit from temozolomide in glioblastoma. *New England Journal of Medicine*, *352*(10), 997–1003.

Hiraoka, M., & Kagawa, Y. (2017). Genetic polymorphisms and folate status. *Congenital Anomalies*, *57*(5), 142–149.

Hirota, T., Date, Y., Nishibatake, Y., Takane, H., Fukuoka, Y., Taniguchi, Y., et al. (2012). Dihydropyrimidine dehydrogenase (DPD) expression is negatively regulated by certain microRNAs in human lung tissues. *Lung Cancer (Amsterdam, Netherlands)*, 77(1), 16–23.

Iparraguirre, L., Gutierrez-camino, A., Umerez, M., Martin-guerrero, I., Astigarraga, I., Navajas, A., et al. (2016). Mir-pharmacogenetics of methotrexate in childhood B-cell acute lymphoblastic leukemia. *Pharmacogenetics and Genomics*, *26*(11), 517–525.

Ivanov, M., Kacevska, M., & Ingelman-Sundberg, M. (2012). Epigenomics and interindividual differences in drug response. *Clinical Pharmacology & Therapeutics*, *92*(6), 727–736.

Johnson, J., Gong, L., Whirl-Carrillo, M., Gage, B., Scott, S., Stein, C., et al. (2011). Clinical pharmacogenetics implementation consortium guidelines for CYP2C9 and VKORC1 genotypes and warfarin dosing. *Clinical Pharmacology and Therapeutics*, *90*(4), 625–629.

Kerb, R., Fux, R., Mörike, K., Kremsner, P. G., Gil, J. P., Gleiter, C. H., et al. (2009). Pharmacogenetics of antimalarial drugs: Effect on metabolism and transport. *The Lancet. Infectious Diseases*, *9*(12), 760–774.

Lai, C. Y., Huang, C. C., Tsai, C. H., Wang, J. Y., Kerr, C. L., Chen, Y. Y., et al. (2017). The DNA methyltransferase 3B -149 genetic polymorphism modulates lung cancer risk from smoking. *Asian Pacific Journal of Cancer Prevention: APJCP*, *18*(10), 2717–2723.

Lauschke, V. M., Barragan, I., & Ingelman-Sundberg, M. (2018). Pharmacoepigenetics and toxicoepigenetics: Novel mechanistic insights and therapeutic opportunities. *Annual Review of Pharmacology and Toxicology*, *58*, 161–185.

Lauschke, V. M., & Ingelman-Sundberg, M. (2016). Precision medicine and rare genetic variants. *Trends in Pharmacological Sciences*, *37*(2), 85–86.

Lee, M.-N., Kang, B., Choi, S. Y., Kim, M. J., Woo, S. Y., Kim, J.-W., et al. (2015). Impact of genetic polymorphisms on 6-thioguanine nucleotide levels and toxicity in pediatric patients with IBD treated with azathioprine. *Inflammatory Bowel Diseases*, *21*(12), 2897–2908.

Li, H., Liu, J., Sun, L., & Yuan, Y. A meta-analysis of the association between DNMT1 polymorphisms and cancer risk, *BioMed Research International* **2017,** 2017, 3971259.

Liao, L., Zhang, H., Lai, M.-P., Chen, S.-L., Wu, M., & Shen, N. (2011). Single-nucleotide polymorphisms and haplotype of CYP2E1 gene associated with systemic lupus erythematosus in Chinese population. *Arthritis Research & Therapy*, *13*(1), R11.

Lima, A., Azevedo, R., Sousa, H., Seabra, V., & Medeiros, R. (2013). Current approaches for *TYMS* polymorphisms and their importance in molecular epidemiology and pharmacogenetics. *Pharmacogenomics*, *14*(11), 1337–1351.

Lin, M., Gu, J., Eng, C., Ellis, L. M., Hildebrandt, M. A., Lin, J., et al. (2012). Genetic polymorphisms in MicroRNA-related genes as predictors of clinical outcomes in colorectal adenocarcinoma patients. *Clinical Cancer Research: An Official Journal of the American Association for Cancer Research*, *18*(14), 3982–3991.

Lin, X., Zhang, W., Lu, Q., Lei, X., Wang, T., Han, X., et al. (2016). Effect of MTHFR gene polymorphism impact on atherosclerosis via genome-wide methylation. *Medical Science Monitor: International Medical Journal of Experimental and Clinical Research*, *22*, 341–345.

Liu, J.-E., Ren, B., Tang, L., Tang, Q.-J., Liu, X.-Y., Li, X., et al. (2016). The independent contribution of miRNAs to the missing heritability in CYP3A4/5 functionality and the metabolism of atorvastatin. *Scientific Reports*, *6* . 26544.

Liu, C., Zhang, F., Li, T., Lu, M., Wang, L., Yue, W., et al. (2012). MirSNP, a database of polymorphisms altering miRNA target sites, identifies miRNA-related SNPs in GWAS SNPs and eQTLs. *BMC Genomics*, *13*, 661.

Lund, E., Güttinger, S., Calado, A., Dahlberg, J. E., & Kutay, U. (2004). Nuclear export of microRNA precursors. *Science (New York, N.Y.)*, *303*(5654), 95–98.

Margaillan, G., Lévesque, É., & Guillemette, C. (2016). Epigenetic regulation of steroid inactivating UDP-glucuronosyltransferases by microRNAs in prostate cancer. *The Journal of Steroid Biochemistry and Molecular Biology*, *155*(Pt. A), 85–93.

Matthaei, J., Brockmöller, J., Tzvetkov, M. V., Sehrt, D., Sachse-Seeboth, C., Hjelmborg, J. B., et al. (2015). Heritability of metoprolol and torsemide pharmacokinetics. *Clinical Pharmacology and Therapeutics*, *98*(6), 611–621.

Mehboob, H., Tahir, I. M., Iqbal, T., Saleem, S., Perveen, S., & Farooqi, A. (2017). Effect of UDP-glucuronosyltransferase (UGT) 1A polymorphism (rs8330 and rs10929303) on glucuronidation status of acetaminophen. *Dose-Response*, *15*(3)1559325817723731.

Meulendijks, D., Henricks, L. M., Amstutz, U., Froehlich, T. K., Largiadèr, C. R., Beijnen, J. H., et al. (2016). Rs895819 in MIR27A improves the predictive value of DPYD variants to identify patients at risk of severe fluoropyrimidine-associated toxicity. *International Journal of Cancer*, *138*(11), 2752–2761.

Meulendijks, D., Henricks, L. M., Sonke, G. S., Deenen, M. J., Froehlich, T. K., Amstutz, U., et al. (2015). Clinical relevance of DPYD variants c.1679T>G, c.1236G>A/HapB3, and c.1601G>A as predictors of severe fluoropyrimidine-associated toxicity: A systematic review and meta-analysis of individual patient data. *The Lancet. Oncology*, *16*(16), 1639–1650.

Miao, Y.-R., Liu, W., Zhang, Q., & Guo, A.-Y. (2017). lncRNASNP2: An updated database of functional SNPs and mutations in human and mouse lncRNAs. *Nucleic Acids Research*, *46*(D1), D276–D280.

Mishra, P. J., Humeniuk, R., Mishra, P. J., Longo-Sorbello, G. S. A., Banerjee, D., & Bertino, J. R. (2007). A miR-24 microRNA binding-site polymorphism in dihydrofolate reductase gene leads to methotrexate resistance. *Proceedings of the National Academy of Sciences of the United States of America*, *104*(33), 13513–13518.

Mohri, T., Nakajima, M., Fukami, T., Takamiya, M., Aoki, Y., & Yokoi, T. (2010). Human CYP2E1 is regulated by miR-378. *Biochemical Pharmacology*, *79*(7), 1045–1052.

Nakano, M., Mohri, T., Fukami, T., Takamiya, M., Aoki, Y., McLeod, H. L., et al. (2015). Single-nucleotide polymorphisms in cytochrome P450 2E1 (CYP2E1) 3'-untranslated region affect the regulation of CYP2E1 by miR-570. *Drug Metabolism and Disposition: The Biological Fate of Chemicals*, *43*(10), 1450–1457.

Offer, S. M., Butterfield, G. L., Jerde, C. R., Fossum, C. C., Wegner, N. J., & Diasio, R. B. (2014). microRNAs miR-27a and miR-27b directly regulate liver dihydropyrimidine dehydrogenase expression through two conserved binding sites. *Molecular Cancer Therapeutics*, *13*(3), 742–751.

Oleson, L., von Moltke, L. L., Greenblatt, D. J., & Court, M. H. (2010). Identification of polymorphisms in the 3′-untranslated region of the human pregnane X receptor (PXR) gene associated with variability in cytochrome P450 3A (CYP3A) metabolism. *Xenobiotica; The Fate of Foreign Compounds in Biological Systems*, *40*(2), 146–162.

Owen, R. P., Gong, L., Sagreiya, H., Klein, T. E., & Altman, R. B. (2010). VKORC1 pharmacogenomics summary. *Pharmacogenetics and Genomics*, *20*(10), 642–644.

Papageorgiou, I., & Court, M. H. (2017a). Identification and validation of microRNAs directly regulating the UDP-glucuronosyltransferase 1A subfamily enzymes by a functional genomics approach. *Biochemical Pharmacology*, *137*, 93–106.

Papageorgiou, I., & Court, M. H. (2017b). Identification and validation of the microRNA response elements in the 3′-untranslated region of the UDP glucuronosyltransferase (UGT) 2B7 and 2B15 genes by a functional genomics approach. *Biochemical Pharmacology, 146*, 199–213.

Pathak, H., Frieling, H., Bleich, S., Glahn, A., Heberlein, A., Haschemi Nassab, M., et al. (2017). Promoter polymorphism rs886205 genotype interacts with DNA methylation of the ALDH2 regulatory region in alcohol dependence. *Alcohol and Alcoholism (Oxford, Oxfordshire), 52*(3), 269–276.

Pellicer, M., García-González, X., García, M. I., Robles, L., Grávalos, C., García-Alfonso, P., et al. (2017). Identification of new SNPs associated with severe toxicity to capecitabine. *Pharmacological Research, 120*, 133–137.

Pérez-Andreu, V., Teruel, R., Corral, J., Roldán, V., García-Barberá, N., Salloum-Asfar, S., et al. (2012). miR-133a regulates vitamin K 2,3-epoxide reductase complex subunit 1 (VKORC1), a key protein in the vitamin K cycle. *Molecular Medicine, 18*(1), 1466–1472.

Quertemont, E. (2004). Genetic polymorphism in ethanol metabolism: Acetaldehyde contribution to alcohol abuse and alcoholism. *Molecular Psychiatry, 9*(6), 570–581.

Ramamoorthy, A., Li, L., Gaedigk, A., Bradford, L. D., Benson, E. A., Flockhart, D. A., et al. (2012). In silico and in vitro identification of microRNAs that regulate hepatic nuclear factor 4α expression. *Drug Metabolism and Disposition: The Biological Fate of Chemicals, 40*(4), 726–733.

Ramamoorthy, A., & Skaar, T. C. (2011). In silico identification of microRNAs predicted to regulate the drug metabolizing cytochrome P450 genes. *Drug Metabolism Letters, 5*(2), 126–131.

Ramos, E. M., Hoffman, D., Junkins, H. A., Maglott, D., Phan, L., Sherry, S. T., et al. (2014). Phenotype–genotype integrator (PheGenI): Synthesizing genome-wide association study (GWAS) data with existing genomic resources. *European Journal of Human Genetics, 22*(1), 144–147.

Rapkins, R. W., Wang, F., Nguyen, H. N., Cloughesy, T. F., Lai, A., Ha, W., et al. (2015). The MGMT promoter SNP rs16906252 is a risk factor for MGMT methylation in glioblastoma and is predictive of response to temozolomide. *Neuro-Oncology, 17*(12), 1589–1598.

Reed, K., Hembruff, S. L., Sprowl, J. A., & Parissenti, A. M. (2010). The temporal relationship between ABCB1 promoter hypomethylation, ABCB1 expression and acquisition of drug resistance. *The Pharmacogenomics Journal, 10*(6), 489–504.

Revathidevi, S., Sudesh, R., Vaishnavi, V., Kaliyanasundaram, M., MaryHelen, K. G., Sukanya, G., et al. (2016). Screening for the 3'UTR polymorphism of the PXR gene in south Indian breast cancer patients and its potential role in pharmacogenomics. *Asian Pacific Journal of Cancer Prevention: APJCP, 17*(8), 3971–3977.

Richardson, K., Nettleton, J. A., Rotllan, N., Tanaka, T., Smith, C. E., Lai, C.-Q., et al. (2013). Gain-of-function lipoprotein lipase variant rs13702 modulates lipid traits through disruption of a MicroRNA-410 seed site. *American Journal of Human Genetics, 92*(1), 5–14.

Ripperger, A., & Benndorf, R. A. (2016). The C421A (Q141K) polymorphism enhances the 3′-untranslated region (3'-UTR)-dependent regulation of ATP-binding cassette transporter ABCG2. *Biochemical Pharmacology, 104*, 139–147.

Schwab, M., Zanger, U. M., Marx, C., Schaeffeler, E., Klein, K., Dippon, J., et al. (2008). Role of genetic and nongenetic factors for fluorouracil treatment-related severe toxicity: A prospective clinical trial by the German 5-FU toxicity study group. *Journal of Clinical Oncology, 26*(13), 2131–2138.

Shen, R., Liu, H., Wen, J., Liu, Z., Wang, L.-E., Wang, Q., et al. (2015). Genetic polymorphisms in the microRNA binding-sites of the thymidylate synthase gene predict risk and survival in gastric cancer. *Molecular Carcinogenesis, 54*(9), 880–888.

Spellicy, C. J., Kosten, T. R., Hamon, S. C., Harding, M. J., & Nielsen, D. A. (2012). The MTHFR C677T variant is associated with responsiveness to disulfiram treatment for cocaine dependency. *Frontiers in Psychiatry*, *3*, 109.

Swart, M., & Dandara, C. (2014). Genetic variation in the 3′-UTR of CYP1A2, CYP2B6, CYP2D6, CYP3A4, NR1I2, and UGT2B7: Potential effects on regulation by micro-RNA and pharmacogenomics relevance. *Frontiers in Genetics*, *5*, 167.

Swart, M., Evans, J., Skelton, M., Castel, S., Wiesner, L., Smith, P. J., et al. (2016). An expanded analysis of pharmacogenetics determinants of efavirenz response that includes 3′-UTR single nucleotide polymorphisms among black south African HIV/AIDS patients. *Frontiers in Genetics*, *6*, 356.

Thomas, L. F., Saito, T., & Sætrom, P. (2011). Inferring causative variants in microRNA target sites. *Nucleic Acids Research*, *39*(16) . e109.

Tremmel, R., Herrmann, K., Engst, W., Meinl, W., Klein, K., Glatt, H., et al. (2017). Methyleugenol DNA adducts in human liver are associated with SULT1A1 copy number variations and expression levels. *Archives of Toxicology*, *91*(10), 3329–3339.

Võsa, U., Esko, T., Kasela, S., & Annilo, T. (2015). Altered gene expression associated with microRNA binding site polymorphisms. *PLoS One*, *10*(10), e0141351.

Wang, L., Chen, J., Zeng, Y., Wei, J., Jing, J., Li, G., et al. (2016). Functional variant in the SLC22A3-LPAL2-LPA gene cluster contributes to the severity of coronary artery disease. *Arteriosclerosis, Thrombosis, and Vascular Biology*, *36*(9), 1989–1996.

Wang, X., Jiang, H., Wu, W., Zhang, R., Wu, L., Chen, H., et al. (2017). An integrating approach for genome-wide screening of MicroRNA polymorphisms mediated drug response alterations. *International Journal of Genomics*, *2017*, 1674827.

Wang, X., Ren, H., Zhao, T., Ma, W., Dong, J., Zhang, S., et al. (2016). Single nucleotide polymorphism in the microRNA-199a binding site of HIF1A gene is associated with pancreatic ductal adenocarcinoma risk and worse clinical outcomes. *Oncotarget*, 7(12), 13717–13729.

Wang, L., Shangguan, S., Chang, S., Yu, X., Wang, Z., Lu, X., et al. (2016). Determining the association between methylenetetrahydrofolate reductase (MTHFR) gene polymorphisms and genomic DNA methylation level: A meta-analysis. *Birth Defects Research. Part A, Clinical and Molecular Teratology*, *106*(8), 667–674.

Wei, R., Yang, F., Urban, T. J., Li, L., Chalasani, N., Flockhart, D. A., et al. (2012). Impact of the interaction between 3′-UTR SNPs and microRNA on the expression of human xenobiotic metabolism enzyme and transporter genes. *Frontiers in Genetics*, *3*, 248.

Welter, D., MacArthur, J., Morales, J., Burdett, T., Hall, P., Junkins, H., et al. (2014). The NHGRI GWAS catalog, a curated resource of SNP-trait associations. *Nucleic Acids Research*, *42*(Database issue), D1001–1006.

Werk, A. N., Bruckmueller, H., Haenisch, S., & Cascorbi, I. (2014). Genetic variants may play an important role in mRNA-miRNA interaction: Evidence for haplotype-dependent downregulation of ABCC2 (MRP2) by miRNA-379. *Pharmacogenetics and Genomics*, *24*(6), 283–291.

Wijayakumara, D. D., Mackenzie, P. I., McKinnon, R. A., Hu, D. G., & Meech, R. (2017). Regulation of UDP-glucuronosyltransferases UGT2B4 and UGT2B7 by MicroRNAs in liver cancer cells. *Journal of Pharmacology and Experimental Therapeutics*, *361*(3), 386–397.

Xu, J., Tian, S., Yin, Z., Wu, S., Liu, L., Qian, Y., et al. (2014). MicroRNA-binding site SNPs in deregulated genes are associated with clinical outcome of non-small cell lung cancer. *Lung Cancer (Amsterdam, Netherlands)*, *85*(3), 442–448.

Yokoi, T., & Nakajima, M. (2013). microRNAs as mediators of drug toxicity. *Annual Review of Pharmacology and Toxicology*, *53*(1), 377–400.

Yu, X., Dhakal, I. B., Beggs, M., Edavana, V. K., Williams, S., Zhang, X., et al. (2010). Functional genetic variants in the 3′-untranslated region of sulfotransferase isoform

1A1 (SULT1A1) and their effect on enzymatic activity. *Toxicological Sciences: An Official Journal of the Society of Toxicology*, *118*(2), 391–403.

Yu, A.-M., Tian, Y., Tu, M.-J., Ho, P. Y., & Jilek, J. L. (2016). MicroRNA pharmacoepigenetics: Posttranscriptional regulation mechanisms behind variable drug disposition and strategy to develop more effective therapy. *Drug Metabolism and Disposition: The Biological Fate of Chemicals*, *44*(3), 308–319.

Zanger, U. M., & Klein, K. (2013). Pharmacogenetics of cytochrome P450 2B6 (CYP2B6): Advances on polymorphisms, mechanisms, and clinical relevance. *Frontiers in Genetics*, *4*, 24.

Zanger, U. M., Klein, K., Thomas, M., Rieger, J. K., Tremmel, R., Kandel, B. A., et al. (2014). Genetics, epigenetics, and regulation of drug-metabolizing cytochrome p450 enzymes. *Clinical Pharmacology and Therapeutics*, *95*(3), 258–261.

Zanger, U. M., & Schwab, M. (2013). Cytochrome P450 enzymes in drug metabolism: Regulation of gene expression, enzyme activities, and impact of genetic variation. *Pharmacology & Therapeutics*, *138*(1), 103–141.

Zhang, G.-H., Lu, Y., Ji, B.-Q., Ren, J.-C., Sun, P., Ding, S., et al. (2017). Do mutations in DNMT3A/3B affect global DNA hypomethylation among benzene-exposed workers in Southeast China?: Effects of mutations in DNMT3A/3B on global DNA hypomethylation. *Environmental and Molecular Mutagenesis*, *58*(9), 678–687.

Zhang, G., & Nebert, D. W. (2017). Personalized medicine: Genetic risk prediction of drug response. *Pharmacology & Therapeutics*, *175*, 75–90.

Zorc, M., Obsteter, J., Dovc, P., & Kunej, T. (2015). Genetic variability of MicroRNA genes in 15 animal species. *Journal of Genomics*, *3*, 51–56.

CHAPTER THREE

Tamoxifen and CYP2D6: A Controversy in Pharmacogenetics

Deirdre P. Cronin-Fenton[*,1], **Per Damkier**[†,‡]
[*]Department of Clinical Epidemiology, Aarhus University, Aarhus, Denmark
[†]Department of Clinical Biochemistry and Pharmacology, Odense University Hospital, Odense, Denmark
[‡]Department of Clinical Research, University of Southern Denmark, Odense, Denmark
[1]Corresponding author: e-mail address: dc@clin.au.dk

Contents

1. Introduction 66
   1.1 Tamoxifen Metabolism 67
   1.2 Tamoxifen Transport 68
2. CYP2D6 and Tamoxifen Metabolism 69
   2.1 Studies on Drug-Induced Inhibition of Tamoxifen Metabolism 71
   2.2 Limitations of the Pharmacoepidemiological Drug–Drug Interaction Studies 73
   2.3 Studies on Pharmacogenetically Reduced Tamoxifen Metabolism 74
   2.4 Comprehensive Genotyping 75
   2.5 Use of Tumor-Infiltrated DNA for Genotyping 77
3. Perspectives 79
   3.1 Comprehensive Genotyping 79
   3.2 Genetically Reduced CYP2D6 Activity May Have Greatest Impact on Tamoxifen Effectiveness in Premenopausal Breast Cancer Patients 80
   3.3 Tamoxifen Transport 81
   3.4 Other Biomarkers May Impact Tamoxifen Effectiveness 82
   3.5 Tamoxifen Analogues 82
4. Conclusion 83
Acknowledgments 83
References 83

Abstract

Tamoxifen reduces the rate of breast cancer recurrence by about one-half. It is converted to more active metabolites by enzymes encoded by polymorphic genes, including cytochrome P450 2D6 (CYP2D6) and transported by ATP-binding cassette transporters. Genetic polymorphisms that confer reduced CYP2D6 activity or concurrent use of CYP2D6-inhibiting drugs may reduce the clinical efficacy of tamoxifen. The issue

Advances in Pharmacology, Volume 83
ISSN 1054-3589
https://doi.org/10.1016/bs.apha.2018.03.001

of the clinical utility of CYP2D6 genotype testing is subject to considerable and ongoing academic and clinical controversy. In this chapter, we outline tamoxifen's clinical pharmacology and give an overview of the research to date on the association between CYP2D6 inhibition and tamoxifen effectiveness. Based on the evidence to date, the impact of drug-induced and/or gene-induced inhibition of CYP2D6 activity is likely to be null or small, or at most moderate in subjects carrying two reduced function alleles. Future research should examine the effect of polymorphisms in genes encoding enzymes in tamoxifen's complete metabolic pathway, should comprehensively evaluate other biomarkers that affect tamoxifen effectiveness, such as the transport enzymes, and focus on subgroups of patients, such as premenopausal breast cancer patients, for whom tamoxifen is the only guideline approved endocrine therapy.

ABBREVIATIONS

ABC	adenosine tyrosine phosphate-binding cassette
AI	aromatase inhibitor
ATAC	Arimidex, Tamoxifen, Alone or in Combination
ATP	adenosine–tyrosine phosphate
BCRP	breast cancer resistance protein
BIG 1-98	Breast International Group 1-98
CYP	cytochrome P450
CYPTAM	cytochrome P450 tamoxifen
DNA	deoxyribonucleotide acid
EM	extensive metabolizer
ERα	estrogen receptor α
ERβ	estrogen receptor β
FFPE	formalin-fixed paraffin-embedded
HWE	Hardy–Weinberg equilibrium
IM	intermediate metabolizer
LOH	loss of heterozygosity
MDR1	multidrug resistance 1
MRP	multidrug resistance protein
P-gp	P-glycoprotein

1. INTRODUCTION

Tamoxifen is a selective estrogen receptor modulator (SERM). For almost 40 years, it has been used in routine clinical practice to target the growth of hormone-responsive breast tumors (Jordan, 2008). Tamoxifen competes with estrogen for binding to the estrogen receptor α (ERα). Tamoxifen is the only endocrine therapy recommended for premenopausal women with breast tumors that express ERα (Jordan et al., 2011; NCCN practice guidelines in oncology, breast cancer—v.2.2014. invasive breast cancer, adjuvant endocrine therapy, 2014). Tamoxifen is an important alternate or sequential treatment to aromatase inhibitors (AIs) among postmenopausal breast cancer patients whose tumors express ERα, depending on their risk of treatment-induced side effects (NCCN practice guidelines in oncology, breast cancer—v.2.2011. invasive breast cancer, adjuvant endocrine therapy, 2010).

Five years of adjuvant tamoxifen therapy reduce the risk of breast cancer recurrence by almost one-half (Early Breast Cancer Trialists, Collaborative Group, 2005; Early Breast Cancer Trialists' Collaborative Group (EBCTCG) et al., 2011; Randomized trial of two versus five years of adjuvant tamoxifen for postmenopausal early-stage breast cancer. Swedish breast cancer cooperative group, 1996) with further long-term survival benefit evident after 10 years of tamoxifen treatment (Davies et al., 2013; Gray et al., 2008). Despite the effectiveness of tamoxifen, patients with identical prognostic factors at diagnosis can vary substantially in their disease clinical course and treatment response. Some patients develop recurrent breast cancer resistant to tamoxifen, and eventually die of their disease.

Intensive international research has investigated mechanisms of resistance to endocrine therapy. However, biomarkers of resistance, beyond ERα, remain elusive. A major challenge to the clinical course of breast cancer and outcomes of the disease is to improve the understanding of mechanisms of endocrine therapy resistance, particularly identifying biomarkers that determine response to tamoxifen treatment, thereby enabling the development of more specific targeted therapies.

1.1 Tamoxifen Metabolism

A series of cytochrome P450 (CYP) enzymes catalyze the conversion of tamoxifen to its more active derivatives—4-hydroxy-tamoxifen, *N*-desmethyltamoxifen, and 4-hydroxy-*N*-desmethyltamoxifen, also called endoxifen (Fig. 1: *metabolic path*) (Jordan, Collins, Rowsby, & Prestwich, 1977; Lien, Solheim, Kvinnsland, & Ueland, 1988; Stearns et al., 2003). Each metabolite has its own specific binding affinity for ERα. The tamoxifen metabolites with the highest binding affinities for the ERα are hydroxylated at tamoxifen's four carbon. The UDP-glucuronosyltransferase enzymes (UGTs, primarily UGT1A8, UGT1A10, UGT2B7, and UGT2B15) (Ahern et al., 2011; Lazarus, Blevins-Primeau, Zheng, & Sun, 2009) and sulfotransferase enzymes (primarily SULT1A1) (Gjerde et al., 2008) catalyze the conversion of the tamoxifen metabolites into excretable forms. All enzymes in tamoxifen's

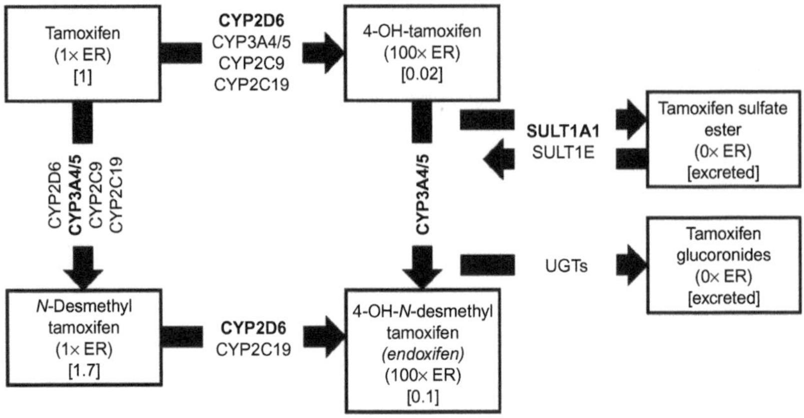

Fig. 1 Tamoxifen metabolic pathway.

metabolic pathway are encoded by polymorphic genes each with distinctive characteristics of allele frequencies and functional significance. Thus, individual differences in tamoxifen metabolism may contribute to variation in the serum metabolite concentration, which may in turn impact tamoxifen effectiveness.

1.2 Tamoxifen Transport

Tamoxifen is transported by members of the ATP-binding cassette (ABC) transporters—ABCB1 (P-glycoprotein or P-gp/MDR1), ABCC1 (breast cancer resistance protein or BCRP), and ABCC2 (multidrug resistance-associated protein 2 or MRP2). ABC transporters are normally expressed at the luminal side of enterocytes, on brain capillary endothelial cells, in the bile canaliculi, and in the proximal tubules of the kidney in germ-line cells. The ABC transporters transport a wide variety of toxins, nutrients, environmental carcinogens, and drugs out of the cells. Given their role in drug efflux, ABC transporters are often overexpressed in cancer cells, where they may mediate drug resistance, and potentially promote cancer cell survival (Amiri-Kordestani, Basseville, Kurdziel, Fojo, & Bates, 2012; International Transporter Consortium et al., 2010; Lai et al., 2012; Leslie, Deeley, & Cole, 2005; Reed & Parissenti, 2011). The primary ER-binding metabolites of tamoxifen–endoxifen and 4-hydroxytamoxifen also bind ABCB1. These metabolites are substrates of the ABCB1 transporter (Iusuf et al., 2011; Teft, Mansell, & Kim, 2011).

Similar to CYP enzymes, polymorphic genes encode the ABC transporters. Polymorphisms that increase the expression of the transporters, enhance drug efflux, and in theory, may reduce the effectiveness of cancer-directed therapy. Yet, the association of genetic polymorphisms in the ABC transporters with tamoxifen effectiveness is poorly understood, as we discuss further later.

Taken together, tamoxifen metabolism and transport is complex and involves multiple enzymes and transporters, all encoded by highly polymorphic genes. Despite this, the majority of studies to date have investigated the association of one enzyme, CYP2D6, and tamoxifen effectiveness. In this chapter, we outline the research to date on the association of CYP2D6 inhibition and tamoxifen effectiveness in breast cancer patients. We highlight some controversies including studies where genotyping results have deviated from Hardy–Weinburg Equilibrium (HWE) and the potential for loss of heterozygosity (LOH) at the CYP2D6 locus, which may result in genotype misclassification. We evaluate studies where researchers have taken a more complete approach to investigating gene-induced tamoxifen inhibition, namely, by comprehensively genotyping enzymes and transporters in the tamoxifen pathway. We also highlight areas that require further investigation including the need for studies specifically focused on premenopausal women, for whom other endocrine therapies, such as AIs are contraindicated (Jordan et al., 2011; NCCN practice guidelines in oncology, breast cancer—v.2.2014. invasive breast cancer, adjuvant endocrine therapy, 2014). Finally, we highlight the need for research on other biomarkers, which may impact tamoxifen effectiveness.

2. CYP2D6 AND TAMOXIFEN METABOLISM

Tamoxifen is sometimes referred to as a prodrug, which implies that it is biologically inactive in its administered form (Goetz, Kamal, & Ames, 2008). However, as administered, tamoxifen has a weak affinity toward the ER, so the term prodrug is not entirely accurate. A number of CYP enzymes convert tamoxifen to its metabolites in complex parallel and serial pathways. Although the metabolites are present at substantially lower concentrations than the administered drug, they have a higher affinity toward the ER. CYP2D6 metabolizes tamoxifen to endoxifen, the most abundant of the high-affinity 4-hydroxylated metabolites. Endoxifen is found at substantially lower concentrations than tamoxifen but has 100-fold higher affinity toward the ERα (Johnson et al., 2004; Lim, Desta, Flockhart, & Skaar, 2005). It is therefore considered the key tamoxifen metabolite and is likely the most biologically active and important molecule among tamoxifen and its myriad of primary and secondary metabolites. Low serum concentrations of endoxifen, but not the other tamoxifen metabolites, have been correlated with an increased risk of recurrent or new primary breast cancer (Madlensky et al., 2011; Saladores et al., 2015). Endoxifen is therefore considered the key metabolite in modulating the estrogen receptor pathway (Madlensky et al., 2011).

The CYP2D6 gene is highly polmorphic. CYP2D6 has over 100 distinct variants, and frequent gene duplications and deletions (http://www.cypalleles.ki.se/cyp2d6.htm). Several CYP2D6 variants can reduce or eliminate enzymatic activity (Hu et al., 2016). This genetic variability results in considerable phenotypical variation in CYP2D6 activity between patients. Thus, theoretically, the effectiveness of tamoxifen may be related to an individual's CYP2D6 activity. With the notable exception of a complete gene deletion (as in the case of *CYP2D6**5*), or the inheritance of two alleles associated with a complete loss of function (most importantly the *CYP2D6**4* allele), substantial controversy surrounds the assignment of functional phenotype according to *CYP2D6* genotype (Hicks, Swen, & Gaedigk, 2014). Based on *CYP2D6* genotype combinations, patients can be classified in four categories. Poor metabolizers (PMs) are those with no or minimal enzymatic activity due to two inactive alleles. Intermediate metabolizers (IMs) have reduced activity owing to two decreased activity alleles or one active and one inactive allele. Extensive metabolizers (EMs) have normal enzymatic activity due to no variants or only one decreased activity allele. Ultrarapid metabolizers have greater than normal enzymatic activity either due to gene duplication or no inactive variants (Zanger, Raimundo, & Eichelbaum, 2004). Metabolic activity correlates with steady-state endoxifen levels (Johnson et al., 2004; Lien et al., 1988). Accordingly, PMs appear to have the lowest plasma endoxifen levels (Helland et al., 2017; Madlensky et al., 2011). EMs have slightly higher *Z*-endoxifen concentrations than IMs (Madlensky et al., 2011).

Some research suggests that the total concentration of tamoxifen and its metabolites is sufficiently high so as to overwhelm and inhibit estrogen binding to the estrogen receptor, irrespective of an individual's CYP2D6 genotype and phenotype (Lash, Lien, Sorensen, & Hamilton-Dutoit, 2009). This may be especially relevant in premenopausal women as they have higher estrogen concentrations compared with their postmenopausal counterparts (Burger, Hale, Dennerstein, & Robertson, 2008; Fan et al., 2009; Freour, Barriere, & Masson, 2017). Accordingly, reduction in tamoxifen metabolite concentrations could potentially reduce the competition with estrogen for binding to ERα (Cronin-Fenton, Damkier, & Lash, 2013).

2.1 Studies on Drug-Induced Inhibition of Tamoxifen Metabolism

Tamoxifen induces mild-to-moderate adverse effects, including hot flashes and vasomotor symptoms, but more rare and more severe adverse reactions including depression, venous thromboembolism, and endometrial cancer have also been reported (Baum et al., 2002; Biglia et al., 2005; Deitcher & Gomes, 2004; Demissie, Silliman, & Lash, 2001; Fisher et al., 2005; Henry et al., 2009; Swerdlow & Jones, 2005). About one-quarter of women who use tamoxifen are coprescribed selective serotonin reuptake inhibitors (SSRIs) to alleviate symptoms of depression and/or to treat the vasomotor side effects associated with tamoxifen therapy. SSRIs inhibit CYP2D6 to varying degrees (Borges et al., 2006; Jin et al., 2005). Concurrent use of SSRIs and tamoxifen can therefore result in competitive or direct inhibition of tamoxifen metabolism. The net effect is a reduced plasma concentration of the tamoxifen metabolite, endoxifen (Jin et al., 2005; Stearns et al., 2003). Substantial reductions in endoxifen plasma concentrations—comparable to those observed in homozygous carriers of the *CYP2D6**4* variant allele—have been observed in patients using strong CYP2D6 inhibitors (i.e., paroxetine or sertraline) concurrent to tamoxifen, but not among those using the weaker CYP2D6 inhibitors citalopram or venlafaxine (Jin et al., 2005). Concerns have therefore been raised regarding the safety of using these drugs concomitant to tamoxifen treatment (Cronin-Fenton, Lash, & Sorensen, 2010; Sideras et al., 2010).

Paroxetine and fluoxetine are the most potent and effective CYP2D6-inhibiting SSRIs. Research suggests that concomitant use of these drugs converts phenotypically extensive or intermediate CYP2D6 metabolizers into PMs—phenotypically equivalent to subjects carrying two nonfunctional *CYP2D6* alleles. In contrast, other SSRIs, citalopram, escitalopram, sertraline, and fluvoxamine, are weak inhibitors of CYP2D6. Women who use paroxetine or fluoxetine concurrent to tamoxifen have lower serum endoxifen concentrations. Intermediate plasma endoxifen concentrations have been observed in women using the weaker CYP2D6 inhibitors, sertraline and citalopram, concurrent to tamoxifen, and little to no impact on endoxifen concentrations associated with concurrent use of the selective serotonin norepinephrine reuptake inhibitor venlafaxine—a weak CYP2D6 inhibitor (Borges et al., 2010, 2006; Jin et al., 2005; Stearns et al., 2003).

The clinical epidemiology studies investigating the association of concurrent use of SSRIs and tamoxifen with breast cancer recurrence have heterogeneous findings. We have previously conducted a quantitative and qualitative review outlining the association of drug-induced inhibition of tamoxifen metabolism with breast cancer recurrence and mortality (Cronin-Fenton et al., 2013). From a total of eight studies of weak CYP2D6 inhibitor drugs, a random effects meta-analytic model suggested little evidence of an association between concurrent use of weak CYP2D6 inhibitors and breast cancer recurrence/survival among tamoxifen-treated women (effect estimate = 1.05, 95% CI = 0.91, 1.22). Likewise, our meta-analysis suggested little evidence of an increased risk of breast cancer recurrence/survival among tamoxifen-treated women who concurrently used strong CYP2D6 inhibitors (effect estimate = 1.03, 95% CI = 0.86, 1.23).

Since the publication of the meta-analysis in 2014, a further four studies (Chubak et al., 2016; Donneyong et al., 2016; Haque et al., 2015; Valachis et al., 2016) investigated the impact of CYP2D6 inhibitor drugs on breast cancer recurrence/survival. However, similar to the preceding studies, the conclusions of these studies are somewhat ambiguous.

In a cohort study based on electronic pharmacy records in the United States, Chubak and colleagues observed an increased rate of breast cancer recurrence among women who used paroxetine concurrent to their tamoxifen (Chubak et al., 2016). In contrast, they found little evidence of an increased recurrence rate associated with use of fluoxetine—a SSRI with CYP2D6 potency equivalent to that of paroxetine. However, the study may be prone to information bias as information on breast cancer recurrence was obtained by medical record review. Also in a US-based cohort of 16,887 survivors of nonmetastatic breast cancer (Haque et al., 2015), Haque and coworkers investigated the association of concurrent use of strong or weak CYP2D6 inhibitors with the risk of new breast cancer—defined as breast cancer recurrence, metastases, or contralateral breast cancer. In a median follow-up of 6 years, they observed little evidence of an increased rate of new breast cancers among concurrent users of tamoxifen and any SSRIs. The null findings remained robust irrespective of the strength of the CYP2D6-inhibiting drug, or the use of other non-SSRI antidepressants. A Swedish nested case–control study by Valachis et al. (2016) also concluded no excess risk of breast cancer-specific mortality associated with concurrent use of SSRIs and tamoxifen. This null finding was evident even among users of strong CYP2D6-inhibiting SSRIs. In an overlapping cohort study, Valachis et al. observed lower adherence to endocrine therapy among patients who used SSRIs either before or after breast cancer, except among those patients who had more than 50% concurrent periods of use of SSRI use and endocrine therapy. Non-adherence to endocrine therapy correlated with poorer survival.

Finally, Donneyong et al. used data from five US databases to investigate the association of potent CYP2D6 inhibitors (paroxetine and fluoxetine) with mortality in breast cancer patients (Donneyong et al., 2016). They stratified SSRI exposure by their CYP2D6-inhibiting potential: patients who used an effective CYP2D6-inhibiting SSRI concurrent to tamoxifen (i.e., paroxetine and fluoxetine), and those who used a moderate or poor CYP2D6 inhibitor (citalopram, escitalopram, fluvoxamine, and sertraline) concurrent to tamoxifen. Their study included two cohorts—6067 patients who initiated SSRI use during tamoxifen treatment, and 8465 patients who were prevalent SSRI users at the time they initiated tamoxifen treatment. Median follow-up time was 2.2 (interquartile range 0.9–4.5) and 2.0 (0.8–3.9) years, respectively. They incorporated propensity scores estimating the probability of exposure to potent vs nonpotent SSRIs, to account for potential confounding. Overall, they observed no evidence of an association of potent SSRI use with outcomes in tamoxifen-treated patients. However, an analysis stratified at age 50—as a proxy for menopausal status—suggested higher mortality associated with effective CYP2D6-inhibiting SSRI use concurrent to tamoxifen among women aged less than 50 at the time of their breast cancer diagnosis.

2.2 Limitations of the Pharmacoepidemiological Drug–Drug Interaction Studies

The pharmacoepidemiology studies have several limitations, which are relevant when investigating the tamoxifen–SSRI interaction using pharmacoepidemiology techniques. An editorial of the Donneyong paper highlighted some of these limitations (Juurlink, 2016). The potential interaction between tamoxifen and SSRIs is not a short-term effect, but may take years to manifest an impact on breast cancer recurrence or mortality. Several papers had relatively short follow-up (Donneyong et al., 2016). Others including a general outcome of mortality, rather than a cancer-specific endpoint, such as recurrence. In addition, other issues including a lack of data on adherence to treatment, the challenge of incorporating information on switching from one SSRI to another, and failure to detect a dose–response effect. Furthermore, few studies have considered the combination of gene-induced and drug-induced inhibition of tamoxifen metabolism, which may be most important to tamoxifen effectiveness. Taken together, these drug–drug interaction studies highlight a need for a greater understanding of the impact of concurrent use of CYP2D6-inhibiting drugs on tamoxifen metabolism using an endpoint of recurrence rather than mortality.

2.3 Studies on Pharmacogenetically Reduced Tamoxifen Metabolism

The association of CYP2D6 genotype and tamoxifen effectiveness is one of the most researched and disputed pharmacogenetic controversies (Cronin-Fenton et al., 2013). Myriad studies conducted in observational settings, clinical series, or nested within clinical trials have investigated the putative association between *CYP2D6* genotype and tamoxifen effectiveness. In our aforementioned meta-analysis (Cronin-Fenton et al., 2013), we also comprehensively reviewed the studies of CYP2D6 genotype variants and associations to outcomes in breast cancer patients among studies published through March 2013. The findings from the published studies were highly discordant, with effect estimates ranging from a 50% decrease in the risk of recurrence or mortality, to a 12-fold increase in the risk of breast cancer recurrence or mortality among carriers of variant *CYP2D6*. Based on the evidence, we concluded that the impact of genetically reduced CYP2D6 activity on tamoxifen effectiveness was likely null or small, or at best moderate among carriers of two reduced function alleles.

Studies were very heterogeneous with respect to design, study population, specific CYP2D6 allele coverage, genotyping methodology, and deoxyribonucleotide acid (DNA) source material. As outlined in our meta-analysis, the published research had substantial limitations. These include small sample size yielding imprecise estimates and retrospective data collection increasing a potential for information bias. Several studies incorrectly classified exposed person-time yielding immortal person-time bias (Kiyotani et al., 2010; Lash et al., 2008; Xu et al., 2008). The *CYP2D6*4* variant is most common among Caucasians, and this allele confers true null activity, i.e., homozygotes have no CYP2D6 activity. The **10* allele which occurs frequently among Asians, however, confers reduced enzyme activity. Clinical data on enzyme activity (phenotype) in subjects carrying two *10 alleles clearly suggest clinically meaningful enzymatic activity. While inferring phenotype and in vivo enzyme activity from IM genotypes has not met absolute scientific consensus, such is also in accordance with the phenotype classification suggested by Hicks, Murray, Powe, Hughes, and Cardwell (2013) and Gaedigk (2013). Despite this, the highest effect estimates were observed in Asian populations evaluating the **10* variant—counterintuitive to the underlying biologic rationale (Cronin-Fenton et al., 2013). In addition, it seems plausible that overall tamoxifen effectiveness would depend on the activity of all the enzymes in the entire pathway, and their interaction, rather than on polymorphisms in a single gene. A widespread limitation of the research to date is a failure to comprehensively genotype the complete tamoxifen metabolic pathway. Taken together, we were unable to detect a consistent anomaly, which could explain the discrepant findings.

For the aforementioned meta-analysis, we used PubMed to retrieve articles on "tamoxifen" and "CYP2D6" and searched the reference lists of the retrieved papers, including those that had cited those previously published. Since the publication of our meta-analysis, using the same search criteria through November 2017 (Cronin-Fenton et al., 2013), over 20 additional published studies have investigated the impact of *CYP2D6* genetic polymorphisms on breast cancer prognosis (Argalacsova, Slanar, Bakhouche, & Pertuzelka, 2017; Chamnanphon et al., 2013; De Ameida Melo et al., 2016; Dezentje et al., 2015, 2013; Goetz et al., 2017; Hertz et al., 2017; Johansson et al., 2016; Lei et al., 2016; Marcath et al., 2017; Markkula, Hjertberg, Rose, Ingvar, & Jernstrom, 2014; Martins, Vidal, Souza, Brusaca, & Brito, 2014; Mwinyi et al., 2014; Powers et al., 2016; Sanchez Spitman et al., 2017; Sanchez-Spitman et al., 2017; Sensorn et al., 2013; Zhang et al., 2015). Most suggest little evidence of an association of the *CYP2D6**4* or **10* variant with recurrence and mortality in tamoxifen-treated breast cancer patients. Here, we provide some highlight some of these studies.

Several of the more recently published studies were restricted to considering one variant or a limited number of variants in a single gene. De Ameida Melo et al. (2016) reported no correlation of *CYP2D6**4*, **10*, or **17* with breast cancer prognosis among 40 ER+ nonmetastatic patients and 40 metastatic patients (De Ameida Melo et al., 2016). Martins et al. also showed no correlation of CYP2D6 (*3, *4, *10) with recurrence/mortality in a cohort of 58 patients, 47% of whom were premenopausal at the time of breast cancer diagnosis (Martins et al., 2014). Yazdi et al. genotyped the CYP2D6*4 variant and used this to predict phenotype (Yazdi et al., 2015). In a study of 101 patients followed for a minimum of 3 years, they observed a decreased risk of recurrence among CYP2D6 EM patients with HER2+ tumors. However, for all three studies, sample size was quite small consequently yielding imprecise estimates and questionable statistical power.

2.4 Comprehensive Genotyping

Up to recently, the only study to comprehensively genotype the enzymes relevant to the tamoxifen metabolic pathway was conducted in the cancer prevention setting. Borges et al. evaluated polymorphisms in the genes encoding the entire tamoxifen metabolic path among women at high risk of breast cancer (Borges et al., 2010). Overall, the study failed to observe a strong association of single *CYP2D6* variants and breast cancer incidence. *CYP2D6* was identified as a key node in the metabolic path, interacting with several variant alleles in other tamoxifen-metabolizing genes.

More recently, studies conducted in the treatment setting have increasingly integrated more comprehensive genotyping—recognizing that tamoxifen effectiveness is likely to hinge on multiple variants in several genes, rather than on single SNPs. A population-based cohort study by Hertz et al. genotyped six CYP2D6 variants and copy number variants among 500 tamoxifen-treated patients and 500 ER+ patients who did not undergo systemic therapy (Hertz et al., 2017). The design of the study is commendable and somewhat similar to a previously published case–control study design (Lash et al., 2011). The tamoxifen-treated cohort aimed to address the utility of CYP2D6 as a *predictor* of tamoxifen effectiveness (i.e., *a determinant of response to tamoxifen treatment*). On the other hand, the ER+ nontamoxifen-treated cohort aimed to elucidate the utility of CYP2D6 as a *prognostic* indicator (i.e., *a determinant of breast cancer prognosis in the absence of tamoxifen treatment*). The Hertz study showed no correlation between *CYP2D6* polymorphisms and recurrence risk in tamoxifen-treated patients in univariate analyses. Adjusted analyses suggested an increased risk of recurrence among patients with increased, rather than the hypothesized decreased, CYP2D6 activity. Furthermore, among the nontreated ER+ patients, higher CYP2D6 activity correlated with prolonged recurrence-free survival. These conflicting findings do not align well to the suggested biologic rationale and preclude any inference of a true association of *CYP2D6* genotype with outcomes in breast cancer patients.

A study by Markkula et al. also took a more comprehensive approach to genotyping, examining the association of *CYP2D6* genotypes *(*3, *4, *6, *10, *41)* with second breast events (recurrence, contralateral breast cancer, or death) among 634 patients, 333 of whom had ER+ tumors and received tamoxifen therapy (Markkula et al., 2014). Blood samples drawn at the time of breast cancer diagnosis were used as a source of DNA for genotyping. In a median follow-up of 4.9 years, they also concluded that there was no evidence of an association between *CYP2D6* genotype and second breast events.

Several studies have studied prediction of CYP2D6 functional status from genotype combinations (Dezentje et al., 2013; Hertz et al., 2017; Johansson et al., 2016; Karle et al., 2013; Marcath et al., 2017; Sanchez Spitman et al., 2017). A study by Marcath et al., including 302 tamoxifen-treated patients, predicted phenotype based on genotypes of 19 enzymes and transporters and correlated these with endoxifen concentration (Marcath et al., 2017). CYP2C9 was the only gene that appeared to correlate with endoxifen concentrations. In contrast, Sanchez Spitman studied the combined impact of CYP2D6 genotypes, CYP3A4*22 and CYP3A5*3 on tamoxifen metabolite concentrations in the sera of 667 women enrolled in the CYPTAM study (Sanchez Spitman et al., 2017). They found little evidence of a meaningful role of the studied CYP3A4 variant alleles. Highest tamoxifen metabolite concentrations were observed among carriers of the CYP3A4*22 variant. However, the effect was small and deemed unlikely of clinical relevance.

Johansson et al. pooled data from four randomized breast cancer prevention trials, including 367 patients followed for a median of 11 years (Johansson et al., 2016). They genotyped 13 SNPs in the *CYP2D6* gene and used these to predict functional metabolizer status. They observed lower recurrence rates in rapid metabolizers compared with slow metabolizers. They also observed higher endoxifen and 4-hydroxytamoxifen levels associated with decreased insulin-like growth factor I—making an important inference that other biomarkers may also impact tamoxifen effectiveness.

We have not focused on the association of the pharmacogenetics of tamoxifen and survival in metastatic patients. However, three recent studies suggest a correlation of CYP2D6 mutations with decreased progression-free survival in patients with advanced breast cancer (De Ameida Melo et al., 2016; Goetz et al., 2017; Karle et al., 2013). However, the studies included fewer than 100 patients, thus estimates were imprecise. In addition, the clinical significance of investigating the association of CYP2D6 polymorphisms and prognosis in *metastatic* breast cancer patients remains unclear, as these patients are likely to have treatment-refractory disease.

2.5 Use of Tumor-Infiltrated DNA for Genotyping

Source DNA for the study of the pharmacogenetics of tamoxifen remains a divisive issue (Goetz et al., 2014; Pharoah, Abraham, & Caldas, 2012; Stanton, 2012). From a practical standpoint, formalin-fixed and paraffin-embedded (FFPE) tissue represent an important resource in most settings, but careful considerations on the quality of the extracted DNA should be made (Wheeler, Maitland, Dolan, Cox, & Ratain, 2013).

A major controversy particularly pertinent to *CYP2D6* polymorphisms and tamoxifen effectiveness is the validity of using DNA derived from tumor tissue rather than genomic DNA. Two studies nested within two prospective clinical trials—Breast International Group (BIG 1-98) and the Arimidex, Tamoxifen, Alone or in Combination (ATAC) trial—genotyped seven and eight CYP2D6 variant alleles, respectively (Rae et al., 2012; Regan et al., 2012). Although the results of both studies were highly anticipated, neither study reported a positive association between reduced CYP2D6 function and breast cancer recurrence. However, the validity of the genotyping in both studies has been questioned as the *CYP2D6* allele frequencies departed substantially from HWE. Deviations from HWE can occur due to sampling error, nonrandom mating, or population admixture due to the inclusion of multiethnic genotype frequencies. The latter may be particularly relevant to the BIG 1-98 and ATAC trials, which were included patients from multiple countries (Deng, 2001). Deviations from HWE may imply genotyping error.

In addition, BIG 1-98 and the ATAC trial studies used DNA derived from FFPE tumor tissue, which some believe may lead to important genotyping error (Goetz et al., 2014; Pharoah et al., 2012; Stanton, 2012). Use of tumor-derived DNA may lead to germ-line genotype misclassification from LOH at the *CYP2D6* locus (chromosome 22q13). Approximately 40% of ER+ breast tumors show a LOH near the *CYP2D6* locus (Ellsworth et al., 2003; Goetz et al., 2014; Hirano et al., 2001; Johnson, Hamadeh, & Langaee, 2015; Sheng et al., 1996). LOH can arise from chromosomal instability in tumor tissue leading to loss of an allele in the tumor DNA, and incorrect genotype assignment. Genotyping tumor-derived DNA can therefore inflate the proportion of homozygotes and underestimate the proportion of heterozygotes in the germ-line DNA. However, except for microdissected tumor tissue, DNA extracted from tumor-infiltrated tissue is likely to contain germ-line information from surrounding stromal and immune cells. As tamoxifen is primarily metabolized in the liver, it is the germ-line genotype, and not the tumor genotype, that potentially determines the impact of *CYP2D6* polymorphisms on tamoxifen effectiveness.

Several concordance studies have compared *CYP2D6* genotype in DNA derived from tumors with that from blood or adjacent marginal or nonmalignant tissue (Ahern et al., 2010; Goetz et al., 2005; Rae et al., 2003, 2013; Schneider et al., 2006; Thompson et al., 2011; Xie et al., 2006). These validation studies report near perfect concordance, with the exception of a study by Goetz et al. (2005) that observed LOH at the *CYP2D6* locus and 20% genotyping misclassification between the FFPE tumor and nontumor tissue. Goetz et al. concluded that tumor-derived DNA was not representative of germ-line DNA at the *CYP2D6* locus. The reasons underlying the discordance in the Goetz study vs the concordance observed in the previously published studies are unclear. In accordance with suggestions made by Berry (2013, 2014) we investigated the extent of potential misclassification by conducting a quantitative bias analysis on the 31 studies that investigated the impact of *CYP2D6* genotype and breast cancer outcomes. We observed little evidence of bias by discordant genotype, and no variation to the overall effect estimates, with or without bias adjustment (Ahern et al., 2017). This is a landmark finding and suggests that studies using archived FFPE tumor tissue as a source of DNA are valid for genotyping the *CYP2D6* locus.

To date, one study that investigated CYP2D6 and breast cancer outcomes incorporated a sensitivity analysis to assess the potential impact of LOH due to the use of FFPE tumor-derived DNA (Dezentje et al., 2013). The study was nested within the tamoxifen exemestane adjuvant multinational trial and genotyped five *CYP2D6* (*CYP2D6*3*, **4*, **6*, **14*, **41*) alleles in 731 tamoxifen-treated patients. *CYP2D6* genotype and functional phenotype were correlated with disease-free survival (time from tamoxifen randomization to tamoxifen discontinuation). Three microsatellite markers adjacent to the *CYP2D6* locus were assessed for potential LOH, resulting in the exclusion of 14 (2%–3%) patients due to suspected LOH. Although overall genotype frequencies deviated from HWE, the frequencies were consistent with others reported in the literature. Notably, *CYP2D6* genotype did not correlate with disease-free survival, irrespective of the inclusion or exclusion of patients with potential LOH.

3. PERSPECTIVES

Several critically important yet sparsely researched issues require consideration to substantiate a better understanding of the interaction between CYP2D6 genotypes and tamoxifen efficacy.

3.1 Comprehensive Genotyping

CYP2D6 is, while arguably the most important, just one enzyme in an intricate metabolic pathway of parallel and serial enzymatic conversions of tamoxifen and its metabolites. Further understanding of the contribution and impact of all polymorphic genes in tamoxifen's metabolic path is therefore urgently needed. Up to recently, the statistical models required to evaluate complex gene–gene interactions had not been well developed (Baurley, Conti, Gauderman, & Thomas, 2010). However, Bayesian pathway modeling offers an approach to better understand and identify the interaction of multiple metabolites with different affinities for ERα. Incorporating empirical Bayes shrinkage methods could reduce the potential for false-positive interactions due to multiple comparisons. Methods such as the Algorithm for Learning Pathway Structure, which incorporates Bayesian analysis, can provide an estimate of the effect of the tamoxifen metabolic pathway on breast cancer recurrence.

3.2 Genetically Reduced CYP2D6 Activity May Have Greatest Impact on Tamoxifen Effectiveness in Premenopausal Breast Cancer Patients

Tamoxifen is the sole guideline-recommended endocrine treatment for premenopausal women. Despite this, studies to date have for the most part included postmenopausal women or, included a low prevalence of premenopausal patients. As premenopausal women account for about one-third of all breast cancer patients, and more than half of them have tumors that express the ERα (Saladores et al., 2015; Sherman, Chapler, Crickard, & Wycoff, 1979), it is essential to fully evaluate the impact of gene-induced and drug-induced inhibition on tamoxifen effectiveness.

The tamoxifen metabolites—4-hydroxy-tamoxifen and 4-hydroxy-*N*-desmethyl-tamoxifen—have approximately the same affinity for ERα as the naturally occurring estrogen, estradiol. Premenopausal women have over 10-fold higher serum estradiol levels compared with their postmenopausal counterparts. As tamoxifen treatment can further increase estradiol concentration (Sherman et al., 1979), premenopausal women may require a higher tamoxifen dose to counter their inherently higher estradiol levels. Impaired tamoxifen metabolism by either genetic polymorphism or CYP inhibition from concomitant drugs may therefore have the greatest impact on recurrence risk in premenopausal women, where the full production of tamoxifen metabolites is necessary to compete with the abundant estrogen.

A study by Saladores et al. focused exclusively on tamoxifen metabolism, metabolite concentrations, and disease-free survival in premenopausal women (Saladores et al., 2015). They combined three cohorts including multiple ethnicities. In a median follow-up of 5.5 years, they observed lower endoxifen concentrations among women with low CYP2D6 activity scores, and poorer disease-free survival. When we stratified our meta-analytic models (Cronin-Fenton et al., 2013) by menopausal status (<20% vs over 20% of premenopausal women), we observed an increased risk of recurrence in studies that had a higher proportion of premenopausal women.

We observed summary hazard ratios of 1.25 (95% CI = 0.91, 1.71) in 9 studies of predominantly postmenopausal women (0%–9% premenopausal, median 0%) and of 1.54 (95% CI = 1.09, 2.18) in 16 studies with at least 20% premenopausal women (20%–80% premenopausal, median 43%) (Cronin-Fenton et al., 2013). These findings strongly suggest that clinically meaningful effects resulting from CYP2D6 genotype and phenotype status on tamoxifen effectiveness may be limited to premenopausal women. Thus, studies of the significance of CYP2D6 pharmacogenetics and inhibition by concomitant administration of other drugs in this particular insufficiently studied population demands attention and clarification.

3.3 Tamoxifen Transport

Few studies have investigated how interindividual differences in tamoxifen transport may influence tamoxifen effectiveness. Highly polymorphic genes also encode the ABC transporters. Yet in contrast to the drug-metabolizing enzymes, studies on the potential impact of ABC transporters and breast cancer outcomes remain scarce. Expression of ABCB1 in breast tumors correlates with clinical outcome in breast cancer patients, regardless of the receipt of adjuvant chemotherapy (Sukasem et al., 2012). In a study of 105 breast cancer patients, where about two-thirds of patients received tamoxifen, higher expression of ABCB1 was associated with higher grade, lymph node involvement, and shorter survival (Xu et al., 2008). In contrast, a study of 516 breast cancer patients (nested in a clinical intervention study of 1099 patients randomized to either tamoxifen/goserelin or cyclophosphamide/methotrexate/fluorouracil chemotherapy) suggested that tumor cell expression of ABCB1 correlated with poorer relapse-free and overall survival, except among tamoxifen-treated patients (Teh et al., 2012). However, the impact of tamoxifen in the study was difficult to determine given its coadministration with goserelin.

Genetic variation in ABC transporters may influence outcomes in breast cancer patients. Kiyotani et al. examined 52 different genomic tag-SNP variants of ABC transporters among 282 postmenopausal breast cancer patients undergoing tamoxifen monotherapy (Kiyotani et al., 2010, 2008). Carriers of the *ABCC2* variant allele (rs3740065) had 10-fold higher rates of recurrence, and estimates were imprecise and were prone to immortal person-time bias (Kiyotani et al., 2010; Lash et al., 2008; Lash & Cole, 2009). A study of 30 Thai patients suggested that ABCB1 may impact recurrence rates (Sensorn et al., 2013), while a US-based study of 116 patients suggested that impaired ABCB1 combined with intermediate metabolism of CYP2D6 correlated with lower endoxifen concentrations (Powers et al., 2016). In contrast, a study by Teh et al. of 95 breast cancer patients treated with tamoxifen found no association between two genetic polymorphisms in *ABCB1* and breast cancer recurrence (Teh et al., 2012). However, when they examined the combined effect of polymorphisms in *ABCB1* and *CYP2D6*, they found an increased risk of breast cancer recurrence. Finally, a study of 196 patients by Teft et al. reported no association of functional polymorphisms in ABCB1 and ABCG2 (BCRP) with endoxifen levels (Teft et al., 2011). A universal limitation of the studies that investigated the association of the pharmacogenetics of ABC transporters with tamoxifen effectiveness is small sample size and imprecise estimates. Clinical data are few, are prone to bias, and are inconsistent regarding the possible impact on breast cancer outcomes. Transporter expression and genomic variants in transporter encoding genes require detailed analysis for their role in tamoxifen effectiveness.

3.4 Other Biomarkers May Impact Tamoxifen Effectiveness

To be effective, tamoxifen and its metabolites must compete with estrogen to overwhelm the estrogen receptor. Yet all clinical epidemiology studies of tamoxifen inhibition have considered one side of this competition—namely, the profile of tamoxifen metabolites. No studies have investigated the impact of estrogen production and the expression levels of estrogen receptors (ERα and ERβ) on tamoxifen effectiveness.

3.5 Tamoxifen Analogues

Several studies have assessed the efficacy of other SERMs—raloxifene (Buzdar et al., 2006; Buzdar, Marcus, Holmes, Hug, & Hortobagyi, 1988; Gradishar et al., 2000), droloxifene (Buzdar et al., 2002), arzoxifene (Deshmane, Krishnamurthy, Melemed, Peterson, & Buzdar, 2007), toremifene (Hayes et al., 1995; International Breast Cancer Study Group et al., 2004)—but all failed to improve upon the effectiveness of tamoxifen. Based on the evidence that tamoxifen may not have equivocal efficacy in all patients, *Z*-endoxifen was developed. Orally administered *Z*-endoxifen potently inhibits tumor growth in vitro and displays substantial bioavailability in mouse models. A recent phase I clinical trial assessed the efficacy of *Z*-endoxifen and prognosis in 38 endocrine-refractory metastatic breast cancer patients (Goetz et al., 2017). The trial aimed to determine the toxicity profile of *Z*-endoxifen, maximum tolerated dose, and the potential clinical effectiveness. Findings suggest minimal toxicity and substantial antitumor activity in women with endocrine-refractory disease. A follow-on phase II trial is ongoing, comparing endoxifen (80 mg/day) with tamoxifen (20 mg/day) in women who have progressed during AI therapy. It may take several years for the clinical utility of *Z*-endoxifen to be fully assessed and for this molecule to receive regulatory approval.

4. CONCLUSION

Despite almost 50 studies, the clinical significance of the pharmacogenetics to tamoxifen effectiveness remains controversial and incompletely understood. Nonetheless, based on the current evidence, we believe regulatory bodies are appropriately recommending against routine *CYP2D6* genotype testing for patients assigned to tamoxifen therapy. The current evidence does not suggest that SSRI inhibition of CYP2D6 reduces the effectiveness of tamoxifen.

The pharmacogenomics of tamoxifen therapy requires further clarification using a comprehensive approach to assessment of the involved metabolic pathways and special attention to premenopausal women with breast cancer.

ACKNOWLEDGMENTS

This work was supported by grants from the US National Institutes of Health, National Cancer Institute (R01CA166825), and the Lundbeck Foundation (R167-2013-15861). The funding agencies had no role in the writing of the chapter or the decision to submit the chapter for publication.

CONFLICT OF INTEREST

The authors declare no conflicts of interest.

REFERENCES

Ahern, T. P., Christensen, M., Cronin-Fenton, D., Lunetta, K. L., Rosenberg, C. L., Sorensen, H. T., et al. (2010). Concordance of metabolic enzyme genotypes assayed from paraffin-embedded, formalin-fixed breast tumors and normal lymphatic tissue. *Clinical Epidemiology*, *2*, 241–246.

Ahern, T. P., Christensen, M., Cronin-Fenton, D. P., Lunetta, K. L., Soiland, H., Gjerde, J., et al. (2011). Functional polymorphisms in UDP-glucuronosyl transferases and recurrence in tamoxifen-treated breast cancer survivors. *Cancer Epidemiology, Biomarkers & Prevention: A Publication of the American Association for Cancer Research, Cosponsored by the American Society of Preventive Oncology*, *20*(9), 1937–1943.

Ahern, T. P., Hertz, D. L., Damkier, P., Ejlertsen, B., Hamilton-Dutoit, S. J., Rae, J. M., et al. (2017). Cytochrome P-450 2D6 (CYP2D6) genotype and breast cancer recurrence in tamoxifen-treated patients: Evaluating the importance of loss of heterozygosity. *American Journal of Epidemiology*, *185*(2), 75–85.

Amiri-Kordestani, L., Basseville, A., Kurdziel, K., Fojo, A. T., & Bates, S. E. (2012). Targeting MDR in breast and lung cancer: Discriminating its potential importance from the failure of drug resistance reversal studies. *Drug Resistance Updates: Reviews and Commentaries in Antimicrobial and Anticancer Chemotherapy*, *15*(1–2), 50–61.

Argalacsova, S., Slanar, O., Bakhouche, H., & Pertuzelka, L. (2017). Impact of ABCB1 and CYP2D6 polymorphisms on tamoxifen treatment outcomes and adverse events in breast cancer patients. *Journal of B.U.ON.: Official Journal of the Balkan Union of Oncology*, *22*(5), 1217–1226.

Baum, M., Budzar, A. U., Cuzick, J., Forbes, J., Houghton, J. H., Klijn, J. G., et al. (2002). Anastrozole alone or in combination with tamoxifen versus tamoxifen alone for adjuvant treatment of postmenopausal women with early breast cancer: First results of the ATAC randomised trial. *Lancet*, *359*(9324), 2131–2139.

Baurley, J. W., Conti, D. V., Gauderman, W. J., & Thomas, D. C. (2010). Discovery of complex pathways from observational data. *Statistics in Medicine*, *29*(19), 1998–2011.

Berry, D. (2013). CYP2D6 genotyping and the use of tamoxifen in breast cancer. *Journal of the National Cancer Institute*, *105*(17), 1267–1269.

Berry, D. A. (2014). Response. *Journal of the National Cancer Institute*, *106*(5). https://doi.org/10.1093/jnci/dju065.

Biglia, N., Torta, R., Roagna, R., Maggiorotto, F., Cacciari, F., Ponzone, R., et al. (2005). Evaluation of low-dose venlafaxine hydrochloride for the therapy of hot flushes in breast cancer survivors. *Maturitas*, *52*(1), 78–85.

Borges, S., Desta, Z., Jin, Y., Faouzi, A., Robarge, J. D., Philip, S., et al. (2010). Composite functional genetic and comedication CYP2D6 activity score in predicting tamoxifen drug exposure among breast cancer patients. *Journal of Clinical Pharmacology*, *50*(4), 450–458.

Borges, S., Desta, Z., Li, L., Skaar, T. C., Ward, B. A., Nguyen, A., et al. (2006). Quantitative effect of CYP2D6 genotype and inhibitors on tamoxifen metabolism: Implication for optimization of breast cancer treatment. *Clinical Pharmacology and Therapeutics*, *80*(1), 61–74.

Burger, H. G., Hale, G. E., Dennerstein, L., & Robertson, D. M. (2008). Cycle and hormone changes during perimenopause: The key role of ovarian function. *Menopause (New York, N.Y.)*, *15*(4 Pt. 1), 603–612.

Buzdar, A., Hayes, D., El-Khoudary, A., Yan, S., Lonning, P., Lichinitser, M., et al. (2002). Phase III randomized trial of droloxifene and tamoxifen as first-line endocrine treatment of ER/PgR-positive advanced breast cancer. *Breast Cancer Research and Treatment*, *73*(2), 161–175.

Buzdar, A., Howell, A., Cuzick, J., Wale, C., Distler, W., Hoctin-Boes, G., et al. (2006). Comprehensive side-effect profile of anastrozole and tamoxifen as adjuvant treatment for early-stage breast cancer: Long-term safety analysis of the ATAC trial. *The Lancet Oncology*, 7(8), 633–643.

Buzdar, A. U., Marcus, C., Holmes, F., Hug, V., & Hortobagyi, G. (1988). Phase II evaluation of Ly156758 in metastatic breast cancer. *Oncology*, *45*(5), 344–345.

Chamnanphon, M., Pechatanan, K., Sirachainan, E., Trachu, N., Chantratita, W., Pasomsub, E., et al. (2013). Association of CYP2D6 and CYP2C19 polymorphisms and disease-free survival of Thai post-menopausal breast cancer patients who received adjuvant tamoxifen. *Pharmacogenomics and Personalized Medicine*, *6*, 37–48.

Chubak, J., Bowles, E. J., Yu, O., Buist, D. S., Fujii, M., & Boudreau, D. M. (2016). Breast cancer recurrence in relation to antidepressant use. *Cancer Causes & Control: CCC*, *27*(1), 125–136.

Cronin-Fenton, D. P., Damkier, P., & Lash, T. L. (2013). Metabolism and transport of tamoxifen in relation to its effectiveness: New perspectives on an ongoing controversy. *Future Oncology*, *10*(1), 107–122.

Cronin-Fenton, D., Lash, T. L., & Sorensen, H. T. (2010). Selective serotonin reuptake inhibitors and adjuvant tamoxifen therapy: Risk of breast cancer recurrence and mortality. *Future Oncology*, *6*(6), 877–880.

Davies, C., Pan, H., Godwin, J., Gray, R., Arriagada, R., Raina, V., et al. (2013). Long-term effects of continuing adjuvant tamoxifen to 10 years versus stopping at 5 years after diagnosis of oestrogen receptor-positive breast cancer: ATLAS, a randomised trial. *Lancet*, *381*(9869), 805–816.

De Ameida Melo, M., De Vasconcelos-Valenca, R. J., Neto, F. M., Borges, R. S., Costa-Silva, D. R., Da Conceicao Barros-Oliveira, M., et al. (2016). CYP2D6 gene polymorphisms in brazilian patients with breast cancer treated with adjuvant tamoxifen and its association with disease recurrence. *Biomedical Reports*, *5*(5), 574–578.

Deitcher, S. R., & Gomes, M. P. (2004). The risk of venous thromboembolic disease associated with adjuvant hormone therapy for breast carcinoma: A systematic review. *Cancer*, *101*(0008-543; 0008-543; 3), 439–449.

Demissie, S., Silliman, R. A., & Lash, T. L. (2001). Adjuvant tamoxifen: Predictors of use, side effects, and discontinuation in older women. *Journal of Clinical Oncology*, *19*(0732-183; 0732-183; 2), 322–328.

Deng, H. W. (2001). Population admixture may appear to mask, change or reverse genetic effects of genes underlying complex traits. *Genetics*, *159*(3), 1319–1323.

Deshmane, V., Krishnamurthy, S., Melemed, A. S., Peterson, P., & Buzdar, A. U. (2007). Phase III double-blind trial of arzoxifene compared with tamoxifen for locally advanced or metastatic breast cancer. *Journal of Clinical Oncology: Official Journal of the American Society of Clinical Oncology*, *25*(31), 4967–4973.

Dezentje, V. O., Opdam, F. L., Gelderblom, H., Hartigh den, J., Van der Straaten, T., Vree, R., et al. (2015). CYP2D6 genotype- and endoxifen-guided tamoxifen dose escalation increases endoxifen serum concentrations without increasing side effects. *Breast Cancer Research and Treatment*, *153*(3), 583–590.

Dezentje, V. O., van Schaik, R. H., Vletter-Bogaartz, J. M., van der Straaten, T., Wessels, J. A., Kranenbarg, E. M., et al. (2013). CYP2D6 genotype in relation to tamoxifen efficacy in a Dutch cohort of the tamoxifen exemestane adjuvant multinational (TEAM) trial. *Breast Cancer Research and Treatment*, *140*(2), 363–373.

Donneyong, M. M., Bykov, K., Bosco-Levy, P., Dong, Y. H., Levin, R., & Gagne, J. J. (2016). Risk of mortality with concomitant use of tamoxifen and selective serotonin reuptake inhibitors: Multi-database cohort study. *BMJ (Clinical Research Ed.)*, *354*, i5014.

Early Breast Cancer Trialists,Collaborative Group. (2005). Effects of chemotherapy and hormonal therapy for early breast cancer on recurrence and 15-year survival: An overview of the randomised trials. *Lancet*, *365*(1474–547; 9472), 1687–1717.

Early Breast Cancer Trialists' Collaborative Group (EBCTCG), Davies, C., Godwin, J., Gray, R., Clarke, M., Cutter, D., et al. (2011). Relevance of breast cancer hormone receptors and other factors to the efficacy of adjuvant tamoxifen: Patient-level meta-analysis of randomised trials. *Lancet*, *378*(9793), 771–784.

Ellsworth, R. E., Ellsworth, D. L., Lubert, S. M., Hooke, J., Somiari, R. I., & Shriver, C. D. (2003). High-throughput loss of heterozygosity mapping in 26 commonly deleted regions in breast cancer. *Cancer Epidemiology, Biomarkers & Prevention: A Publication of the American Association for Cancer Research, Cosponsored by the American Society of Preventive Oncology*, *12*(9), 915–919.

Fan, P., Yue, W., Wang, J. P., Aiyar, S., Li, Y., Kim, T. H., et al. (2009). Mechanisms of resistance to structurally diverse antiestrogens differ under premenopausal and postmenopausal conditions: Evidence from in vitro breast cancer cell models. *Endocrinology*, *150*(5), 2036–2045.

Fisher, B., Costantino, J. P., Wickerham, D. L., Cecchini, R. S., Cronin, W. M., Robidoux, A., et al. (2005). Tamoxifen for the prevention of breast cancer: Current status of the national surgical adjuvant breast and bowel project P-1 study. *The Journal of the National Cancer Institute, 97*(22), 1652–1662.

Freour, T., Barriere, P., & Masson, D. (2017). Anti-mullerian hormone levels and evolution in women of reproductive age with breast cancer treated with chemotherapy. *European Journal of Cancer (Oxford, England: 1990), 74*, 1–8.

Gaedigk, A. (2013). Complexities of CYP2D6 gene analysis and interpretation. *International Review of Psychiatry (Abingdon, England), 25*(5), 534–553.

Gjerde, J., Hauglid, M., Breilid, H., Lundgren, S., Varhaug, J. E., Kisanga, E. R., et al. (2008). Effects of CYP2D6 and SULT1A1 genotypes including SULT1A1 gene copy number on tamoxifen metabolism. *Annals of Oncology, 19*(1), 56–61.

Goetz, M. P., Kamal, A., & Ames, M. M. (2008). Tamoxifen pharmacogenomics: The role of CYP2D6 as a predictor of drug response. *Clinical Pharmacology and Therapeutics, 83*(1), 160–166.

Goetz, M. P., Rae, J. M., Suman, V. J., Safgren, S. L., Ames, M. M., Visscher, D. W., et al. (2005). Pharmacogenetics of tamoxifen biotransformation is associated with clinical outcomes of efficacy and hot flashes. *Journal of Clinical Oncology, 23*(0732-183, 0732-183, 36), 9312–9318.

Goetz, M. P., Suman, V. J., Reid, J. M., Northfelt, D. W., Mahr, M. A., Ralya, A. T., et al. (2017). First-in-human phase I study of the tamoxifen metabolite Z-endoxifen in women with endocrine-refractory metastatic breast cancer. *Journal of Clinical Oncology: Official Journal of the American Society of Clinical Oncology, 35*(30), 3391–3400.

Goetz, M. P., Sun, J. X., Suman, V. J., Silva, G. O., Perou, C. M., Nakamura, Y., et al. (2014). Loss of heterozygosity at the CYP2D6 locus in breast cancer: Implications for germline pharmacogenetic studies. *Journal of the National Cancer Institute, 107*(2). https://doi.org/10.1093/jnci/dju401.

Gradishar, W., Glusman, J., Lu, Y., Vogel, C., Cohen, F. J., & Sledge, G. W., Jr. (2000). Effects of high dose raloxifene in selected patients with advanced breast carcinoma. *Cancer, 88*(9), 2047–2053.

Gray, R. G., Rea, D. W., Handley, K., Marshall, A., Pritchard, M. G., Perry, P.,… (2008). aTTom (adjuvant tamoxifen—To offer more?): Randomized trial of 10 versus 5 years of adjuvant tamoxifen among 6,934 women with estrogen receptor-positive (ER+) or ER untested breast cancer—Preliminary results. [Abstract]. Journal of Clinical Oncology (Meeting Abstracts), 26 513.

Haque, R., Shi, J., Schottinger, J. E., Ahmed, S. A., Cheetham, T. C., Chung, J., et al. (2015). Tamoxifen and antidepressant drug interaction in a cohort of 16,887 breast cancer survivors. *Journal of the National Cancer Institute, 108*(3). https://doi.org/10.1093/jnci/djv337. Print 2016 Mar.

Hayes, D. F., Van Zyl, J. A., Hacking, A., Goedhals, L., Bezwoda, W. R., Mailliard, J. A., et al. (1995). Randomized comparison of tamoxifen and two separate doses of toremifene in postmenopausal patients with metastatic breast cancer. *Journal of Clinical Oncology: Official Journal of the American Society of Clinical Oncology, 13*(10), 2556–2566.

Helland, T., Henne, N., Bifulco, E., Naume, B., Borgen, E., Kristensen, V. N., et al. (2017). Serum concentrations of active tamoxifen metabolites predict long-term survival in adjuvantly treated breast cancer patients. *Breast Cancer Research: BCR, 19*(1), 125.

Henry, N. L., Rae, J. M., Li, L., Azzouz, F., Skaar, T. C., Desta, Z., et al. (2009). Association between CYP2D6 genotype and tamoxifen-induced hot flashes in a prospective cohort. *Breast Cancer Research and Treatment, 117*(3), 571–575.

Hertz, D. L., Kidwell, K. M., Hilsenbeck, S. G., Oesterreich, S., Osborne, C. K., Philips, S., et al. (2017). CYP2D6 genotype is not associated with survival in breast cancer patients treated with tamoxifen: Results from a population-based study. *Breast Cancer Research and Treatment, 166*(1), 277–287.

Hicks, B. M., Murray, L. J., Powe, D. G., Hughes, C. M., & Cardwell, C. R. (2013). Beta-blocker usage and colorectal cancer mortality: A nested case-control study in the UK clinical practice research datalink cohort. *Annals of Oncology: Official Journal of the European Society for Medical Oncology/ESMO, 24*(12), 3100–3106.

Hicks, J. K., Swen, J. J., & Gaedigk, A. (2014). Challenges in CYP2D6 phenotype assignment from genotype data: A critical assessment and call for standardization. *Current Drug Metabolism, 15*(2), 218–232.

Hirano, A., Emi, M., Tsuneizumi, M., Utada, Y., Yoshimoto, M., Kasumi, F., et al. (2001). Allelic losses of loci at 3p25.1, 8p22, 13q12, 17p13.3, and 22q13 correlate with postoperative recurrence in breast cancer. *Clinical Cancer Research: An Official Journal of the American Association for Cancer Research*, 7(4), 876–882.

Hu, X. X., Zhou, Q., Lan, T., Huang, X. X., Liang, B. Q., Dai, D. P., et al. (2016). Functional characterization of 22 novel CYP2D6 variants for the metabolism of tamoxifen. *The Journal of Pharmacy and Pharmacology, 68*(6), 819–825.

International Breast Cancer Study Group, Pagani, O., Gelber, S., Price, K., Zahrieh, D., Gelber, R., et al. (2004). Toremifene and tamoxifen are equally effective for early-stage breast cancer: First results of international breast cancer study group trials 12-93 and 14-93. *Annals of Oncology: Official Journal of the European Society for Medical Oncology, 15*(12), 1749–1759.

International Transporter Consortium, Giacomini, K. M., Huang, S. M., Tweedie, D. J., Benet, L. Z., Brouwer, K. L., et al. (2010). Membrane transporters in drug development. *Nature Reviews. Drug Discovery, 9*(3), 215–236.

Iusuf, D., Teunissen, S. F., Wagenaar, E., Rosing, H., Beijnen, J. H., & Schinkel, A. H. (2011). P-glycoprotein (ABCB1) transports the primary active tamoxifen metabolites endoxifen and 4-hydroxytamoxifen and restricts their brain penetration. *The Journal of Pharmacology and Experimental Therapeutics, 337*(3), 710–717.

Jin, Y., Desta, Z., Stearns, V., Ward, B., Ho, H., Lee, K. H., et al. (2005). CYP2D6 genotype, antidepressant use, and tamoxifen metabolism during adjuvant breast cancer treatment. *The Journal of the National Cancer Institute, 97*(1), 30–39.

Johansson, H., Gandini, S., Serrano, D., Gjerde, J., Lattanzi, M., Macis, D., et al. (2016). A pooled analysis of CYP2D6 genotype in breast cancer prevention trials of low-dose tamoxifen. *Breast Cancer Research and Treatment, 159*(1), 97–108.

Johnson, J. A., Hamadeh, I. S., & Langaee, T. Y. (2015). Loss of heterozygosity at the CYP2D6 locus in breast cancer: Implications for tamoxifen pharmacogenetic studies. *Journal of the National Cancer Institute, 107*(2). https://doi.org/10.1093/jnci/dju437. Print 2015 Feb.

Johnson, M. D., Zuo, H., Lee, K. H., Trebley, J. P., Rae, J. M., Weatherman, R. V., et al. (2004). Pharmacological characterization of 4-hydroxy-N-desmethyl tamoxifen, a novel active metabolite of tamoxifen. *Breast Cancer Research and Treatment, 85*(2), 151–159.

Jordan, V. C. (2008). Tamoxifen: Catalyst for the change to targeted therapy. *European Journal of Cancer (Oxford, England: 1990), 44*(1), 30–38.

Jordan, V. C., Collins, M. M., Rowsby, L., & Prestwich, G. (1977). A monohydroxylated metabolite of tamoxifen with potent antioestrogenic activity. *The Journal of Endocrinology, 75*(2), 305–316.

Jordan, V. C., Obiorah, I., Fan, P., Kim, H. R., Ariazi, E., Cunliffe, H., et al. (2011). The St. Gallen prize lecture 2011: Evolution of long-term adjuvant anti-hormone therapy: Consequences and opportunities. *Breast (Edinburgh, Scotland), 20*(Suppl. 3), S1–S11.

Randomized trial of two versus five years of adjuvant tamoxifen for postmenopausal early stage breast cancer. Swedish breast cancer cooperative group (1996). *Journal of the National Cancer Institute, 88*(21), 1543–1549.

Juurlink, D. (2016). Revisiting the drug interaction between tamoxifen and SSRI antidepressants. *BMJ (Clinical Research Ed.)*, *354*, i5309.

Karle, J., Bolbrinker, J., Vogl, S., Kreutz, R., Denkert, C., Eucker, J., et al. (2013). Influence of CYP2D6-genotype on tamoxifen efficacy in advanced breast cancer. *Breast Cancer Research and Treatment*, *139*(2), 553–560.

Kiyotani, K., Mushiroda, T., Imamura, C. K., Hosono, N., Tsunoda, T., Kubo, M., et al. (2010). Significant effect of polymorphisms in CYP2D6 and ABCC2 on clinical outcomes of adjuvant tamoxifen therapy for breast cancer patients. *Journal of Clinical Oncology*, *28*(0732-183; 8), 1287–1293.

Kiyotani, K., Mushiroda, T., Sasa, M., Bando, Y., Sumitomo, I., Hosono, N., et al. (2008). Impact of CYP2D6*10 on recurrence-free survival in breast cancer patients receiving adjuvant tamoxifen therapy. *Cancer Science*, *99*(5), 995–999.

Lai, Y., Varma, M., Feng, B., Stephens, J. C., Kimoto, E., El-Kattan, A., et al. (2012). Impact of drug transporter pharmacogenomics on pharmacokinetic and pharmacodynamic variability—Considerations for drug development. *Expert Opinion on Drug Metabolism & Toxicology*, *8*(6), 723–743.

Lash, T. L., Ahern, T. P., Cronin-Fenton, D., Garne, J. P., Hamilton-Dutoit, S., & Sorensen, H. T. (2008). Comment on 'impact of CYP2D6*10 on recurrence-free survival in breast cancer patients receiving adjuvant tamoxifen therapy'. *Cancer Science*, *99*(8), 1706–1707.

Lash, T. L., & Cole, S. R. (2009). Immortal person-time in studies of cancer outcomes. *Journal of Clinical Oncology*, *27*(23), e55–e56.

Lash, T. L., Cronin-Fenton, D., Ahern, T. P., Rosenberg, C. L., Lunetta, K. L., Silliman, R. A., et al. (2011). CYP2D6 inhibition and breast cancer recurrence in a population-based study in Denmark. *The Journal of the National Cancer Institute*, *103*(6), 489–500.

Lash, T. L., Lien, E. A., Sorensen, H. T., & Hamilton-Dutoit, S. (2009). Genotype-guided tamoxifen therapy: Time to pause for reflection? *The Lancet Oncology*, *10*(8), 825–833.

Lazarus, P., Blevins-Primeau, A. S., Zheng, Y., & Sun, D. (2009). Potential role of UGT pharmacogenetics in cancer treatment and prevention: Focus on tamoxifen. *The Annals of the New York Academy of Sciences*, *1155*, 99–111.

Lei, L., Wang, X., Wu, X. D., Wang, Z., Chen, Z. H., Zheng, Y. B., et al. (2016). Association of CYP2D6*10 (c.100C>T) polymorphisms with clinical outcome of breast cancer after tamoxifen adjuvant endocrine therapy in Chinese population. *American Journal of Translational Research*, *8*(8), 3585–3592.

Leslie, E. M., Deeley, R. G., & Cole, S. P. (2005). Multidrug resistance proteins: Role of P-glycoprotein, MRP1, MRP2, and BCRP (ABCG2) in tissue defense. *Toxicology and Applied Pharmacology*, *204*(3), 216–237.

Lien, E. A., Solheim, E., Kvinnsland, S., & Ueland, P. M. (1988). Identification of 4-hydroxy-N-desmethyltamoxifen as a metabolite of tamoxifen in human bile. *Cancer Research*, *48*(8), 2304–2308.

Lim, Y. C., Desta, Z., Flockhart, D. A., & Skaar, T. C. (2005). Endoxifen (4-hydroxy-N-desmethyl-tamoxifen) has anti-estrogenic effects in breast cancer cells with potency similar to 4-hydroxy-tamoxifen. *Cancer Chemotherapy and Pharmacology*, *55*(5), 471–478.

Madlensky, L., Natarajan, L., Tchu, S., Pu, M., Mortimer, J., Flatt, S. W., et al. (2011). Tamoxifen metabolite concentrations, CYP2D6 genotype, and breast cancer outcomes. *Clinical Pharmacology and Therapeutics*, *89*(5), 718–725.

Marcath, L. A., Deal, A. M., Van Wieren, E., Danko, W., Walko, C. M., Ibrahim, J. G., et al. (2017). Comprehensive assessment of cytochromes P450 and transporter genetics with endoxifen concentration during tamoxifen treatment. *Pharmacogenetics and Genomics*, *27*(11), 402–409.

Markkula, A., Hjertberg, M., Rose, C., Ingvar, C., & Jernstrom, H. (2014). No association found between CYP2D6 genotype and early breast cancer events in tamoxifen-treated patients. *Acta Oncologica (Stockholm, Sweden)*, *53*(2), 195–200.

Martins, D. M., Vidal, F. C., Souza, R. D., Brusaca, S. A., & Brito, L. M. (2014). Determination of CYP2D6 *3, *4, and *10 frequency in women with breast cancer in Sao Luis, Brazil, and its association with prognostic factors and disease-free survival. *Brazilian Journal of Medical and Biological Research = Revista Brasileira De Pesquisas Medicas e Biologicas*, *47*(11), 1008–1015.

Mwinyi, J., Vokinger, K., Jetter, A., Breitenstein, U., Hiller, C., Kullak-Ublick, G. A., et al. (2014). Impact of variable CYP genotypes on breast cancer relapse in patients undergoing adjuvant tamoxifen therapy. *Cancer Chemotherapy and Pharmacology*, *73*(6), 1181–1188.

NCCN practice guidelines in oncology, breast cancer—v.2.2011. Invasive breast cancer, adjuvant endocrine therapy. (2010).

NCCN practice guidelines in oncology, breast cancer—v.2.2014. invasive breast cancer, adjuvant endocrine therapy. (2014). Retrieved from http://www.nccn.org/professionals/physician_gls/PDF/breast.pdf.

Pharoah, P. D., Abraham, J., & Caldas, C. (2012). Re: CYP2D6 genotype and tamoxifen response in postmenopausal women with endocrine-responsive breast cancer: The breast international group 1-98 trial and re: CYP2D6 and UGT2B7 genotype and risk of recurrence in tamoxifen-treated breast cancer patients. *Journal of the National Cancer Institute*, *104*(16), 1263–1264. author reply 1266-8.

Powers, J. L., Buys, S. S., Fletcher, D., Melis, R., Johnson-Davis, K. L., Lyon, E., et al. (2016). Multigene and drug interaction approach for tamoxifen metabolite patterns reveals possible involvement of CYP2C9, CYP2C19, and ABCB1. *Journal of Clinical Pharmacology*, *56*(12), 1570–1581.

Rae, J. M., Cordero, K. E., Scheys, J. O., Lippman, M. E., Flockhart, D. A., & Johnson, M. D. (2003). Genotyping for polymorphic drug metabolizing enzymes from paraffin-embedded and immunohistochemically stained tumor samples. *Pharmacogenetics*, *13*(8), 501–507.

Rae, J. M., Drury, S., Hayes, D. F., Stearns, V., Thibert, J. N., Haynes, B. P., et al. (2012). CYP2D6 and UGT2B7 genotype and risk of recurrence in tamoxifen-treated breast cancer patients. *Journal of the National Cancer Institute*, *104*(6), 452–460.

Rae, J. M., Regan, M. M., Thibert, J. N., Gersch, C., Thomas, D., Leyland-Jones, B., et al. (2013). Concordance between CYP2D6 genotypes obtained from tumor-derived and germline DNA. *Journal of the National Cancer Institute*, *105*(17), 1332–1334.

Reed, K., & Parissenti, A. M. (2011). The effect of ABCB1 genetic variants on chemotherapy response in HIV and cancer treatment. *Pharmacogenomics*, *12*(10), 1465–1483.

Regan, M. M., Leyland-Jones, B., Bouzyk, M., Pagani, O., Tang, W., Kammler, R., et al. (2012). CYP2D6 genotype and tamoxifen response in postmenopausal women with endocrine-responsive breast cancer: The breast international group 1-98 trial. *Journal of the National Cancer Institute*, *104*(6), 441–451.

Saladores, P., Murdter, T., Eccles, D., Chowbay, B., Zgheib, N. K., Winter, S., et al. (2015). Tamoxifen metabolism predicts drug concentrations and outcome in premenopausal patients with early breast cancer. *The Pharmacogenomics Journal*, *15*(1), 84–94.

Sanchez Spitman, A. B., Moes, D. J. A. R., Gelderblom, H., Dezentje, V. O., Swen, J. J., & Guchelaar, H. J. (2017). Effect of CYP3A4*22, CYP3A5*3, and CYP3A combined genotypes on tamoxifen metabolism. *European Journal of Clinical Pharmacology*, *73*(12), 1589–1598.

Sanchez-Spitman, A. B., Moes, D. A., Gelderblom, H., Dezentje, V. O., Swen, J. J., & Guchelaar, H. J. (2017). The effect of rs5758550 on CYP2D6*2 phenotype and formation of endoxifen in breast cancer patients using tamoxifen. *Pharmacogenomics*, *18*(12), 1125–1132.

Schneider, B. P., Skaar, T. C., Sledge, G. W., Badve, S., Li, L., & Flockhart, D. A. (2006). Analysis of angiogenesis genes from paraffin-embedded breast tumor and lymph nodes. *Breast Cancer Research and Treatment, 96*(3), 209–215.

Sensorn, I., Sirachainan, E., Chamnanphon, M., Pasomsub, E., Trachu, N., Supavilai, P., et al. (2013). Association of CYP3A4/5, ABCB1 and ABCC2 polymorphisms and clinical outcomes of thai breast cancer patients treated with tamoxifen. *Pharmacogenomics and Personalized Medicine, 6*, 93–98.

Sheng, Z. M., Marchetti, A., Buttitta, F., Champeme, M. H., Campani, D., Bistocchi, M., et al. (1996). Multiple regions of chromosome 6q affected by loss of heterozygosity in primary human breast carcinomas. *British Journal of Cancer, 73*(2), 144–147.

Sherman, B. M., Chapler, F. K., Crickard, K., & Wycoff, D. (1979). Endocrine consequences of continuous antiestrogen therapy with tamoxifen in premenopausal women. *The Journal of Clinical Investigation, 64*(2), 398–404.

Sideras, K., Ingle, J. N., Ames, M. M., Loprinzi, C. L., Mrazek, D. P., Black, J. L., et al. (2010). Coprescription of tamoxifen and medications that inhibit CYP2D6. *Journal of Clinical Oncology, 28*(0732-183; 16), 2768–2776.

Stanton, V., Jr. (2012). Re: CYP2D6 genotype and tamoxifen response in postmenopausal women with endocrine-responsive breast cancer: The breast international group 1-98 trial. *Journal of the National Cancer Institute, 104*(16), 1265–1266. author reply 1266-8.

Stearns, V., Johnson, M. D., Rae, J. M., Morocho, A., Novielli, A., Bhargava, P., et al. (2003). Active tamoxifen metabolite plasma concentrations after coadministration of tamoxifen and the selective serotonin reuptake inhibitor paroxetine. *The Journal of the National Cancer Institute, 95*(23), 1758–1764.

Sukasem, C., Sirachainan, E., Chamnanphon, M., Pechatanan, K., Sirisinha, T., Ativitavas, T., et al. (2012). Impact of CYP2D6 polymorphisms on tamoxifen responses of women with breast cancer: A microarray-based study in Thailand. *Asian Pacific Journal of Cancer Prevention: APJCP, 13*(9), 4549–4553.

Swerdlow, A. J., & Jones, M. E. (2005). Tamoxifen treatment for breast cancer and risk of endometrial cancer: A case-control study. *The Journal of the National Cancer Institute, 97*(5), 375–384.

Teft, W. A., Mansell, S. E., & Kim, R. B. (2011). Endoxifen, the active metabolite of tamoxifen, is a substrate of the efflux transporter P-glycoprotein (multidrug resistance 1). *Drug Metabolism and Disposition: The Biological Fate of Chemicals, 39*(3), 558–562.

Teh, L. K., Mohamed, N. I., Salleh, M. Z., Rohaizak, M., Shahrun, N. S., Saladina, J. J., et al. (2012). The risk of recurrence in breast cancer patients treated with tamoxifen: Polymorphisms of CYP2D6 and ABCB1. *The AAPS Journal, 14*(1), 52–59.

Thompson, A. M., Johnson, A., Quinlan, P., Hillman, G., Fontecha, M., Bray, S. E., et al. (2011). Comprehensive CYP2D6 genotype and adherence affect outcome in breast cancer patients treated with tamoxifen monotherapy. *Breast Cancer Research and Treatment, 125*(1), 279–287.

Valachis, A., Garmo, H., Weinman, J., Fredriksson, I., Ahlgren, J., Sund, M., et al. (2016). Effect of selective serotonin reuptake inhibitors use on endocrine therapy adherence and breast cancer mortality: A population-based study. *Breast Cancer Research and Treatment, 159*(2), 293–303.

Wheeler, H. E., Maitland, M. L., Dolan, M. E., Cox, N. J., & Ratain, M. J. (2013). Cancer pharmacogenomics: Strategies and challenges. *Nature Reviews. Genetics, 14*(1), 23–34.

Xie, B., Freudenheim, J. L., Cummings, S. S., Singh, B., He, H., McCann, S. E., et al. (2006). Accurate genotyping from paraffin-embedded normal tissue adjacent to breast cancer. *Carcinogenesis, 27*(2), 307–310.

Xu, Y., Sun, Y., Yao, L., Shi, L., Wu, Y., Ouyang, T., et al. (2008). Association between CYP2D6 *10 genotype and survival of breast cancer patients receiving tamoxifen treatment. *Annals of Oncology, 19*(8), 1423–1429.

Yazdi, M. F., Rafieian, S., Gholi-Nataj, M., Sheikhha, M. H., Nazari, T., & Neamatzadeh, H. (2015). CYP2D6 genotype and risk of recurrence in tamoxifen treated breast cancer patients. *Asian Pacific Journal of Cancer Prevention: APJCP, 16*(15), 6783–6787.

Zanger, U. M., Raimundo, S., & Eichelbaum, M. (2004). Cytochrome P450 2D6: Overview and update on pharmacology, genetics, biochemistry. *Naunyn-Schmiedebergs Archives of Pharmacology, 369*(1), 23–37.

Zhang, X., Pu, Z., Ge, J., Shen, J., Yuan, X., & Xie, H. (2015). Association of CYP2D6*10, OATP1B1 A388G, and OATP1B1 T521C polymorphisms and overall survival of breast cancer patients after tamoxifen therapy. *Medical Science Monitor: International Medical Journal of Experimental and Clinical Research, 21*, 563–569.

SECTION II

Methods

CHAPTER FOUR

Imaging in Pharmacogenetics

Mikkel H. Vendelbo*,†, Lars C. Gormsen*, Niels Jessen*,†,1
*Aarhus University Hospital, Aarhus, Denmark
†Aarhus University, Aarhus, Denmark
[1]Corresponding author: e-mail address: niels.jessen@biomed.au.dk

Contents

1. Introduction 95
2. Imaging Modalities 96
3. Absorption 99
4. Distribution 100
5. Metabolism 102
6. Elimination 103
7. Conclusion 104
References 104

Abstract

An increasing collection of imaging technologies makes it possible to differentiate treatment responders from nonresponders based on genetic variation. This chapter will review some of the imaging technologies currently available in nuclear medicine to visualize drug absorption, distribution, metabolism, and elimination. Some of the commonly used techniques to detect radiation-emitting compounds are the two-dimensional scintigraphy and the three-dimensional single-photon emission computed tomography (SPECT) which both detect photons using a gamma camera, and the three-dimensional positron emission tomography (PET), which detect the decay of positron-emitting radionuclides. Current examples include visualization of functional effects of genetic variants, and these provide proof of concept for imaging in pharmacogenetics as a tool to improve efficacy and safety of drugs.

1. INTRODUCTION

Traditional evidence-based medicine relies on large randomized control trials and meta-analyses, which ignores individual differences. This reliance on large group analyses is increasingly being challenged by the concept of precision medicine where individual variability in genes, environment,

Advances in Pharmacology, Volume 83
ISSN 1054-3589
https://doi.org/10.1016/bs.apha.2018.02.002

and lifestyle for each person is taken into account (Sankar & Parker, 2017). Tools to differentiate treatment responders from nonresponders based on genetic makeup of patients are therefore in demand. At least in part, this request can be met by an increasing collection of imaging technologies. The ability to visualize absorption, distribution, metabolism, and elimination of drugs with noninvasive human imaging is evolving rapidly, and in the postgenomic era, these imaging technologies can be combined with information on genetic variation and thereby improve the predictive value for a drug's efficacy and safety. This chapter will review some of the imaging technologies currently available in nuclear medicine to visualize drug biotransformation and elimination pathways (pharmacokinetics).

2. IMAGING MODALITIES

Several imaging techniques to examine biological processes noninvasively are an integrated part of modern drug discovery and development in both preclinical and clinical stages. Magnetic resonance imaging (MRI) and computed tomography (CT) provide important information about anatomical structures in high resolution. These imaging techniques can also provide functional information, but detection of radiation-emitting compounds is often a superior technique for biological imaging. Radiolabeled compounds are therefore often used to characterize organ functions, metabolism, and molecular markers, but they are especially superior in connection with visualization of drug biodistribution and kinetics. Among the most commonly used techniques to detect radiation-emitting compounds are the two-dimensional scintigraphy and the three-dimensional single-photon emission computed tomography (SPECT) which both detect photons using a gamma camera, and the three-dimensional positron emission tomography (PET), which detect the decay of positron-emitting radionuclides.

The majority of radiation-emitting isotopes used to generate radiopharmacological compounds are produced in reactors or cyclotrons, of which the latter is often an integrated part of research-oriented imaging facilities. Some isotopes can be eluted from a radionuclide generator, which consist of a parent–daughter radionuclide pair. The parent radionuclide is produced in a nuclear reactor and decays to the daughter radionuclide within the generator. The generators are sold by specialized companies and shipped to imaging institutions, where tracers and drugs subsequently are labeled with the daughter radionuclide. However, most positron-emitting isotopes, listed in Table 1, are produced by on-site cyclotrons at

Table 1 Positron-Emitting Radionuclides Used in Nuclear Medicine

Radionuclide	Half-Life (min)	Maximum β^+ Energy (MeV)	Production
^{11}C	≈20	0.96	Cyclotron
^{13}N	≈10	1.19	Cyclotron
^{15}O	≈2	1.72	Cyclotron
^{18}F	≈110	0.64	Cyclotron
^{64}Cu	≈762	0.58	Cyclotron
^{89}Zr	≈4752	0.90	Cyclotron
^{124}I	≈6048	1.50	Cyclotron
^{68}Ga	≈68	1.90	Generator (68Ge)
^{82}Rb	≈1	3.35	Generator (82Sr)

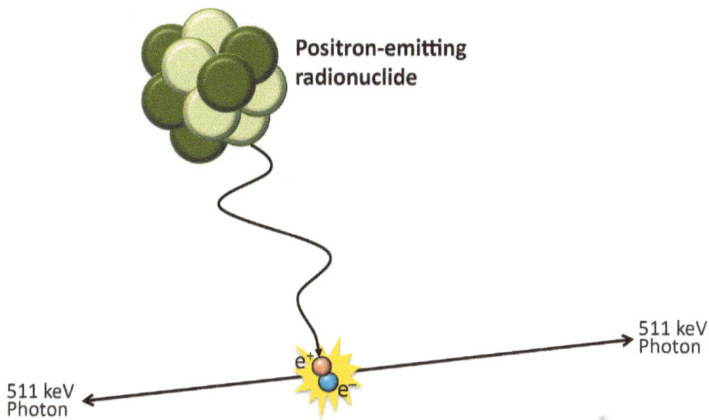

Fig. 1 Two photons with opposite direction are formed when a positron and an electron undergo annihilation after decay of a positron-emitting radionuclide.

larger imaging facilities. After decay of a positron-emitting radionuclide, the positron undergoes annihilation by collision with an electron. This results in a simultaneous emission of two 511 keV photons with 180-degree opposing directions as visualized in Fig. 1. ^{18}F, ^{68}Ga, and ^{11}C are the most commonly used positron-emitting radionuclides and their half-life is short (Table 1). Limiting the time of labeling of compounds to administration into subjects is therefore necessary to obtain high-specific activity. The most often-used gamma emitter in clinical nuclear medicine is Technetium-99m (^{99m}Tc) with a half-life of 6 h. It is extracted from a Molybdenum-99 (^{99}Mo)/^{99m}Tc

generator, where the ^{99}Mo is a fission product from a nuclear reactor. ^{111}Indium, ^{123}Iodine, ^{131}Iodine, and ^{75}Selenium are other longer-lived isotopes that are also used.

Decay of the positron-emitting isotopes and their annihilation products is detected by the ring-shaped PET scanner. The PET ring consists of an inner layer of scintillation detectors, which interact with the 511 keV photons releasing visible light. The next layer in the ring consists of photomultipliers, which when activated produce an electrical pulse, and the opposing direction of the photons is therefore ultimately used to localize a line origin where the annihilation event took place, as visualized in Fig. 2A. By contrast, gamma camera images are generated from collimator linearized single photons producing an image with spatial resolution. In brief, this is essentially a grid structure allowing only gamma rays traveling perpendicular to a single rectangular scintillation detector to be detected. The gamma rays not absorbed in the collimator interact with the scintillation detector, and visible light is released in a manner similar to the PET scanner (visualized in Fig. 2B).

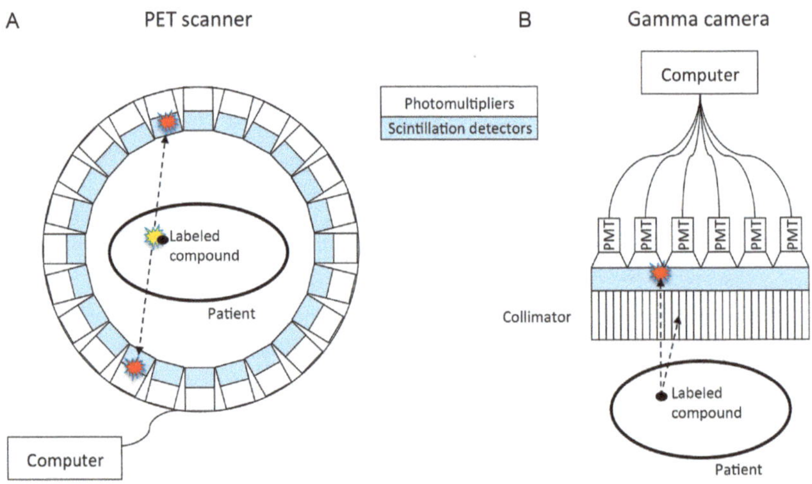

Fig. 2 Two photons with opposite direction are formed after decay of a positron-emitting radionuclide, and light is formed when they interact photoelectrically with the scintillation material in the PET scanner. The light is then used to localize a line of origin and an image can be generated (A). In the gamma camera is a single photon detected when it interacts with a scintillation material as in the PET scanner. A grid structure, called a collimator, is placed in front of the detector, and it is responsible for spatial resolution in the image because it only let gamma rays traveling perpendicular to the scintillation material pass (B).

Finally, the photomultiplier signal is converted to a digital signal and an image of radiotracer decay can be reconstructed. This image is most often fused with a CT or MRI image to produce simultaneous visualization of morphology, anatomical localization, and function. The design of the PET scanner makes it possible to produce both static (tissue activity at a single time point) and dynamic (tissue activity time series) three-dimensional (3D) images. The gamma camera can also be used to produce dynamic scans with two-dimensional (2D) planar images, as exemplified by clinical renography. In addition, the limited spatial resolution of 2D images can be significantly improved by rotating the gamma camera heads around the patient producing a tomographic 3D image of radiotracer decay, SPECT. However, the rotation during a SPECT-scan is time-consuming, and SPECT scans therefore cannot be used to produce time-activity curves of radionuclide distribution (Cherry, Sorenson, & Phelps, 2012).

The metabolic fate of radiotracers (kinetics) can be determined by simultaneous measurements of the tissue input (activity in blood samples or from volumes drawn in the aorta) and tissue time-activity curves. Rate constants describing the transfer of radiotracer between the circulation and intracellular compartments can be calculated by fitting the experimental data to a physiologically meaningful multicompartmental model, which is described by a series of differential equations. In practice, this is often done by commercially available software packages (Carson, 2003; Cherry et al., 2012).

3. ABSORPTION

Basic physical characteristics, including molecular size, electrical charge, and hydrophobicity, are key determinants for drug absorption after oral administration. Cell membranes are rapidly passed by many lipophilic compounds, while hydrophilic molecules only slowly penetrate these barriers, and many drugs interact with membrane transporters during distribution in the body (Benet, Cummins, & Wu, 2004). Genetic variation with functional importance has been demonstrated in genes encoding both ATP-binding cassette (ABC) transporters and genes encoding solute carriers (SLC) (Huang, 2007).

The inaccessibility of the portal vein for blood sampling makes direct assessments of transport from the intestinal lumen to the circulation demanding. Drug absorption has therefore traditionally been determined by posthepatic blood sampling. Several factors affect drug concentrations at this level, most notably first-passage metabolism by the liver. This complicates

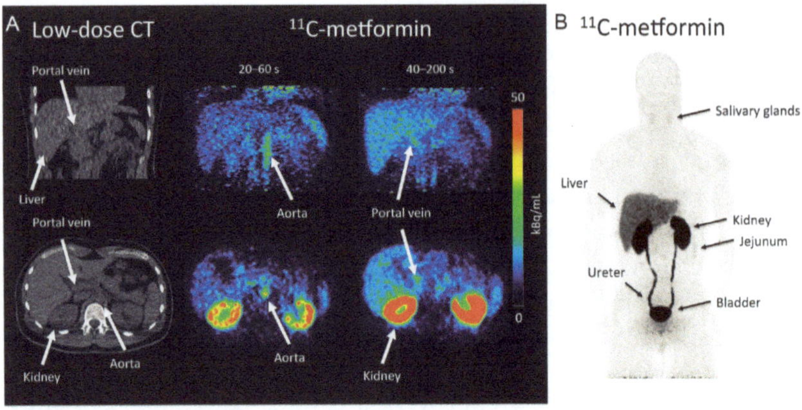

Fig. 3 During a dynamic PET scan it is under optimal conditions possible to create a volume of interest in the portal vein and prehepatic kinetics of a radiolabeled drug can be evaluated (A). Tissue efflux and influx of metformin depends on transporters, and biodistribution of radiolabeled metformin can be visualized in humans with PET imaging (B).

the quantification of specific contributions of genetic variation in membrane transporters, but in some cases it is possible to overcome this challenge by imaging of labeled compounds. Intestinal transit of drugs based on tissue concentrations can be determined using gamma scintigraphy (Kimura & Higaki, 2002; Wilson et al., 2009; Yuen, 2010). Recently, PET imaging has been applied to investigate the oral absorption process using ^{18}F-FDG (Shingaki et al., 2012). Oral ingestion of lipophilic compounds can also be quantified in the thoracic duct (Labbe et al., 2011). In contrast, the compressed anatomy in the portal region makes it difficult to draw a VOI representing only the portal vein during the entire dynamic PET-scanning. Too much movement of the test subject during the scan will significantly hamper correct assessment of drug or tracer metabolism. However, under optimal conditions portal vein activity can be measured by a VOI drawn in the portal vein (visualized in Fig. 3A) (Sundelin et al., 2017), allowing for a noninvasive assessment of prehepatic pharmacokinetics of radiolabeled drugs.

4. DISTRIBUTION

Drugs that depend on interaction with specific transport proteins for the passage of membranes can display restricted distribution based on expressions patterns of the transporter protein. This is evident for uptake into specific tissue but also crossing membrane barriers as the blood–brain barrier and blood–testis barrier. Imaging technologies combined with arterial sampling offer excellent opportunities for quantifying transporter activity in vivo. After administration, the drug is distributed in different compartments of the body in a time-dependent manner. Distribution rate of the drug or metabolite in different compartments depends on the characteristics of the drug and genetic differences in expression of transporters. Distribution of a radiolabelled compound is to the same degree time varying and depends on tracer delivery, vascular extraction, receptors binding, diffusion into cells, metabolism, and excretion. As an example, the fatty acid PET-tracer ^{11}C-palmitate has been used to demonstrate that CD36 Pro90Ser mutation influence fatty acid distribution in vivo (Hames, Vella, Kemp, & Jensen, 2014). A range of nonendogenous compounds, termed radioligands, have also been developed for a multitude of receptors and cell-surface markers. The biodistribution of these radioligands can potentially be affected by genotypes as exemplified by the 18-kDa translocator protein (TSPO), which is highly expressed in the brain during inflammation and is an important marker of activated microglia. Radioligands toward this protein have been developed in order to detect its in vivo expression (Mizrahi et al., 2012), and metabolism of the TSPO radioligand, ^{18}F-FEPPA (Wilson et al., 2008), has been found to be affected in platelets from subjects with the TSPO rs6971 (Ala147Thr) polymorphism (Owen et al., 2012). Similarly, human carriers of the polymorphism have altered brain uptake and whole body biodistribution of the radioligand (Mizrahi et al., 2012, 2013).

Analogous to radioligands, biodistribution of specific drugs has been visualized directly using radiolabeling. Thus, metformin labeled with ^{11}C was initially developed to study the function of multidrug and toxin extrusion proteins (MATEs) (Hume et al., 2013). Using ^{11}C-labeled-metformin, it has been shown that MATE1 and OCT1 are the major hepatic efflux and influx transporters in rodents (Jakobsen et al., 2016; Jensen et al., 2016; Shingaki et al., 2015). As shown in Fig. 3A and B, we have translated these findings to a human setting (Gormsen et al., 2016) and have determined metformin tissue distribution and intracellular fate of the radiopharmaceutical in healthy subjects (Gormsen et al., 2016). We have subsequently extended these findings and have investigated the impact of genetic variants in SLC22A1 associated with impaired organic cation transporter (OCT) function. In line with our hypothesis, we observed reduced hepatic exposure to metformin in homozygote carriers of rs12208357 and rs72552763 after IV-administration (Sundelin et al., 2017). Interestingly, this reduced function of OCT1 was more pronounced after oral administration of ^{11}C-metformin, indicating that OCT1 is involved in both intestinal absorption and hepatic uptake of metformin (Sundelin et al., 2017).

5. METABOLISM

Observations that genetic variation in drug response is due to differences in drug metabolism dates back to the 1950s (Kalow, 1964). Today, new drugs are routinely screened for their dependency on metabolism by specific enzyme systems characterized by a high degree of genetic variability. In clinical practice, variation in drug metabolism can in some instances be overcome by performing therapeutic drug monitoring. However, in many cases the impact of genetic variation in drug metabolism remains to be resolved, and imaging techniques can facilitate this process. However, scanners can only detect the radionuclide and not the molecule to which it is bound. It is therefore not possible to differentiate between intact and metabolized fractions of the labeled compound. This can pose a challenge for mathematical modeling of tracer kinetics. The distribution of the antidementia drug Donepezil can be visualized using (^{11}C)-Donepezil (Gjerloff et al., 2014). The drug is metabolized in a process that includes CYP2D6 (Noetzli et al., 2014), and genetic variation in CYP2D6 function may affect the ratio between intact drug and metabolites. It is therefore important to validate the content of metabolites of Donepezil in plasma before performing mathematical modeling of drug distribution. CYP2D6 is highly expressed in several regions of the brain where it is involved in metabolism of various psychoactive drugs in addition to Donepezil. Functional MRI (fMRI) can be used to examine functional activity in the brain in vivo and using this technique it has been shown that genetic polymorphism of CYP2D6 affects resting brain perfusion and neural activation during cognitive tasks (Kirchheiner et al., 2011; Stingl et al., 2012). Visualization of the pharmacologic response by fMRI has been termed pharmacological MRI (Leslie, 2000). This allows for determination of brain activation after drug distribution and thereby concomitantly measure metabolism and perfusion. These pharmacodynamic measurements can be performed noninvasively in carriers of several genetic variants, and this exiting technology is extensively reviewed by Viviani, Lehmann, and Stingl (2014).

Newly developed spectroscopy techniques have the potential to directly assess drug metabolism in vivo and will perhaps in the future be applied in imaging of pharmacogenetics. MR spectroscopy in combination with dynamic nuclear polarization provides organ-specific metabolic information in a minimally invasive form. The sensitivity of his technology is more than 10,000 times above conventional MR-spectroscopy (Ardenkjaer-Larsen et al., 2003) but only for a very limited time (relaxation times of 20–60 s) (Golman, Ardenkjaer-Larsen, Petersson, Mansson, & Leunbach, 2003; Kurhanewicz et al., 2011), and it has been demonstrated to provide in vivo quantification of hepatic substrate metabolism (Lee et al., 2013). This is likely to be an important technology in the future for assessing metabolism of compounds that can be hyperpolarized.

6. ELIMINATION

Several genes, including SLC22A2, SLC22A6, and SLC22A8, encoding transport proteins are involved in renal elimination of drugs and active metabolites of drugs. Numerous genetic variants in SLC22A2 have been identified and some, as rs316019, have allele frequencies >5% (Lai et al., 2012). SLC22A2 encodes OCT2 which is responsible for hepatic elimination of metformin, but the functional importance of variants in SLC22A2 including rs316019 remains to be determined and conflicting data from in vivo and in vivo studies have been published (Chen et al., 2009; Song et al., 2008; Zolk, Solbach, Konig, & Fromm, 2009). ^{11}C-metformin PET imaging has been used to assess OCT2 function and renal elimination of metformin in an animal model of chronic kidney disease (Pedersen et al., 2016). Visualizing OCT2 function may clarify if genetic variants in SLC22A2 have functional importance for renal elimination of drugs transported by OCT2 as metformin and cisplatin.

In the liver, the organic anion ^{99m}Tc-N-[2-[(3-bromo-2,4,6-trimethylphenyl)-amino]-2-oxoethyl]-*N*-(carboxymethyl)-glycine (^{99m}Tc-mebrofenin) and its analogs are widely used for imaging of bile canalicular transport (de Graaf, van Lienden, van Gulik, & Bennink, 2010). ^{99m}Tc-mebrofenin is predominantly excreted by hepatobiliary transport through multidrug resistance-associated protein 2 (MRP2) encoded by the ABCC2 gene (Bhargava et al., 2009). MRP2 is also responsible for biliary clearance of pravastatin (Kivistö & Niemi, 2007), and observational studies suggest that genetic variation in ABCC2 may affect the pharmacokinetic properties of pravastatin (Niemi et al., 2006). Expression of MRP2 is not confined to the liver and the protein is also involved in, e.g., intestinal efflux (Dahan & Amidon, 2009). The phenotype of carriers of ABCC2 variants is therefore complex, and ^{99m}Tc-mebrofenin imaging may be beneficial to determine tissue-specific MRP2 function.

7. CONCLUSION

Emerging technologies within nuclear medicine allow for investigation of tissue distribution of drugs and for assessment of membrane transporter activity in vivo. If translated to bedside use, this would allow for determination of a specific drug present at its target site. Example of such use today is ^{89}Zr-Trastuzumab in breast cancer patients (Munnink, 2009), and future applications within oncology are likely. In addition, derivative drug effects can be visualized using fMRI and PET scans which allow for determination of pharmacodynamics effects of a specific drug at the individual level. Clinical use of these techniques has potential to greatly improve personalized treatment and in that way be cost-effective (Reddy & Haris, 2015). The investigations include determination of functional importance of genetic variants, and thereby provide proof of concept for imaging in pharmacogenetics as a tool to improve efficacy and safety of drugs.

CONFLICT OF INTEREST

The authors have no conflict of interest to declare.

REFERENCES

Ardenkjaer-Larsen, J. H., Fridlund, B., Gram, A., Hansson, G., Hansson, L., Lerche, M. H., et al. (2003). Increase in signal-to-noise ratio of >10,000 times in liquid-state NMR. *Proceedings of the National Academy of Sciences of the United States of America, 100*(18), 10158–10163. https://doi.org/10.1073/pnas.1733835100.

Benet, L., Cummins, C., & Wu, C. (2004). Unmasking the dynamic interplay between efflux transporters and metabolic enzymes. *International Journal of Pharmaceutics, 277*(1–2), 3–9. https://doi.org/10.1016/j.ijpharm.2002.12.002.

Bhargava, K. K., Joseph, B., Ananthanarayanan, M., Balasubramaniyan, N., Tronco, G. G., Palestro, C. J., et al. (2009). Adenosine triphosphate-binding cassette subfamily C member 2 is the major transporter of the hepatobiliary imaging agent (99m)Tc-mebrofenin. *Journal of Nuclear Medicine: Official Publication, Society of Nuclear Medicine, 50*(7), 1140–1146. https://doi.org/10.2967/jnumed.109.062448.

Carson, R. E. (2003). Tracer kinetic modeling in PET. In *Positron emission tomography: Basic science and clinical practice* (pp. 147–179). Springer.

Chen, Y., Li, S., Brown, C., Cheatham, S., Castro, R. A., Leabman, M. K., et al. (2009). Effect of genetic variation in the organic cation transporter 2 on the renal elimination of metformin. *Pharmacogenetics and Genomics, 19*(7), 497–504. https://doi.org/10.1097/FPC.0b013e32832cc7e9.

Cherry, S. R., Sorenson, J. A., & Phelps, M. E. (2012). *Physics in nuclear medicine* (4th ed.). Elsevier.

Dahan, A., & Amidon, G. L. (2009). Small intestinal efflux mediated by MRP2 and BCRP shifts sulfasalazine intestinal permeability from high to low, enabling its colonic targeting. *American Journal of Physiology. Gastrointestinal and Liver Physiology*, *297*(2), G371–7. https://doi.org/10.1152/ajpgi.00102.2009.

de Graaf, W., van Lienden, K. P., van Gulik, T. M., & Bennink, R. J. (2010). (99m)Tc-mebrofenin hepatobiliary scintigraphy with SPECT for the assessment of hepatic function and liver functional volume before partial hepatectomy. *Journal of Nuclear Medicine: Official Publication, Society of Nuclear Medicine*, *51*(2), 229–236. https://doi.org/10.2967/jnumed.109.069724.

Gjerloff, T., Jakobsen, S., Nahimi, A., Munk, O. L., Bender, D., Alstrup, A. K. O., et al. (2014). In vivo imaging of human acetylcholinesterase density in peripheral organs using 11C-donepezil: Dosimetry, biodistribution, and kinetic analyses. *Journal of Nuclear Medicine*, *55*(11), 1818–1824. https://doi.org/10.2967/jnumed.114.143859.

Golman, K., Ardenkjaer-Larsen, J. H., Petersson, J. S., Mansson, S., & Leunbach, I. (2003). Molecular imaging with endogenous substances. *Proceedings of the National Academy of Sciences of the United States of America*, *100*(18), 10435–10439. https://doi.org/10.1073/pnas.1733836100.

Gormsen, L. C., Sundelin, E. I., Jensen, J. B., Vendelbo, M. H., Jakobsen, S., Munk, O. L., et al. (2016). In vivo imaging of human 11C-metformin in peripheral organs: Dosimetry, biodistribution, and kinetic analyses. *Journal of Nuclear Medicine*, *57*(12), 1920–1926. https://doi.org/10.2967/jnumed.116.177774.

Hames, K. C., Vella, A., Kemp, B. J., & Jensen, M. D. (2014). Free fatty acid uptake in humans with CD36 deficiency. *Diabetes*, *63*(11), 3606–3614. https://doi.org/10.2337/db14-0369.

Huang, Y. (2007). Pharmacogenetics/genomics of membrane transporters in cancer chemotherapy. *Cancer and Metastasis Reviews*, *26*(1), 183–201. https://doi.org/10.1007/s10555-007-9050-6.

Hume, W. E., Shingaki, T., Takashima, T., Hashizume, Y., Okauchi, T., Katayama, Y., et al. (2013). The synthesis and biodistribution of [11C]metformin as a PET probe to study hepatobiliary transport mediated by the multi-drug and toxin extrusion transporter 1 (MATE1) in vivo. *Bioorganic & Medicinal Chemistry*, *21*(24), 7584–7590. https://doi.org/10.1016/j.bmc.2013.10.041.

Jakobsen, S., Busk, M., Jensen, J. B., Munk, O. L., Zois, N. E., Alstrup, A. K. O., et al. (2016). A PET tracer for renal organic cation transporters, 11C-metformin: Radiosynthesis and preclinical proof-of-concept studies. *Journal of Nuclear Medicine*, *57*(4), 615–621. https://doi.org/10.2967/jnumed.115.169292.

Jensen, J. B., Sundelin, E. I., Jakobsen, S., Gormsen, L. C., Munk, O. L., Frøkiær, J., et al. (2016). [11C]-Labeled metformin distribution in the liver and small intestine using dynamic positron emission tomography in mice demonstrates tissue-specific transporter dependency. *Diabetes*, *65*(6), 1724–1730. https://doi.org/10.2337/db16-0032.

Kalow, W. (1964). Pharmacogenetics and anesthesia. *Anesthesiology*, *25*, 377–387. Retrieved from http://www.ncbi.nlm.nih.gov/pubmed/14156579.

Kimura, T., & Higaki, K. (2002). Gastrointestinal transit and drug absorption. *Biological & Pharmaceutical Bulletin*, *25*(2), 149–164. Retrieved from http://www.ncbi.nlm.nih.gov/pubmed/11853157.

Kirchheiner, J., Seeringer, A., Godoy, A. L., Ohmle, B., Maier, C., Beschoner, P., et al. (2011). CYP2D6 in the brain: Genotype effects on resting brain perfusion. *Molecular Psychiatry*, *16*(3), 333–341. https://doi.org/10.1038/mp.2010.42.

Kivistö, K. T., & Niemi, M. (2007). Influence of drug transporter polymorphisms on pravastatin pharmacokinetics in humans. *Pharmaceutical Research*, *24*, 239–247. https://doi.org/10.1007/s11095-006-9159-2.

Kurhanewicz, J., Vigneron, D. B., Brindle, K., Chekmenev, E. Y., Comment, A., Cunningham, C. H., et al. (2011). Analysis of cancer metabolism by imaging hyperpolarized nuclei: Prospects for translation to clinical research. *Neoplasia (New York, NY)*, *13*(2), 81–97. Retrieved from http://www.ncbi.nlm.nih.gov/pubmed/21403835.

Labbe, S. M., Grenier-Larouche, T., Croteau, E., Normand-Lauziere, F., Frisch, F., Ouellet, R., et al. (2011). Organ-specific dietary fatty acid uptake in humans using positron emission tomography coupled to computed tomography. *American Journal of Physiology: Endocrinology and Metabolism*, *300*(3), E445–E453. https://doi.org/10.1152/ajpendo.00579.2010.

Lai, Y., Varma, M., Feng, B., Stephens, J. C., Kimoto, E., El-Kattan, A., et al. (2012). Impact of drug transporter pharmacogenomics on pharmacokinetic and pharmacodynamic variability—Considerations for drug development. *Expert Opinion on Drug Metabolism & Toxicology*, *8*(6), 723–743. https://doi.org/10.1517/17425255.2012.678048.

Lee, P., Leong, W., Tan, T., Lim, M., Han, W., & Radda, G. K. (2013). In vivo hyperpolarized carbon-13 magnetic resonance spectroscopy reveals increased pyruvate carboxylase flux in an insulin-resistant mouse model. *Hepatology (Baltimore, Md.)*, *57*(2), 515–524. https://doi.org/10.1002/hep.26028.

Leslie, R. (2000). Pharmacological magnetic resonance imaging: A new application for functional MRI. *Trends in Pharmacological Sciences*, *21*(8), 314–318. https://doi.org/10.1016/S0165-6147(00)01507-8.

Mizrahi, R., Rusjan, P. M., Kennedy, J., Pollock, B., Mulsant, B., Suridjan, I., et al. (2012). Translocator protein (18 kDa) polymorphism (rs6971) explains in-vivo brain binding affinity of the PET radioligand [^{18}F]-FEPPA. *Journal of Cerebral Blood Flow & Metabolism*, *32*(6), 968–972. https://doi.org/10.1038/jcbfm.2012.46.

Mizrahi, R., Rusjan, P. M., Vitcu, I., Ng, A., Wilson, A. A., Houle, S., et al. (2013). Whole body biodistribution and radiation dosimetry in humans of a new PET ligand, [18F]-FEPPA, to image translocator protein (18 kDa). *Molecular Imaging and Biology*, *15*(3), 353–359. https://doi.org/10.1007/s11307-012-0589-4.

Munnink, T. O. (2009). HER-2-PET imaging with 89Zr-trastuzumab in metastatic breast cancer patients. *Journal of Clinical Oncology*, *27*(15S), 1045.

Niemi, M., Arnold, K. A., Backman, J. T., Pasanen, M. K., Gödtel-Armbrust, U., Wojnowski, L., et al. (2006). Association of genetic polymorphism in ABCC2 with hepatic multidrug resistance-associated protein 2 expression and pravastatin pharmacokinetics. *Pharmacogenetics and Genomics*, *16*(11), 801–808. https://doi.org/10.1097/01.fpc.0000230422.50962.91.

Noetzli, M., Guidi, M., Ebbing, K., Eyer, S., Wilhelm, L., Michon, A., et al. (2014). Population pharmacokinetic approach to evaluate the effect of CYP2D6, CYP3A, ABCB1, POR and NR1I2 genotypes on donepezil clearance. *British Journal of Clinical Pharmacology*, *78*(1), 135–144. https://doi.org/10.1111/bcp.12325.

Owen, D. R., Yeo, A. J., Gunn, R. N., Song, K., Wadsworth, G., Lewis, A., et al. (2012). An 18-kDa translocator protein (TSPO) polymorphism explains differences in binding affinity of the PET Radioligand PBR28. *Journal of Cerebral Blood Flow & Metabolism*, *32*(1), 1–5. https://doi.org/10.1038/jcbfm.2011.147.

Pedersen, L., Jensen, J. B., Wogensen, L., Munk, O. L., Jessen, N., Frøkiær, J., et al. (2016). Renal PET-imaging with (11)C-metformin in a transgenic mouse model for chronic kidney disease. *EJNMMI Research*, *6*(1), 54. https://doi.org/10.1186/s13550-016-0211-x.

Reddy, R., & Haris, M. (2015). Imaging technologies from bench to bedside. *Journal of Translational Medicine*, *13*(1), 97. https://doi.org/10.1186/s12967-015-0449-5.

Sankar, P. L., & Parker, L. S. (2017). The precision medicine initiative's all of us research program: An agenda for research on its ethical, legal, and social issues. *Genetics in Medicine*, *19*(7), 743–750. https://doi.org/10.1038/gim.2016.183.

Shingaki, T., Hume, W. E., Takashima, T., Katayama, Y., Okauchi, T., Hayashinaka, E., et al. (2015). Quantitative evaluation of mMate1 function based on minimally invasive measurement of tissue concentration using PET with [11C]metformin in mouse. *Pharmaceutical Research*, *32*(8), 2538–2547. https://doi.org/10.1007/s11095-015-1642-1.

Shingaki, T., Takashima, T., Wada, Y., Tanaka, M., Kataoka, M., Ishii, A., et al. (2012). Imaging of gastrointestinal absorption and biodistribution of an orally administered probe using positron emission tomography in humans. *Clinical Pharmacology and Therapeutics*, *91*(4), 653–659. https://doi.org/10.1038/clpt.2011.267.

Song, I. S., Shin, H. J., Shim, E. J., Jung, I. S., Kim, W. Y., Shon, J. H., et al. (2008). Genetic variants of the organic cation transporter 2 influence the disposition of metformin. *Clinical Pharmacology and Therapeutics*, *84*(5), 559–562. https://doi.org/10.1038/clpt.2008.61.

Stingl, J. C., Esslinger, C., Tost, H., Bilek, E., Kirsch, P., Ohmle, B., et al. (2012). Genetic variation in CYP2D6 impacts neural activation during cognitive tasks in humans. *NeuroImage*, *59*(3), 2818–2823. https://doi.org/10.1016/j.neuroimage.2011.07.052.

Sundelin, E., Gormsen, L., Jensen, J., Vendelbo, M., Jakobsen, S., Munk, O., et al. (2017). Genetic polymorphisms in organic cation transporter 1 attenuates hepatic metformin exposure in humans. *Clinical Pharmacology & Therapeutics*, *102*(5), 841–848. https://doi.org/10.1002/cpt.701.

Viviani, R., Lehmann, M. L., & Stingl, J. C. (2014). Use of magnetic resonance imaging in pharmacogenomics. *British Journal of Clinical Pharmacology*, 77(4), 684–694. https://doi.org/10.1111/bcp.12197.

Wilson, A. A., Garcia, A., Parkes, J., McCormick, P., Stephenson, K. A., Houle, S., et al. (2008). Radiosynthesis and initial evaluation of [18F]-FEPPA for PET imaging of peripheral benzodiazepine receptors. *Nuclear Medicine and Biology*, *35*(3), 305–314. https://doi.org/10.1016/j.nucmedbio.2007.12.009.

Wilson, C. G., O'Mahony, B., Connolly, S. M., Cantarini, M. V., Farmer, M. R., Dickinson, P. A., et al. (2009). Do gastrointestinal transit parameters influence the pharmacokinetics of gefitinib? *International Journal of Pharmaceutics*, *376*(1–2), 7–12. https://doi.org/10.1016/j.ijpharm.2009.04.008.

Yuen, K.-H. (2010). The transit of dosage forms through the small intestine. *International Journal of Pharmaceutics*, *395*(1–2), 9–16. https://doi.org/10.1016/j.ijpharm.2010.04.045.

Zolk, O., Solbach, T. F., Konig, J., & Fromm, M. F. (2009). Functional characterization of the guman organic cation transporter 2 variant p.270Ala > Ser. *Drug Metabolism and Disposition*, *37*(6), 1312–1318. https://doi.org/10.1124/dmd.108.023762.

CHAPTER FIVE

Pharmacoepidemiology in Pharmacogenetics

Thomas P. Ahern[1]
Department of Surgery, The Robert Larner, M.D. College of Medicine, University of Vermont, Burlington, VT, United States
Department of Biochemistry, The Robert Larner, M.D. College of Medicine, University of Vermont, Burlington, VT, United States
[1]Corresponding author: e-mail address: thomas.ahern@med.uvm.edu

Contents

1. Introduction 109
2. Study Design 110
   2.1 Experimental and Observational Cohort Studies 111
   2.2 Case–Control Studies 114
   2.3 Assessing Interaction in Epidemiologic Studies 117
3. Bias and Validity 121
   3.1 Confounding 122
   3.2 Selection Bias and Matching in Case–Control Studies 124
   3.3 Information Bias 126
   3.4 Reverse Causation 128
4. Conclusion 128
Further Reading 128
References 129

Abstract

Epidemiologic methods provide rigorous means by which to study the interplay between genetic factors and drug response. In this chapter, we describe the differences between experimental and observational study designs, and illustrate how to implement the highly efficient case–control study design. We discuss analytic approaches to evaluating gene–drug interactions within typical study designs and review sources of bias that must be assessed and accounted for in epidemiologic analyses.

1. INTRODUCTION

Epidemiology is the science of elucidating causes of disease, with the overarching goal of motivating and evaluating improvements in public

Advances in Pharmacology, Volume 83
ISSN 1054-3589
https://doi.org/10.1016/bs.apha.2018.04.001

health and clinical practice. While epidemiologists have diverse interests with respect to the diseases and potential risk factors they study, they are unified by their approaches to study design, analysis, and causal inference. Epidemiologic studies can be broadly classified as either descriptive or analytic in nature. *Descriptive studies* serve to characterize the prevalence, distribution, or temporal trend of specific diseases or risk factors in one or more populations, with the goal of targeting public health and research resources to areas in greatest need. *Analytic studies* can be parsed into those that attempt to predict occurrence (or presence) of a disease and those that attempt to identify determinants (or risk factors) for a disease. Most analytic pharmacoepidemiology studies are designed to evaluate the effects—intended and otherwise—of pharmaceuticals on disease outcomes in clinical populations. Predictive studies aim to develop models for estimating an individual's risk of experiencing a particular health outcome, based on a set of readily measured characteristics. Such models are often deployed in clinical settings to guide disease diagnosis, or to select the most appropriate treatment course for a given patient. In contrast, risk factor studies aim for valid and precise measurements of the association between some exposure and some disease, with the ultimate goal of identifying causes of disease.

In this chapter, we will cover the rudiments of epidemiologic methods as they pertain to pharmacogenetic risk factor studies. We will begin with the basics of epidemiologic study design, focusing on case–control studies because of their frequent application to pharmacogenetic hypotheses. We will then cover ways in which epidemiology studies evaluate the interaction between two exposures, such as a medication and a genetic factor that might modify response to that medication. We will then discuss threats to study validity, including selection bias, information bias, and confounding, and introduce methods for the assessment and control of these systematic errors.

2. STUDY DESIGN

Suppose we want to determine whether a common prescription drug increases the risk of cancer. To do so, we would need to compare how often cancer is diagnosed between groups of people with different drug exposures. There are several options for how we can set up this comparison. The first choice we face is whether to conduct an *experimental study* or an *observational study*. The difference between these two approaches is best illustrated by explaining the concept of *cohort studies*.

2.1 Experimental and Observational Cohort Studies

Cohort studies enroll samples of participants from a source population (also called the study base), assign or characterize exposure, and track participants through time for the occurrence of disease. In experimental cohort studies, participants from the study base are randomly assigned to different exposure groups. In our hypothetical example, we would use a random process (such as a coin toss) to assign each participant to either drug treatment or no treatment. Randomizing exposures in this way improve the balance of participant characteristics between exposure groups, making it less likely that one or more of those characteristics distorts the apparent association between the exposure and outcome. In observational cohort studies, we do not manipulate participants' exposure status as we would in an experimental study. Instead, we simply measure their exposure status, which is either self-selected (for example, whether they use nonprescription analgesics) or the result of medical decision-making (for example, whether they are prescribed a statin to treat hypercholesterolemia). Without random allocation to exposure, other participant characteristics are more likely to be correlated with exposure. For example, statin users tend to be older and have a higher prevalence of cardiovascular risk factors than nonusers. If these same characteristics are also associated with the outcome being studied, then the apparent association between exposure and outcome may be biased.

Table 1 summarizes data from a hypothetical observational cohort study of drug exposure and cancer incidence over 10 years. Out of 230 participants, 80 are exposed and 150 are unexposed. Over the 10-year follow-up period, 20 exposed subjects and 30 unexposed subjects developed cancer. The first step in calculating a measure of association between exposure and disease is to calculate a measure of *disease frequency* in each exposure category. Measuring disease frequency requires a denominator that represents the experience of each exposure group. Two types of denominator are reported in Table 1. The first is simply the total number of participants in each exposure group (n_1 in the exposed and n_2 in the unexposed), which permit calculation of the *risk* or *incidence proportion* in each group, which is simply the proportion of subjects who develop the outcome over follow-up. The second type of denominator is *person-time*, which is the sum of follow-up time contributed by the study participants, while they were at risk for the study outcome (PT_1 in the exposed and PT_2 in the unexposed). Person-time denominators permit calculation of the *incidence rate* in each exposure group, which is interpreted as the number of cases that occurred per unit time.

Table 1 Hypothetical Cohort Study of Drug Exposure in Relation to Cancer Incidence Over a 10-Year Follow-Up Period

	Exposed to Drug	**Not Exposed**	**Total**
Cancer cases	$a=20$	$b=30$	50
Noncases	$c=60$	$d=120$	180
Total	$n_1=80$	$n_2=150$	230
Person-time	$PT_1=750$	$PT_2=1485$	
Risk	=20/80 =0.25, or 25% over 10 years	=30/150 =0.20, or 20% over 10 years	
Risk ratio	=risk in exposed/risk in unexposed =0.25/0.20 =1.25 25% higher cancer risk associated with exposure		
Risk difference	=risk in exposed—risk in unexposed =0.25–0.20 =0.05 Exposure is associated with 5 more cases per 100 people		
Rate	=20/750 =0.0266 cases per person-year =26.6 cases per 1000 person-years	=30/1485 =0.0202 cases per person-year =20.2 cases per 1000 person-years	
Rate ratio	=rate in exposed/rate in unexposed =(20/750)/(30/1485) =1.32 32% higher rate of cancer incidence associated with exposure		
Rate difference	=rate in exposed—rate in unexposed =(20/750)–(30/1485) =0.0065 =Exposure is associated with 6.5 more cases per 1000 person-years of follow-up		

2.1.1 Calculating Risk-Based Measures of Disease Frequency and Association

In Table 1, the risk in the exposed group equaled 0.25, or 25%, over the 10 years of follow-up. Expressed in plain language, this means that 25% of the exposed group developed cancer over the follow-up period. The unexposed group had 30 cancer cases over follow-up. The risk in the unexposed was therefore 0.20, or 20%, over 10 years. We can now calculate an estimate of the *association* between exposure and disease by comparing the measures of disease frequency between exposure groups. We can calculate an association on the *relative scale* by taking the ratio of the two risks. The *risk ratio* calculated in Table 1 indicates that exposure is associated with a 1.25-fold higher risk of cancer, compared with no exposure. An equivalent way to express this is to say that exposure was associated with a 25% increase in the risk of cancer. We can also calculate an association on the *absolute scale* by taking the difference of the two risks; the *risk difference* calculated in Table 1 tells us that exposure is associated with 5 more cancer cases per 100 people (or 50 more cases per 1000 people, and so on), compared with no exposure.

2.1.2 Calculating Rate-Based Measures of Disease Frequency and Association

Table 1 reports that the 80 subjects in the exposed group contributed a total of 750 person-years of follow-up time to the study. Twenty cases occurred during follow-up of the exposed, yielding an *incidence rate* of 0.02666 cases per person-year, which is more conveniently expressed as 26.7 cases per 1000 person-years. The corresponding rate in the unexposed group is 20.2 cases per 1000 person-years. Just as we did with the risks in each exposure group, we can estimate associations between exposure and disease incidence by taking either the ratio or the difference of the exposed and unexposed incidence rates. The *incidence rate ratio* for the data in Table 1 is 1.32, indicating a 32% increase in the rate of disease incidence associated with exposure. The *incidence rate difference* is 0.0065, which indicates that exposure is associated with 6.5 more cases occurring per 1000 person-years in the exposed, compared with the unexposed.

In the Table 1 data, both the ratio- and difference-based measures indicate that there is a positive association between exposure and disease. Had there been no association between exposure and disease (that is, equal risks or rates in both exposure groups), the ratio measures would have equaled 1, and the difference measures would have equaled 0—these are the values for *null associations* on the relative and difference scales, respectively. Exposures may also be associated with reduced risks or rates of disease, in which case relative measures of association will be less than 1, and absolute measures of association will be negative.

While cohort studies are straightforward and effective for conducting risk factor research, they often require exposure measurement on a large sample of the study base, most of whom will not go on to develop the outcome of interest. Cohort studies also require long-term follow-up to ascertain disease occurrence in the exposure groups. In the context of pharmacogenetic studies, where exposure measurement typically involves costly biochemical assays, then the cohort design may be prohibitively expensive. In addition, if the disease or outcome of interest is rare, then a cohort design would require enrollment and long-term follow-up of many subjects from the study base to yield a sufficient number of disease cases for statistically precise estimation of the association. These inefficiencies can be remedied by opting for the case–control study design.

2.2 Case–Control Studies

Instead of enrolling a large sample of individuals from a study base and following them through time, case–control studies use sampling strategies to maximize the information extracted from a study base while keeping the total number of enrollees manageable. We will illustrate case–control sampling by conceptualizing the hypothetical cohort data in Table 1 as a study base. Case–control studies enumerated from existing cohorts are common and are known as *nested case–control studies*. We will use a nested case–control study to illustrate important concepts of the case–control design. To convert the hypothetical cohort study into a nested case–control study, we first include all the cases that were diagnosed over the cohort's follow-up period. Since cases are usually less common than noncases in epidemiologic studies, each one of them is information-dense. Specifically, each contributes critical information about the distribution of exposure among the participants who developed the outcome. In the hypothetical cohort there were 50 cases—20 from the exposed group and 30 from the unexposed group—and we will include all 50 in the case–control study. Before we can calculate an association between exposure and disease, we also require an estimate of the exposure distribution in the study base—the source population from which the cases arose. This brings us to the topic of control selection.

2.2.1 Strategies for Sampling Controls

When selecting controls, the investigator must consider how many individuals should be selected, which of the various sampling approaches to use, and whether controls should be matched to cases on one or more characteristics. The choice of number of controls to sample can be guided by power and sample size calculations for case–control data, which are easily implemented in packaged statistical software. Very often, investigators will select the same number of controls as there are cases in a study. However, study precision can be preserved by sampling controls at ratios higher than 1:1—for example, by selecting 10 controls for every case (Rothman, Greenland, & Lash, 2008b). The efficiencies of the case–control study design come with the trade-off of reduced precision compared with cohort studies that enroll a census of the study population rather than a sample. All the same, sampling 4 or more controls per case will recover most of the precision that is lost to sampling.

After settling on the number of controls to sample, the investigator must choose how to sample those controls from the study base. When sampling from a defined cohort, there are three main approaches to control sampling, and each relates to a different portion of follow-up in the underlying study population (Rothman et al., 2008b). Under the first approach, known as *cumulative sampling*, the investigator samples controls from the set of participants who had not developed the study outcome by the end of follow-up. In our hypothetical cohort, 180 participants did not develop cancer by the end of the study. Let us say that we decide to sample 75 controls from the group of noncases. Given the exposure distribution among all of the noncases in Table 1 (1/3 exposed), we would expect 25 of the 75 controls to be exposed, yielding the data in Table 2 under cumulative control sampling.

The second approach to sampling controls is referred to as *case–cohort sampling* or *base sampling*. Under this approach, controls are sampled from all of the at-risk subjects at baseline. Note that some of these at-risk subjects will go on to become cases during follow-up. It is therefore possible that some individuals who are sampled as controls will also appear as cases in the study. While this may seem problematic or counterintuitive, it is wholly appropriate. Recall that the purpose of the controls is to inform us about

Table 2 Example of a Case–Control Study Enrolled From the Hypothetical Cohort From Table 1

	Exposed	Unexposed	Odds Ratio	Measure of Association Estimated by the Odds Ratio
Cases	20	30		
Controls (cumulative sampling, 75 controls)	25	50	=(20/25)/(30/50) =1.33	Incidence odds ratio
Controls (case–cohort sampling, 50% of study base)	40	75	=(20/40)/(30/75) =1.25	Risk ratio

the exposure distribution in the study base (the source population that gave rise to the cases). Since all cases begin the study as members of the study base, they should be eligible for inclusion in a representative sample of that population. If we do not mind having cases both in the numerator and the denominator of a risk, then we should not mind sampling controls who later become cases. To illustrate this sampling approach using the hypothetical cohort, let us assume that we sample half of the study base to serve as controls. We would end up with 115 subjects and would expect 40 to be exposed and 75 to be unexposed based on the exposure distribution among all subjects in the cohort. This yields the case–control data in Table 2 under case–cohort sampling.

The third approach to control selection involves sampling subjects from the study base in proportion to their person-time at risk over follow-up. Under this approach, a subject who contributes a lot of follow-up time to the cohort will have a higher probability of being selected as a control than a subject who contributes very little follow-up time to the cohort. The dependency of selection probability on the length of time a subject is followed in a study results in a set of controls that represents the distribution of exposed and unexposed person-time in the study base. This sort of sampling, known as *incidence density sampling*, can be accomplished by special techniques that account for the relative length of subjects' time at risk, or by the process of *risk-set sampling*. In risk-set sampling, a group of subjects from the study base who are still at risk for the outcome is enumerated each time a case is diagnosed during follow-up. Controls are then selected at random from each case's risk set. This has the effect of matching controls to cases on their follow-up time, which must be properly accounted for in the analysis (see Section 3.2 that describes matching in case–control studies). When case–control studies are enumerated from a dynamic population (instead of a defined cohort), density sampling is the only feasible method of control selection (Vandenbroucke & Pearce, 2012).

2.2.2 Calculating Associations in Case–Control Studies

Since controls only represent a sample of the underlying denominator in a study base, we cannot use case–control data to calculate measures of disease frequency within exposure strata, unless we are fortunate enough to have reliable estimates of the fraction of the study base that was selected as controls. This is another limitation of the case–control design that must be considered against the efficiencies of the design. However, we can calculate a measure of association between exposure and disease known as the *odds ratio*. The odds ratio is a relative measure of association calculated by taking the ratio of cases to controls in the exposed group and dividing it by the ratio of cases to controls in the unexposed group.

The odds ratio from a case–control study will estimate different measures of association depending on which control sampling strategy was applied in the design. When cumulative sampling is used, the controls will represent the exposure distribution in the subjects who remain disease-free until the end of follow-up, and the odds ratio will estimate the *incidence odds ratio* in the underlying cohort. This measure is not used in practice when analyzing cohort studies, where complete denominators (either the total number of participants at risk or the cumulative person-time at risk) are available. Nonetheless, we can calculate the incidence odds ratio from the hypothetical cohort by taking the ratio of cases to noncases in the exposed and dividing it by the ratio of cases to noncases in the unexposed [$OR_{\text{cohort}} = (20/60)/(30/120) = 1.33$]. If we calculate the odds ratio using the case–control data for cumulative sampling in Table 2, we get the same point estimate [$OR_{\text{cumulative}} = (20/25)/(30/50) = 1.33$]. If controls are sampled under the case–cohort approach, they will represent the exposure distribution on the study base, and the odds ratio will estimate the risk ratio. In Table 1, the risk ratio in the hypothetical cohort equals 1.25, and the odds ratio from the case–cohort study in Table 2 also equals 1.25 [$OR_{\text{case–cohort}} = (20/40)/(30/75) = 1.25$]. Had we selected controls from the study base in proportion to subjects' follow-up time, the odds ratio from the case–control study would estimate the incidence rate ratio in the underlying cohort. The discrepancy between the odds ratio under cumulative control sampling and the odds ratio under case–cohort control sampling arises because the risk of disease in the underlying cohort is relatively high in at least one exposure group. If disease is relatively rare in all exposure groups (rare is usually considered to be a risk of $<10\%$), then the risk ratio will be more closely approximated by the odds ratio under cumulative sampling. This phenomenon underlies the common misconception that disease risk must be rare in order for case–control studies to yield valid estimates of the risk ratio. As we have seen, case–cohort sampling will yield estimates of the risk ratio without the caveat of rare outcomes in all exposure groups (Greenland, 1987).

2.3 Assessing Interaction in Epidemiologic Studies

The topic of interactions between risk factors is complicated by the different terminology and approaches that have been taught over the years. Most courses in biostatistics define interaction as the presence of *effect measure modification*, wherein the measure of association between a risk factor and disease is different within levels of a third variable. For example, in a gene–drug interaction study, one could generate multiple 2 × 2 tables to associate drug exposure with disease incidence according to whether or not subjects carry a variant allele in a drug-metabolizing enzyme. If the measure of association within genetic strata is calculated on the absolute scale (e.g., using the risk difference), then the investigator is evaluating *effect modification on the difference scale.* And if the measure of association within genetic strata is calculated on the relative scale (e.g., using the risk ratio), then the investigator is evaluating *effect modification on the ratio scale.* Interaction is considered present if the measures of association are substantially different between the strata. Though highly prevalent in the literature, this approach to evaluating interaction is somewhat arbitrary. It has been demonstrated that if both the exposure and the modifier have nonzero effects on disease incidence, then there will be effect modification on either or both the additive and ratio scales (Greenland, Lash, & Rothman, 2008). It is therefore important to specify which measure of association was used to evaluate effect modification, since the judgment of interaction is dependent on that choice. If you are unsettled by how fickle this assessment of interaction is, we will later discuss an approach to interaction assessment that is reliably interpretable in more concrete terms.

2.3.1 Case-Only Studies

Case-only studies are a variation of the traditional case–control design that are suitable for exploring interaction between genetic factors and drug exposures in relation to disease risk, without requiring a sample of controls. In the simplest scenario, both the exposure and the genetic factor are classified dichotomously—for example, presence of at least one functional polymorphism in a gene of interest and current use vs nonuse of a drug whose effect may be modified by the gene. Case-only studies assume that the exposure and genetic factor are not correlated in the source population, meaning that the presence of the genetic factor does not affect the probability that a subject is exposed. Importantly, case-only studies cannot be used to measure main associations between the exposure or the genetic factor and disease incidence. Instead, case-only studies evaluate whether the factors interact with each other on the multiplicative scale to modify disease risk. Case-only data are organized into a 2 × 2 table like the example in Table 3, from which the case-only odds ratio is calculated. If the exposure and genetic factor do not interact, then the case-only odds ratio is expected to be null (i.e., $OR_{\text{case-only}} = 1.0$). If the exposure and genetic factor synergize to increase disease incidence

Table 3 Data Table for a Case-Only Study of Gene–Environment Interaction

	Drug Exposure Present	Drug Exposure Absent
Genetic factor present	A_{11}	A_{01}
Genetic factor absent	A_{10}	A_{00}
	Case-only odds ratio $OR_{\text{case-only}}=(A_{11}/A_{10})/(A_{01}/A_{00})$	

Internal cells give the number of cases for each combination of drug exposure and the presence of a genetic factor.

(that is, their interaction yields an association greater than the product of their individual effects), then the case-only odds ratio is expected to be greater than unity ($OR_{\text{case-only}} > 1$). It is also possible for the exposure and genetic factor to antagonistically, in which case the case-only odds ratio would be less than 1 ($OR_{\text{case-only}} < 1$). While the case-only design provides a cost-efficient technique to evaluate gene/drug interactions without requiring controls, it also carries some noteworthy limitations. First, it constrains evaluation of interactions to the multiplicative scale. As we will see below, it is often desirable to measure interaction on the additive scale. Also, while it may seem that most genetic factors and environmental exposures would be independent of one another (a key supposition of the case-only method), even slight correlations between genetic status and exposure status can induce substantial bias in case-only studies (Liu, Fallin, & Kao, 2004). And as with all genetic studies, case-only studies are susceptible to bias from population admixture (i.e., confounding by race/ethnicity) and genotype misclassification (Liu et al., 2004).

2.3.2 Biologic Interaction

The presence of interaction in an epidemiologic analysis should ideally be a function of the individual and combined effects between two risk factors, not a function of which association measure happens to be selected for the evaluation. Fortunately, interaction can be formally described in the context of an established model of disease causation—the *counterfactual susceptibility model,* also referred to as the *potential outcomes model.* The complexities of this model are beyond the scope of this chapter but are covered elsewhere (Greenland & Brumback, 2002; Greenland et al., 2008). In the case of two binary exposures, the counterfactual model can be used to delineate 16 unique response types that each individual may fall into. For example, one of the response types is that neither of the two exposures causes or prevents disease; that is, a subject would remain disease-free under any combination of the two exposures. Because each subject in a study will only experience one combination of exposures, and we would not know what their disease experience would be under a different combination, we refer to their outcomes under different exposure combinations as *counterfactual* or *potential outcomes*. As with the assessment of effect modification, assessing interaction within the counterfactual framework is evaluated within stratified tables. Table 4 illustrates the concept using cohort notation. Consider the stratification factor Z to be a genetic factor that might modify response to drug X. We can use the number of cases and the total persons followed within each combination of Z and X to calculate observed disease risks in each joint stratum. For example, the risk in the doubly unexposed ($Z=X=0$) is calculated as $R_{00}=(a_{z=0}/N_{00})$. We can think of the risk in the doubly exposed (R_{11}, when $Z=X=1$) as having three components: (1) the baseline risk of disease, in the absence of both exposures, which equals R_{00}; (2) the change in risk due to X, which equals the difference in risk comparing $X=1$ with $X=0$ when Z is absent (i.e., $R_{01}-R_{00}$); and (3) the change in risk due to Z, which equals the difference in risk comparing $Z=1$ with $Z=0$ when X is absent (i.e., $R_{10}-R_{00}$). We can use these components to estimate the *interaction contrast*, a measure of the excess (or deficit) of disease incidence that arises from biological interaction between X and Z.

Eq. (1) shows how to calculate the interaction contrast using the notation from Table 4. While it may seem counterintuitive to *add* R_{00} to the other terms, realize that the risks due to each exposure (R_{10} and R_{01}) both harbor the baseline risk, and so that risk is essentially subtracted twice, and therefore must be added back. In the absence of biological interaction between X and Z, the interaction contrast will equal zero—meaning that interplay between the two exposures did not yield any extra disease risk beyond their individual effects. If the interaction contrast is greater than zero, we say that

Table 4 Data Table Illustrating Calculation of the Interaction Contrast With Cohort Data

	$Z=0$		$Z=1$	
	$X=0$	$X=1$	$X=0$	$X=1$
Cases	$a_{z=0}$	$b_{z=0}$	$a_{z=1}$	$b_{z=1}$
Total	N_{00}	N_{01}	N_{10}	N_{11}
Risk	$R_{00}=a_{z=0}/N_{00}$	$R_{01}=b_{z=0}/N_{01}$	$R_{10}=a_{z=1}/N_{10}$	$R_{11}=b_{z=1}/N_{11}$
Common *RR*	1. Ref	$RR_{01}=R_{01}/R_{00}$	$RR_{10}=R_{10}/R_{00}$	$RR_{11}=R_{11}/R_{00}$

there is *superadditivity*, meaning the two exposures interacted to increase disease risk beyond their added independent effects. If the interaction contrast is less than zero, we say that there is *subadditivity*, meaning the two exposure interaction to *decrease* disease risk compared with their added independent effects. The interaction contrast is therefore a scale-independent measure of interaction with foundations in an established model of disease causation and is therefore preferable to the practice of evaluating effect modification. Note, however, that the interaction contrast can also be expressed as the difference in risk differences within strata of Z [that is, $\text{IC} = (R_{11} - R_{10}) - (R_{01} - R_{00})$]. Therefore, the presence of effect modification on the difference scale corresponds to a nonzero interaction contrast.

Note that the interaction contrast requires calculation of measures of disease frequency within joint exposure strata, so it cannot be calculated directly using case–control data. However, a variant of the interaction contrast is estimable with case–control data when control selection yields estimates of risk or rate ratios. This is illustrated in the bottom row of Table 4, in which risk ratios are calculated in all strata, using the doubly unexposed as a common reference group. In a case–control study, one would instead calculate odds ratios using the doubly unexposed as a common referent. The scaled interaction contrast (sometimes called the "relative excess risk due to interaction"), IC/R_{00} can be calculated from the common risk or odds ratios: $IC/R_{00} = RR_{11} - RR_{10} - RR_{01} + 1$ (Greenland et al., 2008). If the interaction contrast equals 0, then the scaled interaction contrast will also equal zero. The scaled interaction contrast will also have the same sign as the underlying interaction contrast, so we can use the former quantity to evaluate whether interaction is superadditive or subadditive. Furthermore, if we have a reliable estimate of the risk in the doubly unexposed (perhaps from a cohort study in a similar source population), we can use that estimate to place the scaled interaction contrast in the context of a denominator, which provides a sense of the actual magnitude of the interaction.

Eq. (1) calculating the interaction contrast.

$$IC = R_{11} - R_{10} - R_{01} + R_{00} \tag{1}$$

3. BIAS AND VALIDITY

In epidemiology, the term *bias* refers to systematic errors that arise in the design and conduct of studies that can distort measures of association between exposure and disease. Unlike *random error*, which can be reduced by increasing the size of a study, *systematic error* cannot be attenuated by enrolling more subjects. Selection bias, information bias (misclassification), and confounding are the three broad categories of systematic error, and each can deflect observed associations away from the truth, either toward or away from the null.

3.1 Confounding

We introduced the concept of confounding earlier, when comparing experimental study designs with observational study designs. We said that when an exposure is randomly allocated to study participants, characteristics of those participants (e.g., age, sex, smoking status, adiposity) become balanced between the exposure groups as the number of subjects increases. This is advantageous because, if another characteristic is both correlated with exposure and able to influence disease risk, then the measured association between exposure and disease can be distorted by that characteristic. Such distortion is the essence of *confounding*, and it is especially troublesome in observational studies, where exposures are not randomly assigned. Consider an observational study of the association between use of a statin drug and incidence of stroke (Fig. 1). One might enroll a group of statin users and a group of nonusers, follow them through time, and compare stroke incidence between the two groups. Because the indications for statin prescription tend to afflict older adults, we would expect age to be associated with statin use (the statin users will be older, on average, than the nonusers). Advancing age is also a risk factor for stroke, so the observed association between statin use and stroke would be partially driven by the difference in age distribution between exposure groups. These relationships are codified in Fig. 1. Since age is positively associated with statin use and positively associated with stroke, confounding by age would serve to increase the value of the statins/stroke association that is measured from the study. If the statins/stroke association is truly protective (i.e., risk ratio < 1 or risk difference < 0), confounding by age would make the association look less protective. A variable, like age in this example, that

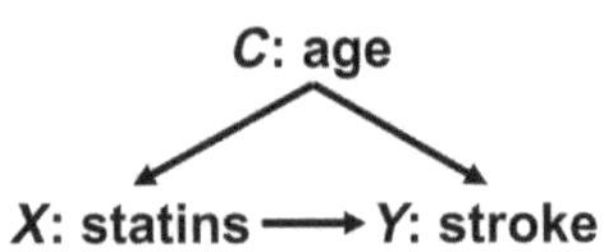

Fig. 1 Diagram of confounding by age, in a study of the association between statin use and stroke incidence.

confounds a particular association between exposure and disease is referred to as a *confounder*. Fig. 1 shows the basic structural features of a confounder (C): it must be a common cause of both the exposure (X) and the outcome (Y), and it must not lie along the causal pathway between X and Y (that is, it should not be a mediator of the effect of X on Y). Fig. 1 is a very simple example of a *directed acyclic graph* (DAG). DAGs (or *causal diagrams*) provide a graphical technique, grounded in the counterfactual susceptibility model that aids in the identification of potential confounders among the complex constellation of variables that surround most exposure–disease relationships (Greenland, Pearl, & Robins, 1999). Candidate confounders are then used to build stratified analyses or to specify multivariable models to reduce confounding bias (Greenland, 1989). DAGs are also helpful for preventing harmful adjustments that lead to increased net bias, and for preventing unnecessary adjustments that do not reduce net bias (Schisterman, Cole, & Platt, 2009).

When a variable (or set of variables) has been flagged as a potential confounder, there are several options for evaluating and addressing the bias. The investigator may *restrict* a study to include only subjects at one level of a confounder, which enforces a uniform distribution of the confounder across exposure strata. The investigator may also *match* exposed and unexposed subjects on levels of one or more confounders. In cohort studies, unexposed subjects can be matched to exposed subjects on selected factors that are also associated with disease occurrence. The matching ensures that exposed and unexposed will have the same distribution of those factors, thus breaking their association with exposure and eliminating confounding bias. Matching works differently in case–control studies, which we will cover below under the topic of selection bias. Restriction and matching can both be implemented in the design phase of the study, or in the analytic phase (an example of the latter is matching exposed to unexposed based on propensity scores). Confounding can also be addressed in the analysis phase of a study, through either *stratified analysis* or *multivariable regression*. In stratified analysis, exposure and disease are tabulated within groups of one or more potential confounders. The result is similar to what happens with restriction, wherein the confounders do not vary substantially within groups (or strata), and therefore cannot distort the stratum-specific exposure–disease associations. The stratum-specific estimates of association can then be pooled or standardized to yield a single estimate adjusted for the stratification variables. While stratified analysis is straightforward and entails few statistical assumptions, it fails when the number of potential confounders generates sparse strata with the available data. It also requires that continuous variables, like age, be collapsed into categories to define strata.

The degree to which continuous confounders vary within strata may lead to incomplete control for bias known as *residual confounding*. If control for confounding involves many variables—or if categorizing one or more of the potential confounders is undesirable—the investigator can turn to *multivariable regression* for their analysis (Bender, 2009). As we discussed in the introduction, models can be developed either to predict an outcome (i.e., explain as much variance in the outcome as possible) or to achieve a valid and precise estimate of an association between an exposure and an outcome. In the latter case, the goal of regression modeling is to retain only those variables that are necessary for attenuating bias. One may start with a large set of candidate confounders for a particular exposure/outcome association (ideally identified through a DAG), but the data at hand may not support a regression model with so many independent variables. Model specification strategies that evaluate the magnitude of change in the exposure variable's regression coefficient upon adjustment for each candidate confounder can guide variable selection in such cases, so that only variables with a substantial impact on bias are retained in the final model (Greenland, 1989).

Pharmacoepidemiology studies are susceptible to a particular type of confounding bias called *confounding by indication*. It occurs when the root cause for the drug exposure (e.g., hypercholesterolemia among statin-treated patients) also influences risk of the outcome. It is therefore challenging to disentangle the effect of the indication from the effect (if any) of the highly correlated drug exposure. Techniques such as propensity score matching, instrumental variable analysis, and use of an active treatment comparison group can help to attenuate confounding by indication (McMahon, 2003; Yoshida, Solomon, & Kim, 2015), but the bias is difficult to eliminate altogether (Bosco et al., 2010).

3.2 Selection Bias and Matching in Case–Control Studies

Selection bias occurs when participation in a study is jointly influenced by exposure and disease status. In a cohort study, selection bias can occur when losses to follow-up are a function of both exposure and disease. In case–control studies, selection bias occurs when selection of controls is not independent of exposure. The practice of matching in case–control studies illustrates this concept. Unlike in cohort studies, matching in case–control studies entails selection of controls who match cases on one or more potentially confounding factors. We might accomplish this matching through risk-set sampling where, instead of enumerating risk sets from the entire study base, we enumerate risk sets of subjects from the study base who happen to have the same matching factor profile as the case. One or more controls are then selected at random from the matched risk set for each case. Recall that the cardinal rule of control selection is that selection must be kept independent of exposure, the reason being that controls must reflect the distribution of exposure in the study base. When we match controls to cases, however, we are creating an artificial similarity between the representatives of the study base (the controls) and the cases of disease that arose from that base. If one or more of the chosen matching factors correlates with exposure, then the exposure distribution in the matched controls will become less like the distribution in the study base and more like the distribution in the cases. The result is that the calculated association between exposure and disease will be biased, unless the matching factors are accounted for in the analysis. Therefore, unlike in cohort studies, matching alone does not attenuate bias due to confounding in case–control studies. Rather, it induces a selection bias (inclusion is a function of both exposure—via correlation with matching factors—and disease) that must be removed by carrying out a *matched analysis*. Matched analysis can be performed by standardizing or pooling odds ratios across joint strata of the matching factors, or by adjustment for the matching factors in multivariable regression models (Greenland & Rothman, 2008). Conditional logistic models account for matching factors by identifying case–control strata instead of requiring that all matching factors be included as independent variables (Greenland & Rothman, 2008).

Given the negative consequences of matching controls to cases, it is natural to wonder why an investigator would choose to match in case–control studies at all. While matching alone does not address confounding in case–control studies, it does guarantee that there will be a balanced number of cases and controls within strata of the matching factors to permit efficient statistical adjustment for those factors. The investigator essentially induces selection bias to enable efficient control of confounding. The induced selection bias is removed along with confounding by the matched analysis.

Another source of selection bias in pharmacoepidemiology studies, called *prevalent user bias*, occurs when the exposed group is comprised of individuals who have been exposed to the pharmaceutical of interest for some period of time before the study. Prevalent users enrolled in a study will have experienced some amount of exposed time without being diagnosed with the disease of interest. Subjects who had been taking the drug and who developed the event of interest—and therefore would not be eligible for enrollment in a study—would be selected out of the prevalent user group. Therefore, groups of prevalent users may be enriched for subjects who are resilient to any influence that the drug exerts on disease risk, thus biasing the association between exposure and disease. This bias can be avoided by adopting an exposure definition that counts only incident use of a drug during follow-up, starting with study population that is uniformly unexposed at time zero (Danaei, Tavakkoli, & Hernan, 2012). So-called *new initiator designs* allow for the entire period of exposed time at risk to be observed. Unfortunately, these designs are sometimes impractical and have limitations that must be balanced against their potential benefits (Vandenbroucke & Pearce, 2015).

3.3 Information Bias

Information bias refers to systematic errors that occur when study variables (exposure, disease, modifiers, and confounders) are measured imperfectly. Misclassification errors are said to be *differential* or *nondifferential,* according to whether error rates differ between groups. As an example, outcome misclassification (imperfect measurement of disease status) is *nondifferential* if the degree of imperfection is the same for both exposed and unexposed subjects. If the degree of imperfection is better or worse in one group, then the outcome misclassification is *differential.* Similar logic applies to the definition of differential vs nondifferential exposure misclassification, which is based on measurement error rates in diseased and nondiseased subjects. Pharmacoepidemiology studies, which often rely on prescription claims data, are frequently faced with exposure misclassification, particularly through poor adherence with prescribed regimens (Fischer et al., 2010).

Pharmacoepidemiology studies are susceptible to *detection bias,* a form of information bias in which exposed subjects have more frequent contact with the medical system than unexposed subjects, and may therefore be under better surveillance for health outcomes. This is a form of differential outcome misclassification, in which the *sensitivity* of disease detection is potentially higher among the exposed. When collecting data for an epidemiology study, the goal should be to keep misclassification errors to a minimum, and to keep error rates similar between case and noncases (or exposed and unexposed). The reason for the latter goal is that nondifferential misclassification has a tendency to bias association measurements toward the null. The impact of nondifferential misclassification is therefore more predictable, and it is less likely to generate false-positive findings (Jurek, Greenland, Maldonado, & Church, 2005). In contrast, differential misclassification can bias estimates of association in any direction (Rothman et al., 2008a).

The degree of misclassification in an epidemiology study can is evaluated through a *validation study,* in which exposure and/or disease measurements using the original instrument are compared with measurements using a *gold standard*. For example, in a study of gestational weight gain in relation to perinatal outcomes, the investigators were concerned about the accuracy of maternal prepregnancy body mass index reported on birth certificates (Bodnar et al., 2016). They conducted an internal validation study to compare body mass index data from birth certificates with body mass index data from medical records (the gold standard) for a subset of the participants (Bodnar et al., 2014). The results of validation studies not only inform the degree of misclassification but can also be used to correct information bias. *Validation parameters* (including sensitivity and specificity, and positive and negative predictive values) estimated from validation studies can be used for *probabilistic bias analysis*, in which corrected study data are simulated based on drawing validation parameters from a probability distribution and using the selected values to back-calculate the expected truth (Lash, Fox, & Fink, 2009). The distribution of association estimates from many simulated datasets is then used to characterize a new point estimate and a *simulation interval*, which portrays uncertainty due to sampling error and due to the selection of bias parameters used to correct the data. In the gestational weight gain study, the investigators saw that prepregnancy body mass index was poorly classified on birth certificates. They applied the predictive values calculated from their validation study to a probabilistic bias analysis, generating 100,000 copies of their study data with weight corrected for misclassification. The summary estimate and simulation interval from the bias analysis confirmed the main findings from their conventional analysis (Bodnar et al., 2016). Probabilistic bias analysis methods extend to modeling the impact of unmeasured confounders, residual confounding, and selection bias (Lash et al., 2009).

In pharmacogenetic studies, genotyping errors are a potential source of information bias. Performance of genotyping assays in population-based studies is evaluated with the Hardy–Weinberg equilibrium (HWE) test, which calculates a chi-squared test statistic based on comparison of observed genotype frequencies with those expected under conditions of random mating and lack of genetic admixture in the tested population. If the chi-squared test is deemed statistically significant based on a selected type I error rate, the genotypes are declared inconsistent with HWE. If the above assumptions for equilibrium are expected to be true in the study population, then departure from HWE may signal genotyping error. It is recommended, however, to look beyond the *P*-value for the HWE test and focus on the magnitude of the differences between observed and expected frequencies. A statistically significant chi-squared test in a large dataset may arise from fairly trivial differences in observed and expected frequencies, in which case the strict hypothesis testing paradigm would be misrepresent the actual likelihood of bias.

3.4 Reverse Causation

Reverse causation, sometimes called *protopathic bias* in pharmacoepidemiology, refers to the phenomenon whereby early onset of the study outcome influences drug exposure. This can lead to apparent associations that might be falsely attributed to a drug effect. Reverse causation bias can be avoided by *lagging* exposure in regression models, so that events are modeled as a function of past exposure status, which is less likely influenced by incipient disease. Selection of an appropriate *lag period* (i.e., how far back in time exposure status should be characterized) depends upon the specific drug/outcome pair being studied and should be consistent with known biology regarding disease induction processes.

4. CONCLUSION

Throughout the design and analysis of epidemiology studies, careful attention must be paid to the sources of bias outlined earlier. Novel methods for bias analysis now permit quantitative assessment and control for systematic errors beyond the traditional focus on sampling error and confounding in typical regression models. A thorough understanding of the principles outlined in this chapter will help investigators to maximize the validity and precision of the evidence from pharmacogenetic studies.

FURTHER READING

The design, analysis, and evaluation of epidemiologic studies are critical for effective contributions to the field of pharmacogenetics. Naturally, a field so large and diverse cannot be covered thoroughly in a single chapter. For readers seeking deeper coverage of basic principles of study design, bias, and causal inference, we recommend *Epidemiology: An Introduction* by Rothman—a slender volume that nonetheless conveys a solid grasp of fundamental concepts (Rothman, 2012). Those who are ready to tackle nuances and advanced topics are directed to *Modern Epidemiology* (Rothman et al., 2008c). For those whose interests tend toward predictive studies, we recommend *The Statistical Evaluation of Medical Tests for Classification and Prediction* (Pepe, 2003). Discussion of advanced topics pertinent to pharmacoepidemiology can be found in Strom's *Pharmacoepidemiology* (Strom, 2005). And finally, an overview of bias analysis methods to quantify and adjust for systematic errors is provided by *Applying Quantitative Bias Analysis to Epidemiologic Data* (Lash et al., 2009).

CONFLICT OF INTEREST

The author has no conflict of interest to declare.

REFERENCES

Bender, R. (2009). Introduction to the use of regression models in epidemiology. *Methods in Molecular Biology*, *471*, 179–195. https://doi.org/10.1007/978-1-59745-416-2_9.

Bodnar, L. M., Abrams, B., Bertolet, M., Gernand, A. D., Parisi, S. M., Himes, K. P., et al. (2014). Validity of birth certificate-derived maternal weight data. *Paediatric and Perinatal Epidemiology*, *28*(3), 203–212. https://doi.org/10.1111/ppe.12120.

Bodnar, L. M., Pugh, S. J., Lash, T. L., Hutcheon, J. A., Himes, K. P., Parisi, S. M., et al. (2016). Low gestational weight gain and risk of adverse perinatal outcomes in obese and severely obese women. *Epidemiology*, *27*(6), 894–902. https://doi.org/10.1097/EDE.0000000000000535.

Bosco, J., Silliman, R., Thwin, S., Geiger, A., Buist, D., Prout, M., et al. (2010). A most stubborn bias: No adjustment method fully resolves confounding by indication in observational studies. *Journal of Clinical Epidemiology*, *63*(1), 64–74. https://doi.org/10.1016/j.jclinepi.2009.03.001.

Danaei, G., Tavakkoli, M., & Hernan, M. A. (2012). Bias in observational studies of prevalent users: Lessons for comparative effectiveness research from a meta-analysis of statins. *American Journal of Epidemiology*, *175*(4), 250–262. https://doi.org/10.1093/aje/kwr301.

Fischer, M. A., Stedman, M. R., Lii, J., Vogeli, C., Shrank, W. H., Brookhart, M. A., et al. (2010). Primary medication non-adherence: Analysis of 195,930 electronic prescriptions. *Journal of General Internal Medicine*, *25*(4), 284–290. https://doi.org/10.1007/s11606-010-1253-9.

Greenland, S. (1987). Interpretation and choice of effect measures in epidemiologic analyses. *American Journal of Epidemiology*, *125*(5), 761–768.

Greenland, S. (1989). Modeling and variable selection in epidemiologic analysis. *American Journal of Public Health*, *79*(3), 340–349.

Greenland, S., & Brumback, B. (2002). An overview of relations among causal modelling methods. *International Journal of Epidemiology*, *31*(5), 1030–1037.

Greenland, S., Lash, T. L., & Rothman, K. J. (2008). Concepts of interaction. In K. J. Rothman, S. Greenland, & T. L. Lash (Eds.), *Modern epidemiology* (3rd ed., pp. 71–83). Philadelphia: Wolters Kluwer/Lippincott Williams & Wilkins.

Greenland, S., Pearl, J., & Robins, J. (1999). Causal diagrams for epidemiologic research. *Epidemiology*, *10*(1), 37–48.

Greenland, S., & Rothman, K. J. (2008). Introduction to stratified analysis. In K. J. Rothman, S. Greenland, & T. L. Lash (Eds.), *Modern epidemiology* (3rd ed., pp. 258–282). Philadelphia, PA: Lippincott Williams & Wilkins.

Jurek, A., Greenland, S., Maldonado, G., & Church, T. (2005). Proper interpretation of non-differential misclassification effects: Expectations vs observations. *International Journal of Epidemiology*, *34*(3), 680–687. https://doi.org/10.1093/ije/dyi060.

Lash, T. L., Fox, M. P., & Fink, A. K. (2009). *Applying quantitative bias analysis to epidemiologic data*. Dordrecht/New York: Springer.

Liu, X., Fallin, M. D., & Kao, W. H. (2004). Genetic dissection methods: Designs used for tests of gene-environment interaction. *Current Opinion in Genetics and Development*, *14*(3), 241–245. https://doi.org/10.1016/j.gde.2004.04.011.

McMahon, A. D. (2003). Approaches to combat with confounding by indication in observational studies of intended drug effects. *Pharmacoepidemiology and Drug Safety*, *12*(7), 551–558. https://doi.org/10.1002/pds.883.

Pepe, M. S. (2003). *The statistical evaluation of medical tests for classification and prediction*. Oxford, NY: Oxford University Press.

Rothman, K. J. (2012). *Epidemiology: An introduction* (2nd ed.). New York, NY: Oxford University Press.

Rothman, K. J., Greenland, S., & Lash, T. (2008a). Validity in epidemiologic studies. In K. J. Rothman, S. Greenland, & T. L. Lash (Eds.), *Modern epidemiology* (3rd ed., pp. 128–147). Philadelphia: Wolters Kluwer.

Rothman, K. J., Greenland, S., & Lash, T. L. (2008b). Case-control studies. In K. J. Rothman, S. Greenland, & T. L. Lash (Eds.), *Modern epidemiology* (3rd ed., pp. 111–127). Philadelphia: Wolters Kluwer.

Rothman, K. J., Greenland, S., & Lash, T. L. (2008c). *Modern epidemiology* (3rd ed.). Philadelphia: Wolters Kluwer Health/Lippincott Williams & Wilkins.

Schisterman, E., Cole, S., & Platt, R. (2009). Overadjustment bias and unnecessary adjustment in epidemiologic studies. *Epidemiology (Cambridge, Mass)*, *20*(4), 488–495. https://doi.org/10.1097/EDE.0b013e3181a819a1.

Strom, B. L. (2005). *Pharmacoepidemiology* (4th ed.). Chichester/Hoboken, NJ: John Wiley.

Vandenbroucke, J. P., & Pearce, N. (2012). Case-control studies: Basic concepts. *International Journal of Epidemiology*, *41*(5), 1480–1489. https://doi.org/10.1093/ije/dys147.

Vandenbroucke, J., & Pearce, N. (2015). Point: Incident exposures, prevalent exposures, and causal inference: Does limiting studies to persons who are followed from first exposure onward damage epidemiology? *American Journal of Epidemiology*, *182*(10), 826–833. https://doi.org/10.1093/aje/kwv225.

Yoshida, K., Solomon, D. H., & Kim, S. C. (2015). Active-comparator design and new-user design in observational studies. *Nature Reviews. Rheumatology*, *11*(7), 437–441. https://doi.org/10.1038/nrrheum.2015.30.

SECTION III

Special Themes

CHAPTER SIX

Population Diversity in Pharmacogenetics: A Latin American Perspective

Guilherme Suarez-Kurtz*[,1], Esteban J. Parra†
*Instituto Nacional de Câncer and Rede Nacional de Farmacogenética, Rio de Janeiro, Brazil
†University of Toronto at Mississauga, Mississauga, ON, Canada
[1]Corresponding author: e-mail address: kurtz@inca.gov.br

Contents

1. Introduction 134
2. Global Distribution of PGx Variants 139
3. Population Admixture in Latin America: Pharmacogenomic Implications 141
4. Pharmacogenetics of TAC: CYP3A5 Polymorphisms 145
5. Population Diversity and Warfarin Dosing Algorithms 147
6. Conclusion 150
Acknowledgments 151
References 151

Abstract

Pharmacogenetics/pharmacogenomics (PGx) relies on human genetic diversity. In this review we initially examine the PGx implications of human demographic history and genetic diversity, and highlight results from recent studies on the worldwide distribution of common and rare variants in pharmacogenes. The abundance of rare variants implies that a substantial effort will be required to identify their putative functional effects and to develop reliable algorithms for PGx-guided prescription. Furthermore, variants in all pharmacogenes relevant to a drug treatment must be considered. This implies a shift of the current paradigm of PGx-informed prescription based on genotyping a few common variants in selected genes toward comprehensive sequencing approaches. The following sections deal with the impact of population admixture on PGx diversity focusing on Latin America, where a kaleidoscopic combination of individual proportions of Native American, European, and sub-Saharan African ancestries prevails. We illustrate this diversity by contrasting Brazil and Mexico, the two most populous countries in Latin America, and show that population *average* admixture proportions are not predictive of the corresponding proportions at the *individual* level. As a consequence of admixture, the genetic differentiation of common pharmacogenetic

Advances in Pharmacology, Volume 83
ISSN 1054-3589
https://doi.org/10.1016/bs.apha.2018.02.001

variants in Latin Americans is much attenuated in comparison to their most relevant ancestral populations. Finally, we review data for tacrolimus and warfarin to illustrate the opportunities and challenges presented by Latin American populations for PGx studies and clinical implementation.

1. INTRODUCTION

Pharmacogenetics/pharmacogenomics (PGx) relies on human genetic diversity to individualize drug therapy for greater efficacy with minimum or, ideally, no toxicity. In this review we initially examine the PGx implications of human demographic history and genetic diversity, presenting an updated and expanded version of our previous assay on this topic (Parra & Suarez-Kurtz, 2014). To further examine this question, we highlight results from recent studies on the worldwide distribution of common and rare variants in pharmacogenes, based on data from population-scale sequencing projects. The following sections deal with the impact of population admixture on PGx diversity, focusing on Latin America where five centuries of admixture between three major ancestral groups (Native American, European, and sub-Saharan African), resulted in the extensive population heterogeneity observed nowadays.

The remarkable developments in next-generation sequencing technologies have made it possible to characterize human genomic variation with an unprecedented level of detail (Koboldt, Steinberg, Larson, Wilson, & Mardis, 2013). As a result, there have been important advances in our understanding of human demographic history, and this has important implications for the conceptual development and clinical implementation of PGx. Several studies have highlighted aspects of human variation that were poorly understood, such as the abundance of rare variants in the human genome (Fu et al., 2013; Keinan & Clark, 2012; Nelson et al., 2012; Tennessen et al., 2012). As a consequence, we now have a much more complete perspective of the distribution of genetic variation, both common and rare, in our species.

It has long been known that most *common genetic markers* (i.e., with minor allele frequencies [MAF] higher than 5%) are shared across populations (Jakobsson et al., 2008) and also that, on average, the amount of genetic differentiation between continental populations is a small proportion of the total genetic variation (Li et al., 2008). However, there are population differences in some key parameters, such as the amount of genetic diversity (heterozygosity) and the extent of linkage disequilibrium (LD, i.e., the extent of nonrandom association of alleles at two or more loci on the same chromosome) (Jakobsson et al., 2008; Li et al., 2008). This is a reflection of serial founder effects during and after the out-of-Africa (OOA) migrations of anatomically modern humans that started approximately 50–60 thousand years ago. Genetic diversity is highest in African populations and decreases with distance from East Africa. Conversely, LD increases with distance from Africa. In particular, Native American and Melanesian populations show higher levels of LD than other population groups. This is expected under a model with sequential founder effects, which will increase LD at each step of the expansion (Jakobsson et al., 2008; Li et al., 2008).

It should be emphasized that although the genetic differences between populations (often expressed by the F_{ST} statistic; Wright, 1951) are *on average* very small, the distribution of F_{ST} is quite broad, and there is a long tail of markers showing substantial population differentiation (Barreiro, Laval, Quach, Patin, & Quintana-Murci, 2008). This pattern was verified in the F_{ST} distribution among HapMap populations for ~2500 polymorphisms in 42 "Important Pharmacogenomic (PGx) Genes" (Chen, Teo, Toh, & Sung, 2010) and ~2000 single-nucleotide polymorphisms (SNPs) in 19 pharmacogenes included in the DMET Plus chip (Bonifaz-Peña et al., 2014). For example, in the two aforementioned studies the F_{ST} for pairwise comparisons between CEU (European ancestry) and YRI (African ancestry) averaged 0.08 (Chen et al., 2010) and 0.06 (Bonifaz-Peña et al., 2014), which equates with moderate PGx divergence (Wright, 1951). However, large ($F_{ST}=0.19$) and very large ($F_{ST}=0.69$) divergence between CEU and YRI are observed with respect to the clinically relevant *VKORC1* 3673G>A (rs9923231) and *CYP3A5*3* (rs776746) SNPs. Similarly, a hierarchical analysis of molecular variance for the rs9923231 locus among 52 world populations disclosed an unusually high level of geographical differentiation (Ross et al., 2010). This has important PGx consequences, because this SNP is a major determinant of interindividual variability in warfarin dose required for adequate anticoagulation (International Warfarin Pharmacogenetics Consortium et al., 2009).

Differences in allele frequency and in extent of LD across populations impact the ability to identify common genetic markers involved in drug response using genome-wide association (GWA) approaches. This is well illustrated in a GWA study of warfarin dose requirements in African Americans (Perera et al., 2013). The data confirmed the genome-wide significant association of *VKORC1* rs9923231 with warfarin dose, but failed to verify association between warfarin dose and *CYP2C9*2* and *CYP2C9*3*, which had been previously reported in populations of European descent and in Japanese (Cha, Mushiroda, Takahashi, et al., 2011; Cooper et al., 2008; Takeuchi et al., 2009). It was proposed that the low frequency of *CYP2C9*2* and *CYP2C9*3* in African Americans accounted for this discrepancy. After conditioning on these *CYP2C9* alleles and the *VKORC1* locus, a novel genome-wide significant association of warfarin dose with rs12777823, a G>A transition within the *CYP2C* cluster, was disclosed. Although common in African Americans (minor allele frequency=0.25 in the study cohort), Europeans (0.14), and Japanese (0.32), rs12777823 showed no genome-wide significant association with warfarin dose in the latter two populations (Cha et al., 2011; Cooper et al., 2008; Takeuchi et al., 2009). This led Perera et al. (2013) to suggest "that the association in African Americans might not be due to rs12777823 itself, but a causal SNP in LD with rs12777823 in African Americans but not in other populations."

Population variation in the patterns of LD is important not only for the identification of susceptibility regions through GWA efforts, but also for fine-mapping of the regions, which is required to pinpoint the potential causal variants. Typically, in GWA studies focused on individual populations, and more particularly, in populations with extensive LD between markers, the significant regions identified in the study may comprise a substantial number of markers that are in strong disequilibrium, thus complicating efforts to identify the functional variant. A very promising strategy that is being increasingly employed to overcome this issue is to perform *trans*-ethnic meta-analysis. Combining data from populations of diverse ancestry has two important advantages: (1) the increased sample size makes it possible to identify markers with smaller effects and (2) the differential patterns of LD between populations increase the resolution of the regions identified in the meta-analysis, thereby facilitating fine-mapping efforts. *Trans*-ethnic meta-analysis has been employed with notorious success for a number of traits, such as serum protein loci (Franceschini et al., 2012), fasting glucose and insulin (Liu et al., 2016), and erythrocyte traits (van Rooij et al., 2017), but to our knowledge, this strategy has not been used yet in PGx studies. A limiting factor has been that the overwhelming majority of GWA studies have been carried out in individuals of European ancestry (Popejoy & Fullerton, 2016), a trend that only now seems to be changing.

Perhaps one of the most relevant findings of recent sequencing efforts has been the disclosure of extensive amount of *rare variants* (typically described as markers with MAF <1% or <0.5%) in our genome (Keinan & Clark, 2012; Koboldt et al., 2013; Nelson et al., 2012; Tennessen et al., 2012). The abundance of rare variation is primarily due to the recent growth of our species, and more particularly the dramatic acceleration of population growth that started 5000 years ago (Tennessen et al., 2012). The geographic distribution of rare variants, which tend to be recent mutations (Nelson et al., 2012), is remarkably different from the distribution of common variants, which typically predate the OOA expansion. Due to their recent origin there is very little sharing of rare variants among continental populations, in contrast to what is observed for common variants (Keinan & Clark, 2012; Tennessen et al., 2012). In fact, rare variants show limited levels of sharing even within continental populations, and the extent of allele sharing is dependent on geographic distances (Keinan & Clark, 2012). In general, all the large-scale sequencing efforts carried out to date show that the vast majority of coding variants are rare, and also that low-frequency variants are enriched for potentially functional mutations, which is consistent with the action of purifying selection on deleterious mutations (Keinan & Clark, 2012; Koboldt et al., 2013; Nelson et al., 2012; Tennessen et al., 2012). As an example, the NHLBI Exome Sequencing Project (ESP; Nelson et al., 2012) identified more than 1.1 million autosomal coding single-nucleotide variants (SNVs) in the exomes of 6515 individuals (4298 European Americans and 2217 African Americans). Of these, 164,688 (14.4%) were predicted to be deleterious using a conservative majority rule approach. More than 86% of the SNVs classified as deleterious were predicted to have arisen in the past 5000 years (Nelson et al., 2012).

Regarding PGx biomarkers, Kozyra, Ingelman-Sundberg, and Lauschke (2017) combined data from the ESP and the 1000 Genomes (1KG) project (IGSR: International Genome Sample Resource, n.d.) for ~7800 individuals of European and African ancestry to explore the impact of rare genetic variants on drug response. The authors studied 146 genes affecting drug absorption, distribution, metabolism, and elimination (ADME) and identified 12,152 SNVs in exons, most of which were rare (MAF <1%; 92.9%) or vary rare (MAF <0.1%, 82.7%). Importantly, 56.2% of the variants identified were nonsynonymous, and based on statistic and machine-learning approaches, more than 50% were predicted to be putatively functional. The major conclusions drawn were that: (1) approximately 30%–40% of functional variability in pharmacogenes can be attributed to rare variants and (2) genetic variability in clinically relevant pharmacogenes differs considerably between individuals of European and African descent

(Kozyra et al., 2017). More recently, Schärfe, Tremmel, Schwab, Kohlbacher, and Marks (2017) performed an in-depth computational analysis of the prevalence of functional variants in 806 genes involved in ADME processes and drug targets, based on 60,706 human exomes from the exome aggregation consortium (ExAC) dataset (Lek et al., 2016). They identified 61,134 variants with complete loss of function (by affecting splicing sites or stop codons) or predicted to be "damaging" by different algorithms. As many as 98.7% of these putatively functional variants had MAF < 0.1%, and only 0.1% of predicted functional variants occurred with MAF >0.1% across all six populations represented in the ExAC database.

Clarifying the role of rare variants in drug response will pose important challenges to the scientific community. In order to identify associations of rare variants with drug response, the sample sizes required will be very large (Keinan & Clark, 2012), and the restricted geographic distribution of rare variants will result in a dual problem: the potential of false-positives due to fine-scale population structure (O'Connor et al., 2013; Tennessen et al., 2012), and the difficulties to replicate significant findings. Considering the abundance of rare variants in our genomes, it will be critical to develop robust methods to identify the functionally important variants. Additionally, it will be necessary to develop population-specific catalogs of rare variants (Tennessen et al., 2012).

Precision medicine initiatives in which drug treatment is adjusted based on the genetic makeup of the specific patient will be complicated by the potentially large role of rare variants. Strategies based on exome sequencing will not be optimal because they will miss potential regulatory variants located in intronic and intergenic regions. In fact, most of the signals identified in GWA studies for many different traits are located in these regions (ENCODE Project Consortium, 2012). Therefore, having complete genome data coupled to reliable functionality assessment of the variants found would be required. One of the major challenges will be the development of robust prediction algorithms that identify putative functional variants located in exons, introns, and intergenic regions. Furthermore, the functional impact of the extensive genetic variation in *all* pharmacogenes with relevance for a specific drug treatment must be considered. This implies a shift of the current paradigm of PGx-informed prescription based on genotyping a few common variants in selected genes toward comprehensive sequencing approaches coupled to correct functional assignment of the variants identified, both common and rare.

2. GLOBAL DISTRIBUTION OF PGx VARIANTS

It is well known that biogeographical ancestry is a major determinant of genomic variation, and this has been verified for PGx variants in a multiplicity of studies around the world. Here we will highlight results from recently published analyses of worldwide distribution of PGx variants, based on data from population-scale sequencing projects (Hovelson et al., 2017; Schärfe et al., 2017; Zhou, Ingelman-Sundberg, & Lauschke, 2017).

Hovelson et al. (2017) explored exome sequence data for 298 ADME genes in 1432 samples from 19 populations of the 1KG Project, plus Koreans and Japanese from the Northeast Asian Variation Analysis. A total of 8161 ADME-coding variants were identified, of which 62% were nonsynonymous and 43% of these were predicted to be functionally deleterious. There was considerable heterogeneity in frequency distribution of the nonsynonymous variants across populations: the 1KG African samples showed the highest level of variation followed by admixed Americans, Europeans, South Asians, and East Asians. As expected, populations in relatively close geographic proximity shared most common ADME variants at similar frequencies.

Zhou et al. (2017) integrated exome sequencing data from nearly 57,000 individuals provided by the ExAC, with whole genome and linkage information from the 1KG project to derive the frequency distribution of 176 haplotypes in 12 *CYP* genes, among five "aggregated superpopulations" (Europeans, Africans, East Asians, South Asians, and admixed Americans). They reported "drastic extent of genetic variability between major populations, which entail phenotypic consequences on the level of metabolic activity profiles". Importantly, there were "additional layers of genetic variability between specific subpopulations within the aggregated superpopulations," which is consistent with the pivotal study of Lewontin (1972) regarding the partition of genetic diversity in humans. Zhou et al. (2017) stressed the notion that population-specific genetic background must be taken into account for the guidance of personalized drug therapy and in the design of PGx clinical trials.

The aforementioned study of Schärfe et al. (2017) extended the analysis of the ExAC data to 178 ADME and 628 drug target genes in six aggregated populations (African, South Asian, East Asian, Finnish, non-Finnish European, and admixed American) and found that 54% of the predicted functional variants in pharmacogenes were unique to only one of these populations. The authors used a "cumulative allele probability" (CAP) statistic to assess the probability for an individual to carry at least one variant allele in a given gene and showed that 114 pharmacogenes had a CAP score above 1% in all six populations. This was taken as an indication that "there are genes with similar worldwide pharmacogenetic relevance." However, for the same CAP cutoff score, 231 and 298 pharmacogenes had functional variants in the European and African cohorts, respectively, indicating the impact of population diversity on the distribution of functional variants in drug-related genes. To estimate the extent of the effect of functional variants in all genes related to a given drug, Schärfe et al. (2017) defined a drug-specific, "drug risk probability" (DRP) score, by combining the CAP scores for all target genes. Analysis based on a cutoff point of DRP >1% for high risk showed: (i) 312 out of 1236 FDA-approved drugs were of high risk in all six ExAC populations; (ii) 11 (non-Finish Europeans) to 66 (Africans) drugs were of high risk in only one population; (iii) 11–62 drugs were at high risk in 2–5 populations. Again, these data not only point to genes or gene combinations with "similar worldwide PGx relevance" but also verify the impact of population diversity on the PGx on many drugs in clinical use.

Collectively, the studies highlighted in this section reveal multiple patterns in the worldwide distribution of PGx variants, whether common or rare, deleterious or putatively functional. A remarkable example of PGx diversity across populations is the severe, life-threatening toxicity of carbamazepine, in the form of Stevens-Johnson syndrome and toxic epidermal necrolysis, in carriers of the *HLA-B*15:02* haplotype. This haplotype has a very distinct global distribution (Leckband et al., 2013) with highest frequency in Han Chinese; it is also common in some (e.g., Singapore, Hong Kong, Malaysia, Thailand, and Vietnam), but not all, Asian countries and is absent or quite rare in African and European populations. This distribution pattern underlies the FDA recommendation that "patients with ancestry in at-risk populations should be screened for the presence of *HLA-B*15:02* allele prior to starting carbamazepine," while cautioning that it must be "bear in mind that many people may be unaware of or fail to disclose more distant Asian ancestry in their families." Of notice, "at-risk populations" in the FDA recommendation for carbamazepine are inferred from biogeographical ancestry (Leckband et al., 2013).

Partitioning human diversity into continental or subcontinental (e.g., South Asians and East Asians) aggregated populations is common practice in large-scale genomic studies, such as the aforementioned 1KG and ExAc projects, and within-group heterogeneity in individual ancestry is not always fully acknowledged. In the following sections, we will explore PGx implications of population heterogeneity, especially population admixture. Our focus will be Latin America, where a kaleidoscopic combination of individual proportions of Native American, European, and sub-Saharan African ancestries prevails among its 650 million people.

3. POPULATION ADMIXTURE IN LATIN AMERICA: PHARMACOGENOMIC IMPLICATIONS

PGx studies of Latin American populations must take into account ethnic, cultural, socioeconomic, scientific, and technological disparities, but also their diversity and genetic heterogeneity. Although Native American, European, and sub-Saharan African biogeographical ancestries are common to all Latin American countries, the relative proportions of each ancestral root vary across nations, and, most importantly within each nation. We will illustrate this diversity by contrasting Brazil and Mexico, the two most populous countries in Latin America, with over 200 million and nearly 140 million people, respectively. We present data from Brazilians self-identified as White, Brown ("pardo," in Brazilian Portuguese), and Black, according to the race/color categories adopted by the Brazilian Census and from Mexicans self-identified as Mestizo, recruited in five geographically distant regions (Bonifaz-Peña et al., 2014). All individuals were genotyped with the DMET Plus platform, which interrogates 1936 variants across 231 pharmacogenes. From this platform, we identified 71 markers with high degree of differentiation between the relevant ancestral populations, represented by Zapotecas (Native American), HapMap CEU (European), and YRI and LWK (sub-Saharan African) cohorts. The data obtained with these ancestry informative markers were analyzed with the software structure v.2.3.4 (Pritchard, Stephens, & Donnelly, 2000) to estimate the individual admixture proportions, as well as the average admixture proportions in each cohort.

Table 1 shows the *average* African, European, and Native American genetic contributions to the Brazilian and Mexican cohorts. Among Brazilians, European ancestry decreased progressively from self-reported White (0.85) to Brown (0.65) and then to Black individuals (0.38), whereas the opposite trend was observed with respect to African ancestry, which averaged 0.08, 0.25, and 0.54, respectively. The average Native American ancestry remained relatively constant (0.06–0.10) across the three groups. By contrast, in Mexico the combined Native American and European ancestry

Table 1 Biogeographical Ancestry of Brazilians and Mexicans

	Biogeographical Ancestry[a]		
Population	**Native**	**European**	**African**
Brazilian[b]			
Black	0.083	0.381	0.536
Brown	0.100	0.647	0.253
White	0.056	0.846	0.097
Mexican[c]			
Guanajuato	0.546	0.396	0.058
Guerrero	0.744	0.184	0.072
Sonora	0.256	0.701	0.043
Vera Cruz	0.674	0.281	0.045
Yucatan	0.574	0.378	0.048

[a]Average proportions of parental ancestry, based on 71 ancestry informative markers.
[b]Race/color categories of the Brazilian census.
[c]Geographical locations in Mexico.

accounted for 93%–96% of the variation in all geographical regions, while the African contribution was only 4%–7%. Of notice, there was considerable variation in ancestral contribution across the Mexican cohorts, especially between Guerrero and Sonora: the Native American and European proportions in Guerrero averaged 0.74 and 0.18, respectively, compared to 0.26 and 0.70 in Sonora.

Analyses of the *individual* proportions of biogeographical ancestry provide further insight into the complex structure of Latin American populations. The ternary plots in Fig. 1 display the wide range and, most importantly, the *continuous* variation in the individual proportions of African and European ancestry among Brazilians and of Native American and European ancestry in Mexicans. Corollaries to this pattern are: (1) there are no "cutoff points" that allow discrimination among the race/color categories of the Brazilian census, or to distinguish among the geographical origin of the Mexican cohorts; (2) *average* admixture proportions are not predictive of the corresponding proportions at the *individual* level in Brazilians and Mexicans, and most likely, other Latin American peoples. A similar situation might prevail also in admixed, non-Latin American populations: for example, in a detailed study in which genomic variation was analyzed in a large

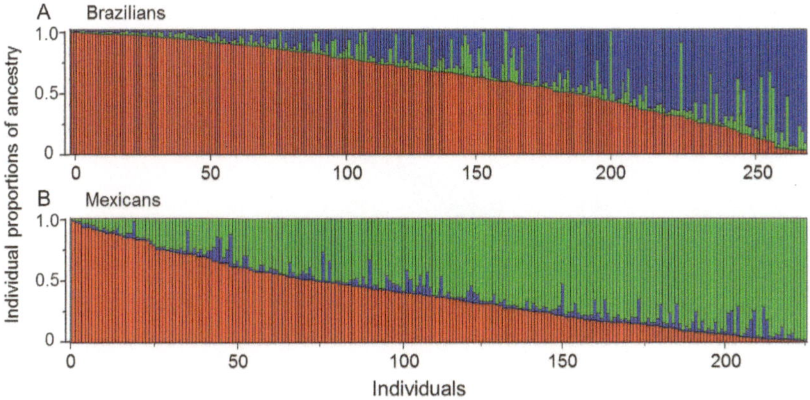

Fig. 1 Assignment of Brazilian and Mexican samples to genetic clusters inferred using a panel of ancestry informative markers and the program STRUCTURE. (A) Data from unrelated, healthy adults, from the Southeast region of Brazil, self-identified as *White* ($n = 89$), *Brown* (90), or *Black* ($n = 89$), according to the color classification adopted by the Brazilian Census. (B) Data from unrelated, healthy, Mestizo Mexicans, from five geographically distant regions. Each individual is represented by a *vertical line*, which is partitioned in three segments corresponding to the estimated membership proportion in the African (*blue*), Amerindian (*green*), and European (*red*) clusters (Bonifaz-Peña et al., 2014).

number of populations from India, the authors reported that most Indian populations have ancestry from two ancient groups, "Ancestral North Indians" and "Ancestral South Indians," and there is a broad range of ancestral proportions from these two groups across India (Reich, Thangaraj, Patterson, Price, & Singh, 2009).

Estimating admixture proportions at the population or individual level can be useful in two respects. At the individual level, ancestry proportions will determine the probability of having genotypes of PGx relevance. At the population level, knowing average admixture proportions permits to infer allele (and genotype) frequencies of relevant variants, which are useful for sample calculations in the design of PGx trials. This is illustrated in Fig. 2 using data from Brazilian and Mexicans (Bonifaz-Peña et al., 2014) for the DMET Plus biomarkers. The predicted MAF in each population was calculated using the expression (Suarez-Kurtz, Paula, & Struchiner, 2014):

Predicted $\mathrm{MAF} = (\mathrm{MAF}_{\mathrm{Zapotecas}} {}^{*} P_{\mathrm{Native\ ancestry}}) + (\mathrm{MAF}_{\mathrm{HapMap\ CEU}} {}^{*} P_{\mathrm{European\ ancestry}}) + (\mathrm{MAF}_{\mathrm{HapMap\ YRI\_LWK}} {}^{*} P_{\mathrm{African\ ancestry}})$, where P is the average proportion of each biogeographical ancestry. The correlation coefficient (R^2) between observed and predicted MAF was 0.97 in Brazilians and 0.95 in Mexicans for 936 and 866 polymorphic markers, respectively.

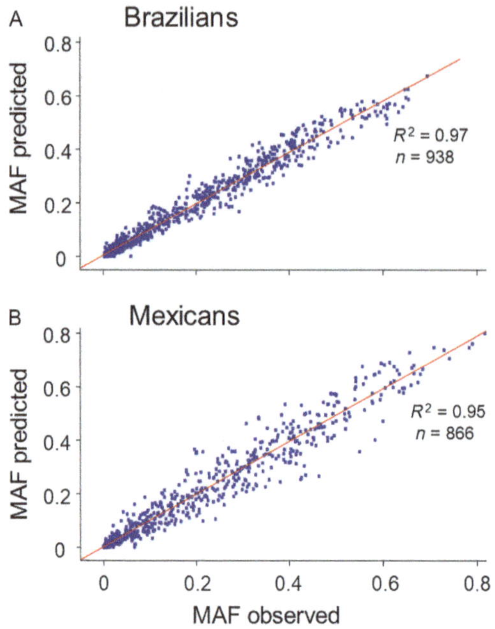

Fig. 2 Prediction of MAF of pharmacogenetic polymorphisms in Brazilians (A) and Mexicans (B). The observed MAFs (>0) are plotted against the corresponding MAFs predicted by the expression described in the text, based on average ancestry proportions and the MAF in the parental populations. *n*, number of SNPs; R^2, regression coefficient. *Original data from Bonifaz-Peña, V., Contreras, A. V., Struchiner, C. J., Roela, R. A., Furuya-Mazzotti, T. K., Chammas, R, et al. (2014). Exploring the distribution of genetic markers of pharmacogenomics relevance in Brazilian and Mexican populations.* PLoS One, *9(11), e112640.*

The F_{ST} statistic was applied to the DMET Plus data to measure the degree of genetic differentiation among Brazilians, Mexicans, and their relevant ancestral populations, represented by the Zapotecas and the HapMap CEU, YRI, and LWK samples (Bonifaz-Peña et al., 2014). The extent of PGx divergence between any two populations is denoted according to Wright's qualitative guidelines (Wright, 1951): F_{ST} values less than 0.05 represent low genetic divergence, values between 0.05 and 0.15 represent moderate divergence, values between 0.15 and 0.25 represent large divergence, and values greater than 0.25 represent very large divergence. Genetic differentiation assessed by the DMET markers was low for Brazilians vs Mexicans (average $Fst = 0.012$) and moderate for paired comparison of the ancestral populations: 0.062 (European vs Native American), 0.059 (European vs African), and 0.085 (Native American vs African). The lower F_{ST} for the

Brazilian–Mexican pair compared to the paired ancestral populations is not surprising in view of the history of admixture in Latin American countries.

Pairwise comparison among the Brazilian race/color cohorts revealed very low genetic differentiation, with average *Fst* values of 0.007 (Black vs Brown), 0.005 (Brown vs White), and 0.015 (White vs Black), consistent with the overlapping ancestry proportions among the three groups shown in Fig. 1. Indeed, comparison of the F_{ST} distribution in paired White vs Black Brazilians with the distribution in Europeans vs Africans reveals that the divergence in the PGx markers is much attenuated in the Brazilian cohorts (Fig. 3). Two distinct examples of this attenuation are *CYP3A5*3* (rs776746) and *VKORC1 3673G>A* (rs9923231), which have F_{ST} values of 0.638 and 0.174, respectively, in paired European vs African, but only 0.155 and 0.018 in paired White vs Black Brazilians. These two SNPs are major determinants of the recommendations in the Clinical Pharmacogenetics Implementation Consortium (CPIC) guidelines for tacrolimus (TAC) (Birdwell et al., 2015) and warfarin (Johnson et al., 2017), respectively, and will be used in Sections 4 and 5 to exemplify the PGx consequences of population admixture in Latin America.

4. PHARMACOGENETICS OF TAC: CYP3A5 POLYMORPHISMS

The CPIC guidelines for TAC, a widely used immunosuppressant drug after solid organ and hematopoietic stem cell transplantation, provide dosing recommendations based on *CYP3A5* phenotype, inferred from the genotypes comprising *CYP3A5*3, *6* (rs10264272), and *7 (rs413003343) SNPs, all of which are nonfunctional alleles. Because of the rarity of *CYP3A5*6* and *CYP3A5**7 in most populations, the guidelines rely mainly on data for *CYP3A5*3*. The wide range of variation in *CYP3A5*3* among the relevant ancestral populations coupled to a broad range of admixture proportions has clear implications for the implementation of the guidelines in Latin American populations. This is illustrated in the surface plot shown in Fig. 4, created by fitting nonlinear piecewise smooth logistic regression models to the CYP3A5*3 frequency and ancestry proportions data for Brazilians and Mexicans, to predict the individual odds of having the *CYP3A5*3* allele.

In addition to *CYP3A5*3*, Latin Americans may also be carriers of the *CYP3A5*6* and *7 alleles, because of their African ancestry. Indeed, in a cohort of 301 Brazilian renal transplant patients, these alleles had frequencies of 2.8% and 2.3%, respectively, while CYP3A5*3 frequency was 72.8% (Santoro et al., 2011). The combined impact of the *CYP3A5*3, *6,* and *7

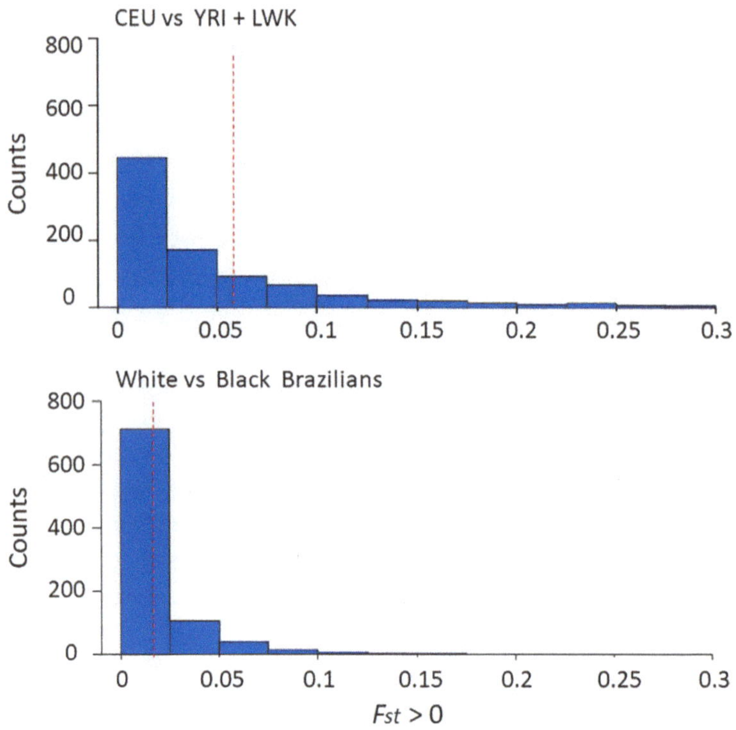

Fig. 3 Distribution of F_{ST} values. Pairwise comparisons for the proxy ancestral European vs African populations and for White vs Black Brazilians. The *dashed vertical lines* correspond to the average *Fst* values. *Original data from Bonifaz-Peña, V., Contreras, A. V., Struchiner, C. J., Roela, R. A., Furuya-Mazzotti, T. K., Chammas, R, et al. (2014). Exploring the distribution of genetic markers of pharmacogenomics relevance in Brazilian and Mexican populations.* PLoS One, *9(11), e112640.*

variant alleles on the daily TAC dose, adjusted to the trough drug concentration in plasma (TAC C_0/dose), revealed a highly significant association ($P < 0.0001$) between the TAC C_0/dose and the number of variant alleles, with increasingly negative regression coefficients as the number of defective alleles decrease from two to one and to zero. This is consistent with the inferred CYP3A5 activity phenotype: as the number of the defective *CYP3A5*3, *6,* and **7* alleles decreases, CYP3A5-mediated TAC clearance increases, requiring higher TAC doses to reach the target C_0 blood levels. This, in turn, leads to lower TAC C_0/dose values.

Association between the *CYP3A5*3* SNP and TAC pharmacokinetics had been previously reported in various populations. However, the study of Santoro et al. (2011) disclosed two novel and important findings: first,

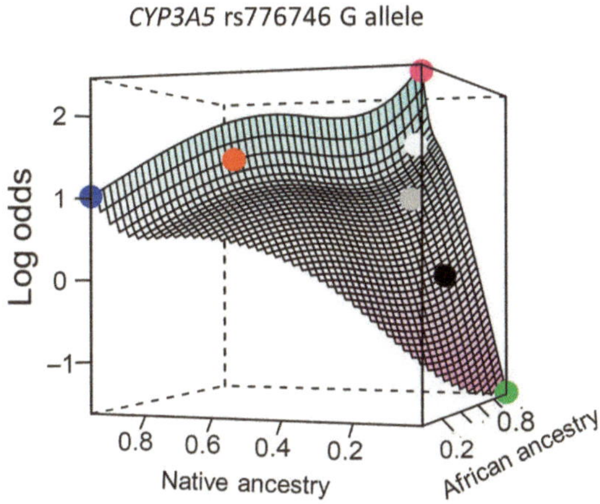

Fig. 4 Surface plot describing the predicted relationship between the distribution of rs776746 (*CYP3A5**3) and parental ancestry, obtained by fitting piecewise smooth logistic regression models to the 268 Brazilians and 224 Mexicans data obtained with DMET Plus array. The plotted surfaces correspond to the natural logarithm of the odds of having the variant rs776746A allele, according to the relative admixture proportions of the parental populations. The *circles* correspond to the average ancestral proportions for Black Brazilians (*black circle*), Brown Brazilians (*gray*), White Brazilians (*white*), Mexicans (*red*), EUR (*purple*), AFR (*green*), and NAT (*blue*). *Original data from Bonifaz-Peña, V., Contreras, A. V., Struchiner, C. J., Roela, R. A., Furuya-Mazzotti, T. K., Chammas, R, et al. (2014). Exploring the distribution of genetic markers of pharmacogenomics relevance in Brazilian and Mexican populations.* PLoS One, *9(11), e112640.*

it extended the PGx association between *CYP3A5* and TAC dose requirement to two other nonfunctional *CYP3A5* alleles, namely, *CYP3A5*6* and *CYP3A5*7* which are common in populations of African descent. A clinically relevant implication is that inference of CYP3A5 metabolic activity in these populations requires genotyping for *CYP3A5*6* and *CYP3A5*7*, in addition to *CYP3A5*3*. Second, the study included patients with the *CYP3A5**1/*1 genotype, which is rare or absent in populations of European or Asian descent, providing the first demonstration of a gene-dose effect of *CYP3A5* polymorphisms on TAC pharmacokinetics.

5. POPULATION DIVERSITY AND WARFARIN DOSING ALGORITHMS

The widely used anticoagulant warfarin combines several characteristics, including a large interindividual variation in dose requirement, that makes it a model case for clinical implementation of PGx. Guidelines for

PGx-guided warfarin dosing were among the first to be published by CPIC and were recently updated (Johnson et al., 2017). The major PGx variables in these guidelines are *CYP2C9* and *VKORC1* polymorphisms, which have been identified in a number of GWAS studies in various populations, including Brazilians (Cha et al., 2011; Cooper et al., 2008; Parra et al., 2015; Takeuchi et al., 2009). Notably, the updated CPIC guideline incorporates distinct recommendations for self-specified continental ancestry, namely, African vs non-African ancestry in adult patients and European vs non-European ancestry in pediatric patients. The guideline recommends that PGx warfarin dosing be accomplished through the Gage (Gage et al., 2008) and IWPC algorithms (International Warfarin Pharmacogenetics Consortium et al., 2009). Both algorithms contain race/color terms, such as White, Asian, Black or African American, Missing, or Mixed Race, which do not capture the heterogeneity of admixed Latin American populations. As illustrated in Fig. 1, most Latin American individuals share Native American, European, and sub-Saharan African ancestry in variable proportions (Bonifaz-Peña et al., 2014; Galanter et al., 2012; Pena et al., 2011; Silva-Zolezzi et al., 2009; Suarez-Kurtz & Pena, 2007). The continuous variation in the individual contribution of these ancestral roots coupled to the tenuous correlation between skin color and biogeographical ancestry (Pena et al., 2011; Suarez-Kurtz & Pena, 2007) are, in our view, major limitations for the implementation of the CPIC recommended warfarin dosing algorithms in Latin American patients.

Nevertheless, Cavallari et al. (2011) studied 50 patients of "Hispanic ethnicity," the majority (89%) of Mexican descent, and concluded that the IWPC and Gage algorithms "derived from mostly non-Hispanic cohorts appear to perform similarly in U.S. Hispanics." However, this was not verified in other Latin American populations, and studies in Brazilian and Puerto Rican patients led to the development of autochthonous PGx dosing algorithms (Botton, Bandinelli, Rohde, Amon, & Hutz, 2011; Duconge et al., 2016; Duconge & Ruaño, 2016; Perini et al., 2008; Santos et al., 2015). The *VKORC1* 3673G>A SNP (or a linked allele) and *CYP2C9* polymorphisms are the major PGx variables in all these algorithms, which are consistent with the outcome of our GWAS study combining Brazilian patients from different institutions (Parra et al., 2015). The PGx algorithms derived by Suarez-Kurtz and colleagues from an admixed cohort of 390 patients performed equally well in self-reported White and Black patients (Perini et al., 2008). One of these algorithms ("Perini algorithm," Perini et al., 2008), when tested in patients from other Brazilian institutions, confirmed its predictive power in an admixed cohort (Santos et al., 2015), but was less effective in patients of exclusive European descent (Botton et al., 2011). The similar performance of this algorithm in self-reported White and Black individuals contrasts markedly with the considerably poorer predictive power of the IWPC and Gage algorithms in African or Black patients compared to European or White patients (Gage et al., 2008; International Warfarin Pharmacogenetics Consortium et al., 2009). Importantly, the covariates in these algorithms differ from the Perini algorithm (Perini et al., 2008) by the inclusion of "race" terms. The fact that despite inclusion of race terms, both algorithms perform poorly in African/Black patients, supports the notion that the complexity of human diversity cannot be simply "adjusted" by numerical coefficients (Suarez-Kurtz & Botton, 2015). Rather, the similar performance of the dosing algorithm in White and Black Brazilians can be explained by the much attenuated difference in MAF of the *VKORC1 3673* SNP (and of *CYP2C9* defective alleles, *2 and *3) between White and Black Brazilians, compared to the European and African HapMap populations, as shown by the F_{ST} statistics (see above). This interpretation is supported by an analysis of the impact of the high level of geographical differentiation of *VKORC1* 3673G>A on the predictive power of the IWPC algorithm (Limdi et al., 2010): although the percentage of variation in warfarin dose explained by *VKORC1* 3673G>A differed substantially across the IWPC populations, possession of the risk allele was associated with similar decreases in individual warfarin dose requirements, irrespective of population (Limdi et al., 2010). In other words, the effect of the risk allele was similar in the different cohorts (e.g., the risk allele changes by a similar amount the required warfarin dose); however, at the population level, the variation in warfarin dose explained by the polymorphism is different, because this depends not only on allele effect but also on allele frequency.

An attempt to incorporate metrics of individual admixture into PGx dosing algorithms was recently reported for Caribbean Hispanics (Duconge et al., 2016). Based on cluster analysis of ancestry informative markers using the STRUCTURE software, a *categorical* admixture index was attributed to "individuals not clearly positioned toward any cluster or vertex of the STRUCTURE triangle plot, but rather located in the middle of the triangle"; individuals distributed in the proximity to each triangle vertex were labeled Europeans, Native Americans, or African ancestry. These categorical variables were incorporated into an "admixture-adjusted" PGx model, which explained more than two-third of the variance in warfarin stable dose in the study cohort, outperforming other clinical and PGx algorithms. The authors noted that theirs was the first PGx study to include a measure of admixture in warfarin dose predictions (Duconge et al., 2016; Duconge & Ruaño, 2016). While agreeing with this statement and also favoring the notion of incorporating admixture variable(s) in warfarin dosing algorithms for Latin American patients, we would argue that a categorical variable does not represent appropriately the complex pattern of admixture among Latin Americans.

6. CONCLUSION

A mi edad y con tantas sangres cruzadas, ya no sé a ciencia cierta de dónde soy... Nadie lo sabe por estos reinos y creo que necesitarán siglos para saberlo (Garcia Márquez, 1994; free translation: At my age and with so much mixed blood, I do not know for sure from where I come .... Nobody knows in these kingdoms and I believe that it will take centuries to learn).

PGx conceptual development and praxis remain contingent upon a better understanding of human genomic diversity and its impact on drug pharmacokinetics and pharmacodynamics. Recognition of population diversity in drug response is relevant to establishment of public health policies, design, and interpretation of clinical trials, implementation of PGx-informed prescription, and identification of drugs with selective or distinct effects in specific populations. This latter aspect is dramatically exemplified by the risk of carbamazepine-induced severe, often fatal toxicity in some Asian populations, which can be avoided by preemptive PGx testing. However, personalized drug therapy, the original promise of PGx, must be based on the recognition of the inherent genetic individuality. This notion is particularly relevant to admixed populations, in which substructure increases further the fluidity of racial/ethnic labels. Because interethnic admixture is either common or increasing at a fast pace in many, if not most populations, extrapolation on a global scale of PGx data from well-defined ethnic groups is plagued with uncertainty. To impact positively on global health, PGx must broaden its scope, with respect to both target and population diversity, and be inclusive of admixed populations with their perceived challenges and advantages. This goal is not likely to be achieved simply by mandates to include subjects from ethnic minorities in clinical drug trials, especially when these groups are represented in relatively small numbers and are labeled by phenotypes which do not accurately reflect genetic ancestry (Suarez-Kurtz, 2007).

ACKNOWLEDGMENTS

We thank Prof. Claudio J. Struchiner for kindly providing the plot shown in Fig. 4 G.S.-K. is funded by Conselho Nacional de Desenvolvimento Científico e Tecnológico (CNPq), Fundação de Amparo à Pesquisa do Estado do Rio de Janeiro (Faperj), and Departamento de Ciência e Teconologia (DECIT)/Ministério da Saúde/Brazil. E.J.P. has received funding from the Canadian Institutes of Health Research (CIHR), the Natural Sciences and Engineering Research Council of Canada (NSERC), the Canada Foundation for Innovation (CFI), the Ontario Innovation Trust (OIT), and the Government of Ontario Early Research Award (ERA).

CONFLICT OF INTEREST

None to declare.

REFERENCES

Barreiro, L. B., Laval, G., Quach, H., Patin, E., & Quintana-Murci, L. (2008). Natural selection has driven population differentiation in modern humans. *Nature Genetics*, *40*, 340–345.

Birdwell, K. A., Decker, B., Barbarino, J. M., Peterson, J. F., Stein, C. M., Sadee, W., et al. (2015). Clinical pharmacogenetics implementation consortium (CPIC) guidelines for CYP3A5 genotype and tacrolimus dosing. *Clinical Pharmacology and Therapeutics*, *98*, 19–24.

Bonifaz-Peña, V., Contreras, A. V., Struchiner, C. J., Roela, R. A., Furuya-Mazzotti, T. K., Chammas, R., et al. (2014). Exploring the distribution of genetic markers of pharmacogenomics relevance in Brazilian and Mexican populations. *PLoS One*, *9*(11), e112640.

Botton, M. R., Bandinelli, E., Rohde, L. E., Amon, L. C., & Hutz, M. H. (2011). Influence of genetic, biological, and pharmacological factors on warfarin dose in a southern Brazilian population of european ancestry. *British Journal of Clinical Pharmacology*, *72*, 442–450.

Cavallari, L. H., Momary, K. M., Patel, S. R., Shapiro, N. L., Nutescu, E., & Viana, M. A. (2011). Pharmacogenomics of warfarin dose requirements in hispanics. *Blood Cells, Molecules & Diseases*, *46*, 147–150.

Cha, P. C., Mushiroda, T., Takahashi, A., et al. (2011). Genome-wide association study identifies genetic determinants of warfarin responsiveness for japanese. *Human Molecular Genetics*, *19*, 4735–4744.

Chen, J., Teo, Y. Y., Toh, D. S. L., & Sung, C. (2010). Interethnic comparisons of important pharmacology genes using SNP databases: Potential application to drug regulatory assessments. *Pharmacogenomics*, *11*, 1077–1094.

Cooper, G. M., Johnson, J. A., Langaee, T. Y., Feng, H., Stanaway, I. B., Schwarz, U. I., et al. (2008). A genome-wide scan for common genetic variants with a large influence on warfarin maintenance dose. *Blood*, *112*, 1022–1027.

Duconge, J., Ramos, A. S., Claudio-Campos, K., Rivera-Miranda, G., Bermúdez-Bosch, L., Renta, J. Y., et al. (2016). A novel admixture-based pharmacogenetic approach to refine warfarin dosing in caribbean hispanics. *PLoS One*, *11*(1), e0145480.

Duconge, J., & Ruaño, G. (2016). Admixture and ethno-specific alleles: Missing links for global pharmacogenomics. *Pharmacogenomics*, *17*, 1479–1482.

ENCODE Project Consortium. (2012). An integrated encyclopedia of DNA elements in the human genome. *Nature*, *489*, 57–74.

Franceschini, N., van Rooij, F. J., Prins, B. P., Feitosa, M. F., Karakas, M., Eckfeldt, J. H., et al. (2012). Discovery and fine mapping of serum protein loci through transethnic meta-analysis. *American Journal of Human Genetics*, *5*, 744–753.

Fu, W., O'Connor, T. D., Jun, G., Kang, H. M., Abecasis, G., Leal, S. M., et al. (2013). Analysis of 6,515 exomes reveals the recent origin of mosthuman protein-coding variants. *Nature, 493*, 216–220.

Gage, B. F., Eby, C., Johnson, J. A., Deych, E., Rieder, M. J., Ridker, P. M., et al. (2008). Use of pharmacogenetic and clinical factors to predict the therapeutic dose of warfarin. *Clinical Pharmacology and Therapeutics, 84*, 326–331.

Galanter, J. M., Fernandez-Lopez, J. C., Gignoux, C. R., Barnholtz-Sloan, J., Fernandez-Rozadilla, C., et al. (2012). Development of a panel of genome-wide ancestry informative markers to study admixture throughout the Americas. *PLoS Genetics, 8*(3), e1002554.

Garcia Márquez, G. (1994). *Del amor y otros demonios*. Bogota, Colombia: Alfred A. Knopf.

Hovelson, D. H., Xue, Z., Zawistowski, M., Ehm, M. G., Harris, E. C., Stocker, S. L., et al. (2017). Characterization of ADME gene variation in 21 populations by exome sequencing. *Pharmacogenetics and Genomics, 27*, 89–100.

IGSR: International Genome Sample Resource. http://www.internationalgenome.org/home.

International Warfarin Pharmacogenetics Consortium, Klein, T. E., Altman, R. B., Eriksson, N., Gage, B. F., Kimmel, S. E., et al. (2009). Estimation of the warfarin dose with clinical and pharmacogenetic data. *The New England Journal of Medicine, 360*(8), 753–764.

Jakobsson, M., Scholz, S. W., Scheet, P., Gibbs, J. R., VanLiere, J. M., Fung, H. C., et al. (2008). Genotype, haplotype, and copy-number variation in worldwide human populations. *Nature, 451*, 998–1003.

Johnson, J. A., Caudle, K. E., Gong, L., Whirl-Carrillo, M., Stein, C. M., Scott, A. S., et al. (2017). Clinical pharmacogenetics implementation consortium (CPIC) guideline for pharmacogenetics-guided warfarin dosing: 2017 update. *Clinical Pharmacology and Therapeutics, 102*, 397–404.

Keinan, A., & Clark, A. G. (2012). Recent explosive human population growth has resulted in an excess of rare genetic variants. *Science, 336*, 740–743.

Koboldt, D. C., Steinberg, K. M., Larson, D. E., Wilson, R. K., & Mardis, E. R. (2013). The next-generation sequencing revolution and its impact on genomics. *Cell, 155*, 27–38.

Kozyra, M., Ingelman-Sundberg, M., & Lauschke, V. M. (2017). Rare genetic variants in cellular transporters, metabolic enzymes, and nuclear receptors can be importante determinants of interindividual differences in drug response. *Genetics in Medicine, 19*, 20–29.

Leckband, S. G., Kelsoe, J. R., Dunnenberger, H. M., George, A. L., Jr., Tran, E., Berger, R., et al. (2013). Clinical pharmacogenetics implementation consortium guidelines for HLA-B genotype and carbamazepine dosing. *Clinical Pharmacology and Therapeutics, 94*, 324–328.

Lek, M., Karczewski, K. J., Minikel, E. V., Samocha, K. E., Banks, E., Fennell, T., et al. (2016). Analysis of protein-coding genetic variation in 60,706 humans. *Nature, 536*, 285–291.

Lewontin, R. C. (1972). The apportionment of human diversity. *Evolutionary Biology, 6*, 381–398.

Li, J. Z., Absher, D. M., Tang, H., Southwick, A. M., Casto, A. M., Ramachandran, S., et al. (2008). Worldwide human relationships inferred from genome-wide patterns of variation. *Science, 319*, 1100–1104.

Limdi, N. A., Wadelius, M., Cavallari, L., Eriksson, N., Crawford, D. C., Lee, M. T., et al. (2010). Warfarin pharmacogenetics: A single VKORC1 polymorphism is predictive of dose across 3 racial groups. *Blood, 115*, 3827–3834.

Liu, C. T., Raghavan, S., Maruthur, N., Kabagambe, E. K., Hong, J., Ng, M. C., et al. (2016). Trans-ethnic meta-analysis and functional annotation illuminates the genetic architecture of fasting glucose and insulin. *American Journal of Human Genetics, 99*, 56–75.

Nelson, M. R., Wegmann, D., Ehm, M. G., Kessner, D., St Jean, P., & Verzilli, C. (2012). An abundance of rare functional variants in 202 drug target genes sequenced in 14,002 people. *Science*, *337*, 100–104.

O'Connor, T. D., Kiezun, A., Bamshad, M., Rich, S. S., Smith, J. D., & Turner, E. (2013). Fine-scale patterns of population stratification confound rare variant association tests. *PLoS One*, *8*, e65834.

Parra, E. J., Botton, M. R., Perini, J. A., Krithika, S., Bourgeois, S., Johnson, T. A., et al. (2015). Genome-wide association study of warfarin maintenance dose in a Brazilian sample. *Pharmacogenomics*, *16*(11), 1253–1263.

Parra, E. J., & Suarez-Kurtz, G. (2014). Demographic history and human genetic diversity: Pharmacogenomic implications. *Pharmacogenomics*, *15*, 253–256.

Pena, S. D., Di Pietro, G., Fuchshuber-Moraes, M., Genro, J. P., Hutz, M. H., et al. (2011). The genomic ancestry of individuals from different geographical regions of brazil is more uniform than expected. *PLoS One*, *6*, e17063.

Perera, M. A., Cavallari, L. H., Limdi, N. A., Gamazon, E. R., Konkashbaev, A., Daneshjou, R., et al. (2013). Genetic variants associated with warfarin dose in african-american individuals: A genome-wide association study. *Lancet*, *382*, 790–796.

Perini, J. A., Struchiner, C. J., Silva-Assunção, E., Santana, I. S., Rangel, F., Ojopi, E. B., et al. (2008). Pharmacogenetics of warfarin: Development of a dosing algorithm for Brazilian patients. *Clinical Pharmacology and Therapeutics*, *84*, 722–728.

Popejoy, A. B., & Fullerton, S. M. (2016). Genomics is failing on diversity. *Nature*, *538*, 161–164.

Pritchard, J. K., Stephens, M., & Donnelly, P. (2000). Inference of population structure using multilocus genotype data. *Genetics*, *155*, 945–959.

Reich, D., Thangaraj, K., Patterson, N., Price, A. L., & Singh, L. (2009). Reconstructing Indian population history. *Nature*, *461*, 489–494.

Ross, K. A., Bigham, A. W., Edwards, M., Gozdzik, A., Suarez-Kurtz, G., & Parra, E. J. (2010). Worldwide allele frequency distribution of four polymorphisms associated with warfarin dose requirements. *Journal of Human Genetics*, *55*, 582–589.

Santoro, A., Felipe, C. R., Tedesco-Silva, H., Medina-Pestana, J. O., Struchiner, C. J., Ojopi, E. B., et al. (2011). Pharmacogenetics of calcineurin inhibitors in Brazilian renal transplant patients. *Pharmacogenomics*, *12*, 1293–1303.

Santos, P. C., Marcatto, L. R., Duarte, N. E., Gadi Soares, R. A., Cassaro Strunz, C. M., Scanavacca, M., et al. (2015). Development of a pharmacogenetic-based warfarin dosing algorithm and its performance in Brazilian patients: Highlighting the importance of population-specific calibration. *Pharmacogenomics*, *16*, 865–876.

Schärfe, C. P. I., Tremmel, R., Schwab, M., Kohlbacher, O., & Marks, D. S. (2017). Genetic variation in human drug-related genes. *Genome Medicine*, *9*(1), 117.

Silva-Zolezzi, I., Hidalgo-Miranda, A., Estrada-Gil, J., Fernandez-Lopez, J. C., Uribe-Figueroa, L., et al. (2009). Analysis of genomic diversity in Mexican mestizo populations to develop genomic medicine in Mexico. *Proceedings of the National Academy of Sciences of the United States of America*, *106*, 8611–8616.

Suarez-Kurtz, G. (2007). Synopsis and perspectives. In G. Suarez-Kurtz (Ed.), *Pharmacogenomics in admixed population* (pp. 75–98). Austin, TX: Landes Bioscience.

Suarez-Kurtz, G., & Botton, M. R. (2015). Pharmacogenetics of coumarin anticoagulants in Brazilians. *Expert Opinion on Drug Metabolism & Toxicology*, *11*, 67–79.

Suarez-Kurtz, G., Paula, D. P., & Struchiner, C. J. (2014). Pharmacogenomic implications of population admixture: Brazil as a model case. *Pharmacogenomics*, *15*, 209–219.

Suarez-Kurtz, G., & Pena, S. D. (2007). Pharmacogeneomic studies in the Brazilian population. In G. Suarez-Kurtz (Ed.), *Pharmacogenomics in admixed population* (pp. 75–98). Austin, TX: Landes Bioscience.

Takeuchi, F., McGinnis, R., Bourgeois, S., Barnes, C., Eriksson, N., Soranzo, N., et al. (2009). A genome-wide association study confirms *VKORC1*, *CYP2C9*, and *CYP4F2* as principal genetic determinants of warfarin dose. *PLoS Genetics*, *5*, e1000433.

Tennessen, J. A., Bigham, A. W., O'Connor, T. D., Fu, W., Kenny, E. E., Gravel, S., et al. (2012). Evolution and functional impact of rare coding variation from deep sequencing of human exomes. *Science*, *337*, 64–69.

van Rooij, F. J., Qayyum, R., Smith, A. V., Zhou, Y., Trompet, S., Tanaka, T., et al. (2017). Genome-wide trans-ethnic meta-analysis identifies seven genetic loci influencing erythrocyte traits and a role for RBPMS in erythropoiesis. *American Journal of Human Genetics*, *100*, 51–63.

Wright, S. (1951). The genetic structure of populations. *Annals of Eugenics*, *15*, 323–354.

Zhou, Y., Ingelman-Sundberg, M., & Lauschke, V. M. (2017). Worldwide distribution of cytochrome P450 alleles: A meta-analysis of population-scale sequencing projects. *Clinical Pharmacology and Therapeutics*, *102*, 688–700.

CHAPTER SEVEN

Pharmacogenetics of Adverse Drug Reactions

Orod Osanlou*, Munir Pirmohamed*, Ann K. Daly[†,1]
*Department of Molecular and Clinical Pharmacology, The University of Liverpool, Liverpool, United Kingdom
[†]Institute of Cellular Medicine, Newcastle University, Medical School, Newcastle upon Tyne, United Kingdom
[1]Corresponding author: e-mail address: a.k.daly@ncl.ac.uk

Contents

1. Introduction 156
 1.1 Adverse Drug Reactions 156
 1.2 Pharmacogenetics 157
 1.3 Drug Labels 159
2. Genetic Predisposition to Type A ADRs 161
3. Genetic Predisposition to Type B ADRs 165
 3.1 HLA Associations 165
 3.2 Non-HLA Genetic Risk Factors for ADRs 173
4. Current Examples of Genetic Testing to Prevent ADRs 179
5. Future Prospects 180
6. Conclusion 181
References 182

Abstract

Adverse drug reactions (ADRs) are an important cause of morbidity and mortality. Genetic factors predispose to many ADRs, affecting susceptibility to both type A and type B reactions. The overall contribution of genetics will vary according to drug and ADR, and should be considered when attempting to predict and prevent ADRs. Genetic risk factors are considered in detail for a number of type A ADRs, especially those relating to warfarin and thiopurines, and type B ADRs affecting skin, the liver, and the heart. As the availability of whole genome sequencing increases, it is likely that prospective genotype for particular ADRs prior to drug prescription will become more common in the future. Current examples of genetic testing to prevent ADRs which have already been implemented and future prospects for developments in the field are discussed in detail.

Advances in Pharmacology, Volume 83
ISSN 1054-3589
https://doi.org/10.1016/bs.apha.2018.03.002

ABBREVIATIONS

ADR adverse drug reaction
cLQTS congenital long QT syndrome
CYP cytochrome P450
DILI drug-induced liver injury
diLQTS drug-induced long QT syndrome
GWAS genome-wide association study
HIV human immunodeficiency virus
HLA human leukocyte antigen
LQTS long QT syndrome
MHRA medicines and healthcare products regulatory agency
PI package insert
PIL patient information leaflet
SCAR severe cutaneous adverse reaction
SJS Stevens–Johnson syndrome
SmPc summary of product characteristics
SNP single-nucleotide polymorphism
TEN toxic epidermal necrolysis
TdP torsades de pointes
TPMT thiopurine methyltransferase
VKORC1 vitamin K epoxide reductase complex 1
WHO World Health Organization

1. INTRODUCTION

1.1 Adverse Drug Reactions

For thousands of years, humans have been harnessing the power of nature for their medicinal properties. In the 11th century, Avicenna, a Persian physician, described over 800 drugs of herbal, mineral, or animal origin in the "Canon of Medicine," a primary textbook used by physicians for over 600 years (Buranova, 2015; Moosavi, 2009). Paracelsus, a Swiss alchemist and one of the fathers of toxicology, looked at the harm that these drugs can cause and is quoted as stating "Solely the dose determines that something is not a poison." In other words, all drugs are poisonous, but it is the dose that makes it a poison (Borzelleca, 2000). An example is digitalis, known to cause cardiac toxicity and sudden cardiac death in overdose, but widely used at low dose in the form of digoxin to treat cardiac arrhythmias. Unintended harms such as this are known as adverse drug reactions (ADRs). The World Health Organization (WHO) defines an ADR as:

> *A response to a drug which is noxious and unintended, and which occurs at doses normally used in man for the prophylaxis, diagnosis, or therapy of disease, or for the modifications of physiological function*
>
> ***WHO (2009)***

ADRs came to prominence in the unfortunate thalidomide scandal of the 1960s. Marketed as an antiemetic in pregnancy, and available over the counter, thalidomide resulted in serious teratogenic effects including phocomelia and death that affected thousands of babies. Out of this, in the United Kingdom, the yellow card system of pharmacovigilance was born (Routledge, 1998). Despite significant progress in pharmacovigilance, up to 6.5% of acute hospital admissions are still related to ADRs (Pirmohamed et al., 2004).

Some ADRs are extensions of wanted pharmacological effects, but others are less predictable. They can be broadly categorized into being type A or intrinsic, and type B or idiosyncratic. Type A reactions are those which can readily be predicted from the pharmacology of the drug. These are usually dose-related toxicities and are often identified prior to a drug being licensed. An example is bleeding from warfarin. Type A reactions are responsible for the majority of ADRs. Conversely, type B reactions cannot be predicted easily by the known pharmacology of the drug. There is no clear dose relationship and they are poorly reproduced in animal models. They are less common but can carry high morbidity and mortality. Type B reactions often have an immunological or genetic pathophysiology (Edwards & Aronson, 2000). Due to the nature of type B reactions, and that by the time a drug is licensed, it has only been used on approximately 3000 patients (Alomar, 2014), type B ADRs are often only identified in post-marketing pharmacovigilance. Troglitazone, a drug marketed for use in type II diabetes mellitus, is an example of a drug withdrawn after post-marketing studies identified drug-induced liver injury (DILI) as a serious type B ADR (Henney, 2000). DILI will be considered in more detail later (see Section 3.1.2). As well as reducing harm, being able to predict susceptibility to type B ADRs such as this could potentially save the industry money and help avoid waste of time and resources into drugs that have unacceptable side effect profiles and will eventually be withdrawn.

1.2 Pharmacogenetics

In the 6th century BC, Pythagoras noted that certain individuals suffered a serious adverse reaction to fava beans. It is now known that these individuals show variation in the glucose-6 phosphate dehydrogenase (*G6PDH*) gene; the resulting deficiency in the G6PDH enzyme can induce a fatal hemolytic anemia in affected individuals who eat fava beans (Meletis & Konstantopoulos, 2010). Following the discovery of different perceptions of taste in people following treatment with phenylthiocarbamide in 1959,

German physician Friedrich Vogel coined the term pharmacogenetics (Vogel, 1959). Pharmacogenetics can be described as the study of how genetic variation affects individuals' response to drugs. More recently, the term pharmacogenomics has been introduced. This usually encompasses a wider scope of all genes that are implicated in drug responses. These terms, however, are often used interchangeably (Pirmohamed, 2001).

Candidate gene studies focus on a specific disease and review the association of preselected genes with a specific phenotype. A candidate gene is first selected and then specific single-nucleotide polymorphisms (SNPs) are identified. SNPs are single base pair changes in DNA that occur at a high frequency and are the most common form of genetic variation in the human genome (Bush & Moore, 2012). If a particular allele or SNP is encountered with greater frequency in affected individuals than in unaffected individuals, this provides an association for the candidate gene to that disease outcome. They are relatively quick and inexpensive to perform but rely on some degree of prior knowledge and insight into the disease process and genetic function in question (Kwon & Goate, 2000; Patnala, Clements, & Batra, 2013). There has been some criticism that candidate gene studies have been difficult to reproduce, particularly for pharmacogenetic markers, with small sample sizes and poor phenotyping being among reasons cited that many have stayed in the discovery phase (Pirmohamed, 2014). This type of genetic association study, however, has also had many successes, with notable examples including the discovery of the thiopurine methyltransferase (TPMT) genotype and risk of bone marrow suppression with mercaptopurines (see Section 2) and abacavir hypersensitivity (see Section 3.1.1).

With the advent of the human genome project, genome-wide association studies (GWAS) have become more prominent. GWAS can assess up to 1 million or more SNPs simultaneously. Analyzing DNA sequence variation can allow specific SNPs to be linked with specific phenotypes including diseases (Bush & Moore, 2012). Over the last decade or so, this has resulted in the identification of many variants predisposing to complex diseases. This is also true of ADRs, where both type A and type B ADRs have been investigated with GWAS leading to the identification of novel predisposing loci (beyond those already discovered through candidate gene studies). A major issue with pharmacogenomic GWAS is that large sample sizes are difficult to attain (unlike the situation with complex diseases), which has meant drug response phenotypes represent less than 5% of all GWAS undertaken. Despite this, interestingly, the effect size with pharmacogenomic phenotypes is significantly greater than that seen with complex diseases, and hence it has been possible to identify novel associations using small sample sizes. For example, GWAS using 51 cases of flucloxacillin-associated DILI and 43 cases of carbamazepine-induced maculoapapular exanthema have identified associations with *HLA-B*57:01* and *HLA-A*31:01*, respectively (Daly et al., 2009; McCormack et al., 2011).

1.3 Drug Labels

In 2009, the European Commission released a guideline on the summary of product characteristics (SmPC) (Guideline on summary of product characteristics (SmPC), 2009). It detailed that all available relevant pharmacogenetic information should be included in the SmPC. This includes the risks and benefits of particular genotypes or phenotypes. An example SmPC for warfarin can be found in Fig. 1.

In 2015, Ehmann et al. performed a review of all 517 medicinal products approved for use in the European Union by the European Medicines Agency (EMA) from 1995 to 2014 (Ehmann et al., 2015). They found that almost 15% of medicines contained pharmacogenetic information that directly impacted treatment in their SmPC. The majority of these are listed as "antineoplastic and immunomodulatory agents." Oncological treatments are increasingly targeting somatic mutations in tumors as opposed to hereditary ones, as these are often significant in driving the growth of the cancer and this area is outside the scope of this chapter. However, nononcological treatments also feature pharmacogenetic information in their SmPC. For example, the nucleoside reverse transcriptase inhibitor abacavir used in the treatment of human immunodeficiency virus (HIV) is generally well tolerated but causes a severe hypersensitivity reaction in 4%–8% of patients. This reaction, which can potentially be lethal, is more common in individuals with the *HLA-B*57:01* allele (see Section 3.1.1) (Hughes et al., 2004). The mandatory requirements for testing of individuals for the *HLA-B*57:01* allele can be found in the SmPC and in the patient information leaflet (PIL) which are freely available online (MHRA, 2017). As this information came to light after postauthorization studies, this resulted in an update to the SmPC and PIL. Pharmacogenetic information listed in package inserts (PIs) internationally has also been reviewed, with specific reference to the United States, United Kingdom, and Japan. Of 118 PIs reviewed, 29 provided information on drug targets and 69 on metabolic pathways, demonstrating a high proportion that provided pharmacogenetic data (Shimazawa & Ikeda, 2013). Genetic biomarkers were described in 44 PIs from Japan compared to 71 from the

Summary of product characteristics

1 Name of the medicinal product

Marevan 3 mg tablets

Warfarin 3 mg tablets

2 Qualitative and quantitative composition

Each tablet contains 3 mg warfarin sodium BP
Excipients with known effect:
Lactose: contains 94.500 mg lactose per tablet
For the full list of excipients, see Section 6.1.

3 Pharmaceutical form

Tablet

Blue coloured, flat, circular, bevel-edged uncoated tablets having "M" breakline "3" on one side and plain on other side.

4 Clinical particulars

Genetic information

Genetic variability particularly in relation to CYP2C9 and VKORC1 can significantly affect dose requirements for warfarin. If a family association with these polymorphisms is known extra care is warranted.

Patients with rare hereditary problems of galactose intolerance, the Lapp lactase deficiency, or glucose–galactose malabsorption should not take this medicine.

Fig. 1 Summary of selected product characteristics for warfarin taken from the current UK version (MHRA, 2016).

United Kingdom. This shows that there is intercountry variability in the amount of pharmacogenetic information included by various regulatory bodies. Differences in ethnicity, social cultures, medical practice, dosing regimens, and indication are among the factors that may influence this (Shah & Shah, 2013). However, it is interesting to note that Ehmann et al. have found that the amount of pharmacogenetic information appearing in SmPCs and PILs is increasing and is likely to increase further in the future (Ehmann et al., 2015). This is vital for pharmacovigilance to be able to identify type A and type B ADRs.

2. GENETIC PREDISPOSITION TO TYPE A ADRs

To understand factors determining genetic predisposition to ADRs, it is important to bear in mind the elimination pathways of a drug. Drugs and their active metabolites can either be eliminated from the body unchanged or through biotransformation as metabolites with a higher elimination rate. The liver is the primary site of this biotransformation, with the kidneys, lungs, gastrointestinal tract, muscle, and skin known as other sites of biotransformation (Ionescu & Caira, 2005). The principal enzymatic pathway for phase I drug metabolism is the cytochrome P450 (CYP) family (Zanger & Schwab, 2013). Phase II metabolic pathways are also polymorphic, for example, the UDP-glucuronosyltransferases and arylamine *N*-acetyltransferases. Drugs can also be eliminated via transporters—this can be the primary route of elimination for nonmetabolized drugs, but drugs that undergo metabolism may also be substrates for transporters. Genetic variation is also known to exist for transporter genes.

Most of the studies in the literature on pharmacogenomic variation have focused on the P450 genes. There is considerable variation in the expression of CYP enzymes which is dependent on genetic factors, as well as a range of other factors including sex, age, weight, lipid distribution, hepatic function, hepatic blood flow, disease status, pregnancy status, smoking status, renal function, and polypharmacy (Alomar, 2014; Zanger & Schwab, 2013).

Approximately 40% of P450-catalyzed metabolism is via enzymes encoded by genes where polymorphisms lead to absence of activity in some individuals. For example, *CYP2D6* has over 80 known polymorphisms which lead to over- or underactivity of the enzyme. Individuals can be categorized as poor metabolizers, intermediate metabolizers, extensive metabolizers, and ultrarapid metabolizers. Poor metabolizers carry two alleles with no functionality, intermediate metabolizers two with reduced function, extensive metabolizers are homozygous or heterozygous for wild-type or normal activity alleles, while ultrarapid metabolizers carry duplicated active alleles (Meyer, 2000). For example, some individuals have between 3 and 13 copies of the gene coding for CYP2D6, known as amplification of the gene (Ingelman-Sundberg, Oscarson, & McLellan, 1999). There is also significant interethnic variation in *CYP2D6* polymorphism frequencies. For example, in the Americas, *CYP2D6* deletion is more prevalent than CYP2D6 duplication, whereas in North Africa, the Middle East, and Oceania, the opposite is true

(Johansson & Ingelman-Sundberg, 2008). These variables pose a challenge when dosing patients. In the case of amitriptyline, poor metabolizers risk toxicity with the drug, notably anticholinergic side effects and cardiac toxicity, which can be fatal. Ultrarapid metabolizers, however, have subtherapeutic levels of amitriptyline and supratherapeutic levels of its active metabolites including nortriptyline, making risk assessment of ADRs extremely complicated (Dean, 2017).

Warfarin is a very widely used anticoagulant in clinical practice (Kim et al., 2015). It has a narrow therapeutic index, can result in bleeding, and has been demonstrated to be among the most common cause of ADRs resulting in hospitalization (Pirmohamed et al., 2004). The clinical therapeutic dose of warfarin ranges by a factor of 40, from 0.5 to 20 mg/day (Pirmohamed, 2011). Many variables contribute to this difference including age, weight, disease status, nutrition, concomitant drugs, diet, smoking status, and genetic factors. Warfarin is a mixture of R- and S-enantiomers. S-warfarin is three to five times more potent than R-warfarin and is metabolized by CYP2C9 (Wadelius & Pirmohamed, 2007). Compared with normal wild type, homozygosity for *CYP2C9*2* and *CYP2C9*3* is known to reduce enzyme activity to 12% and 5%, respectively (Kim et al., 2015). *CYP2C9*3* has also been shown in systematic reviews to increase the risk of warfarin-induced bleeding (Jorgensen, FitzGerald, Oyee, Pirmohamed, & Williamson, 2012; Yang et al., 2013). Vitamin K epoxide reductase complex 1 (*VKORC1*) polymorphisms also contribute to interindividual variability in warfarin dose requirement, with the homozygous A-1639 genotype being associated with reduced warfarin dose requirements by up to 3 mg/day (Jorgensen et al., 2012). CYP4F2 contributes to vitamin K metabolism, with some polymorphisms in the gene encoding this protein associated with higher warfarin doses. GWAS have confirmed these associations, with *VKORC1* contributing the most and *CYP4F2* contributing the least to this variability. This understanding has led to the development of genotype-guided warfarin-dosing algorithms, for example, by the International Warfarin Pharmacogenetics Consortium, where the algorithm was validated in over 1000 patients (Klein et al., 2009). *VKORC1* and *CYP2C9* genetic testing prior to dosing has been shown to predict stable warfarin dose requirement more accurately than conventional dosing. Early clinical trials assessed use of genotype and other patient-related factors to set initial warfarin dose (Anderson et al., 2007; Burmester et al., 2011; Caraco, Blotnick, & Muszkat, 2008; Epstein et al., 2010; Johnson et al., 2011; McMillin et al., 2010). These studies did not find any significant improvement with anticoagulation control combined with genetic testing, but they all had limitations including sample size, dosing algorithms, or genotyping strategy. Outcomes of further controlled trials were reported in 2013. These studies, termed EU-PACT and COAG, based in Europe and the United States, respectively, came to differing conclusions (Kimmel et al., 2013; Pirmohamed et al., 2013). EU-PACT found that patients given a genotype-guided warfarin dose remained in the target therapeutic range for a significantly longer time during the first 3 months of treatment than patients treated with a standardized conventional dosing regimen. COAG reported no improvement in time within therapeutic range in the first 4 weeks of treatment. These conflicting findings may be due to differences in study protocol and the participating patients. As suggested elsewhere (Pirmohamed, Kamali, Daly, & Wadelius, 2015), due to use of a maintenance dose algorithm to determine initial dose, it is unlikely that steady state was achieved in most COAG patients by day 4. Recently, the outcome of a further controlled trial, the GIFT study, has been reported (Gage et al., 2017). Genotype-guided dosing showed a better outcome compared with control dosing for several clinical parameters including international normalized ratio above 4, bleeding, and death. These overall findings appear consistent with EU-PACT. The positive findings for genotyping raise the possibility that future patients could be dosed using point-of-care genetic testing prior to loading with warfarin. However, whether this is going to be possible will depend on the degree of competition from the new direct acting oral anticoagulants, and the associated patient and clinician choice.

Codeine is an example of a drug where polymorphic metabolism by both phase I and phase II enzymes has led to regulatory interventions in order to protect public health. Codeine is a widely used opioid analgesic which has been shown to cause serious ADRs in certain populations, especially in children posttonsillectomy. It is metabolized through glucuronidation, N-demethylation to norcodeine, and CYP2D6-mediated O-demethylation to morphine, its active metabolite (Crews et al., 2014). Hence poor codeine metabolizers lack significant analgesic effect with codeine, affecting approximately 7% of Caucasians and 1%–3% of other races (Susce, Murray-Carmichael, & de Leon, 2006). Contrastingly, ultrarapid metabolizers are at risk of opioid toxicity, including respiratory depression and death. In addition to CYP2D6 metabolism, glucuronidation of codeine and its active metabolite, morphine, occurs via UGT2B7, and variability in this gene has also been implicated in predisposing to respiratory depression (Madadi et al., 2013). Children with sleep apnea and airway difficulties are at particular risk of ADRs with codeine. The EMA's Pharmacovigilance Risk Assessment Committee identified multiple deaths in children who had received codeine, the majority of these having undergone a tonsillectomy. Following this, in the United Kingdom, codeine is now contraindicated in all children who have had a tonsillectomy and is only recommended in children aged over 12 and when other analgesics have been ineffective (MHRA, 2013).

Another example of a phase II gene polymorphism leading to significant toxicity is with TPMT which metabolizes thiopurine drugs. These drugs include azathioprine and 6-mercaptopurine which have active metabolites that suppress DNA, RNA, and protein synthesis, giving them cytotoxic and immunosuppressive properties (Lennard, 1992). TPMT catalyzes the S-methylation of these drugs and deficiency of TPMT activity has been associated with dangerously elevated levels of the cytotoxic thioguanine nucleotide metabolites. ADRs for thiopurines include myelosuppression and death. Screening patients for TPMT enzyme activity prior to starting treatment with thiopurines can help to prevent toxicity. *TPMT* is known to have at least 36 genetic polymorphisms, most of which result in reduced or absent TPMT activity. *TPMT*3A* is the most common variant allele in Caucasian populations (5%) and *TPMT*3C* is the most common in Asian populations (2%) (Katara & Kuntal, 2016). Approximately 0.3% of the general population have significantly reduced or no detectable enzyme activity, usually due to a homozygous genotype for alleles *TPMT*2*, *TPMT*3A*, or *TPMT*3C* (Katara & Kuntal, 2016). Both phenotyping and genotyping assays have been used to identify at risk individuals (see Section 4). Interestingly, more recently, other genetic factors predisposing to toxicity from thiopurines have also been identified. For example, in individuals from East Asia, variability in the gene *NUDT15* has been shown to increase the risk of thiopurine-induced leukopenia (Moriyama et al., 2016). How genotyping for *NUDT15* variants will be used in combination with *TPMT* polymorphisms in improving the use of mercaptopurines is unclear at present.

Polymorphisms in drug transporters can also contribute to ADRs. *ABCB1* which encodes MDR1 is the most widely studied efflux transporter gene. This codes for an ATP-dependent P-glycoprotein whose function includes the extracellular transport of drugs. In the case of digoxin, homozygous carriers of the C3435T polymorphism in *ABCB1* have been found to have higher plasma concentrations than noncarriers after a single oral dose, as well as a higher C_{max} after chronic use (Hoffmeyer et al., 2000). Many other drugs including most HIV protease inhibitors and immunosuppressive drugs are also P-glycoprotein substrates (Meyer, 2000) but the overall effect of *ABCB1* genotype on their disposition remains somewhat controversial (Cascorbi, 2011; Dickens, Owen, Alfirevic, & Pirmohamed, 2013).

3. GENETIC PREDISPOSITION TO TYPE B ADRs

3.1 HLA Associations

HLA gene products are important in presenting foreign peptides to T lymphocytes. HLA genes are located on chromosome 6 in an area of the genome referred to as the major histocompatibility complex (MHC) and are divided into two types, class I and II. These genes are subject to a large amount of polymorphism. This probably arose originally to help protect the body from pathogens, but certain HLA alleles are also risk factors for some types of autoimmune disease (e.g., multiple sclerosis, type 1 diabetes) and for ADRs such as DILI. There is increasing evidence that a range of ADRs involve an inappropriate immune response to a drug. This may involve either due to direct interaction of the drug with the HLA molecule followed by an inappropriate T-cell response or formation of a covalent link between the drug and a cellular protein, with HLA gene products likely to contribute by presenting drug-containing peptides from this complex to T-cells.

3.1.1 Drug-Induced Skin Reactions Including Hypersensitivity Reactions

Drug-induced skin reactions are a form of type B ADR, which exists on a spectrum from trivial involvement to severe cutaneous adverse reactions (SCARs) including Stevens–Johnson syndrome (SJS) and toxic epidermal necrolysis (TEN). SJS and TEN are severe mucocutaneous reactions characterized by detachment of the epidermal layer of the skin, including the mucous membranes and the respiratory tract, systemic fever, and hemorrhagic erosions (Harr & French, 2010). Both conditions are life threatening with mortality rates of up to 10% and 30%, respectively (Yip, Alfirevic, & Pirmohamed, 2015). They require immediate withdrawal of the implicated drug and in-patient admission for urgent treatment and monitoring (Devi, George, Criton, Suja, & Sridevi, 2005). As discussed elsewhere (Yip et al., 2015), hypersensitivity syndrome is another type of drug-induced skin reaction which also requires immediate drug withdrawal. There have been a number of studies on genetic factors affecting susceptibility to SJS/TEN and hypersensitivity syndrome due to various drugs, but, as summarized in Table 1, the main associations found to date are with various HLA alleles.

Table 1 HLA Alleles Associated With SJS and TEN

Compound	HLA Allele	Odds Ratio (95% CI) and *P* Value	References
Allopurinol	*B*58:01*	580.3 (34.4–9780.9), $P = 4.7 \times 10^{-24}$	Hung et al. (2005)
Carbamazepine	*B*15:02*	89.25 (19.25–413.83), $P = 3.51 \times 10^{-18}$	Cheung et al. (2013)
	*B*15:11*	9.76 (CI 2.01–47.5), $P = 0.0263$	
	*B*15:18*	*HLA-B*15:18* relative risk 13.58	Kaniwa et al. (2010)
	*B*59:01*	*HLA-B*59:01* relative risk 15.16	Ikeda et al. (2010)
	*C*07:04*	*HLA-C*07:04* relative risk 12.89	
	*A*31:01*	10.8 (5.9–19.6), $P = 3.64 \times 10^{-15}$	Ozeki et al. (2011)
Dapsone	*B*13:01*	54.00 (7.96–366.16), $P = 0.0001$	Tempark et al. (2017)
Lamotrigine	*B*15:02*	5.1 (0.8–33.8), $P = 0.1266$	Hung et al. (2010)
Methazolamide	*B*59:01*	249.8 (13.4–4813.5), $P < 0.001$	Kim et al. (2010)
Methazolamide	*Cw*0102*	22.1 (1.2–414.3), $P = 0.004$	Kim et al. (2010)
Nevirapine	*C*04:01*	5.17 (2.39–11.18)	Carr et al. (2013)
Oxcarbazepine	*B*15:02*	80.7 (3.8–1714.4), $P = 8.4 \times 10^{-4}$	Hung et al. (2010)
Oxicam NSAIDs	*B*73:01*	152 (20–1167), $P = 0.027$	Lonjou et al. (2008)
Phenobarbital	*B*51:01*	16.71 (3.66–83.06), $P = 0.0003$	Kaniwa et al. (2013)
Phenytoin	*B*15:02-B*13:01, Cw*0801* and *DRB1*16:02* (*Cw*0801* is within the haplotype of *B*1502*)	5.1 (1.8–15.1), $P = 0.0041$	Hung et al. (2010)
		4.26 (1.93–9.39), $P < 0.0003$	Cheung et al. (2013)
		OR: 3.0–4.3, $P = 0.0128$–0.0281	Hung et al. (2010)
Sulfonamide–trimethoprim	*B*15:02-C*08:01* haplotype	4.87 (1.48–17.22), $P = 0.0041$	Kongpan et al. (2015)
Zonisamide	*A*02:07*	9.77 (3.07–31.1), $P = 0.0008$	Kaniwa et al. (2013)

Abacavir is a nucleoside analogue reverse transcriptase inhibitor used to treat HIV. Using a candidate gene approach, Mallal et al. demonstrated abacavir hypersensitivity was associated with *HLA-B*57:01* (Mallal et al., 2002). This hypersensitivity, which is generally worse on reexposure, has a prevalence of 4%–8% and can be potentially life threatening. Exclusion of *HLA-B*57:01*-positive patients through pharmacogenetic screening has been shown to reduce the risk of hypersensitivity reactions and to be cost-effective (Hughes et al., 2004; Mallal et al., 2008). The underlying mechanism for the *HLA-B*57:01*/abacavir hypersensitivity is now well understood with data obtained by three independent groups of investigators using different approaches indicating that abacavir binds to the B*57:01 gene product and induces a conformational change in the protein. This results in incorrect recognition of self-peptides as foreign by the immune system, triggering an inappropriate immune response (Illing et al., 2012; Norcross et al., 2012; Ostrov et al., 2012).

Of the more than 100 drugs known to cause TEN and SJS, antiepileptics, NSAIDs, anti-HIV drugs, beta-lactams, and allopurinol are the most frequently implicated. Three drugs warrant further discussion. Carbamazepine-induced SJS and TEN are strongly associated with the *HLA-B*15:02* allele which has a prevalence of around 4%–9% in Han Chinese and Thai populations, while it is found in less than 1% of Europeans (Chung et al., 2004). The association with *HLA-B*15:02* has been found in some South East Asian populations (though not in Japanese or South Koreans), leading to drug label changes which mandate testing for *HLA-B*15:02* in some populations only. These population differences reflect the known differences in frequency of *HLA-B*15:02*. In Europeans, carbamazepine hypersensitivity reactions have been associated with *HLA-A*31:01* instead of *HLA-B*15:02* (McCormack et al., 2011). This association has been replicated in other ethnic groups, and unlike the association with *HLA-B*15:02*, it is not restricted to SJS–TEN, but has also been seen with maculopapular exanthema and drug reaction with eosinophilia and systemic symptoms.

Allopurinol is used for the treatment of gout. It can cause severe cutaneous adverse reactions (SCARs). In 2005, Hung et al. showed that *HLA-B*58:01* was strongly associated with allopurinol-induced SCAR [odds ratio 580, 95% CI 34–9781] (Hung et al., 2005). The association has been replicated in Europeans (Lonjou et al., 2008), Japanese (Kaniwa et al., 2008), Thai (Tassaneeyakul et al., 2009), and South Korean (Kang et al., 2011) patients. A recent prospective evaluation in Taiwan showed that preprescription genotyping prevented the occurrence of allopurinol-induced SCAR when compared with historical controls (Ko et al., 2015; Woolbright et al., 2015). Given that the frequency of *HLA-B*58:01* is higher in South East Asians compared with Caucasians, prospective genotyping for this alleles seems to be cost-effective in some South East Asian countries compared with Northern European countries (Plumpton, Alfirevic, Pirmohamed, & Hughes, 2017).

Phenytoin is an aromatic anticonvulsant associated with a high risk of SCAR. In South East Asian countries, an association between SJS and TEN due to phenytoin and *HLA-B*15:02* has been identified, but it is not as strong as that seen with carbamazepine (Caudle et al., 2014). Interestingly, a recent GWAS involving patients from several South East Asian countries showed a strong association with *CYP2C9*3* and phenytoin-induced SCAR, implicating slower metabolism of phenytoin via CYP2C9 and higher systemic exposure in the predisposition to serious skin reactions (Chung et al., 2014).

3.1.2 Drug-Induced Liver Injury

3.1.2.1 Background

A range of widely prescribed drugs can sometimes be toxic to the liver. In drug development, DILI is one of the most common reasons for drug withdrawal, either at a late stage of the development process or soon after licensing (Wilke et al., 2007). If hepatotoxicity is detected either during preclinical studies or early in clinical development, it is likely to be a concentration-dependent (type A) event. The best example of a concentration-dependent intrinsic DILI is that which can develop following acetaminophen overdose. The majority of such overdoses are treated successfully with *N*-acetylcysteine and DILI does not develop, but a recent estimate from Spain suggests approximately 7% of overdose patients show hepatotoxicity, representing an incidence of approximately 2 per 100,000 population (Tong et al., 2015). In the United Kingdom, there are approximately 50,000 hospital admissions annually for paracetamol overdose (Narayan et al., 2015). If a similar incidence of hepatotoxicity to the Spanish study is assumed, this would give an incidence of approximately 6 cases per 100,000 population. Estimates from the United Kingdom suggest that 57% of all cases of acute liver failure annually are due to acetaminophen overdose compared with approximately 11% due to idiosyncratic DILI (Bernal & Wendon, 2013). In spite of their relatively low contribution to cases of acute liver failure, idiosyncratic type B ADRs affecting the liver are more common than class A and can be caused by a range of different drugs. A recent study estimated an incidence of 19 cases per 100,000 individuals annually

(Bjornsson, Bergmann, Bjornsson, Kvaran, & Olafsson, 2013). There are several relatively recent examples of drugs withdrawn from the market due to causing idiosyncratic DILI such as troglitazone. Despite these withdrawals, many drugs that occasionally cause idiosyncratic DILI remain on the market with warnings on the drug label. Common examples of drugs that can cause type B idiosyncratic DILI are listed in Table 2. As discussed in detail elsewhere, population surveys worldwide suggest that for between 27% and 65% of all idiosyncratic DILI cases, antiinfective agents are implicated as the cause (Nicoletti et al., 2017). Genetic risk factors for idiosyncratic DILI can be divided into HLA and non-HLA risk factors. In the case of the HLA risk factors for DILI discussed in this section, there is some overlap with other type B ADRs and these are relevant to ADRs affecting the skin (see Section 3.1.1) in addition to the liver. Genetic studies have provided some information on the underlying mechanism of idiosyncratic DILI and this aspect will also be considered.

As discussed in Section 2, the liver is the main site of metabolism of many drugs and reactions involving CYPs and other metabolizing enzymes may result in the production of reactive metabolites which bind to cellular proteins. These complexes may cause cellular damage directly or trigger an inappropriate immune response which may also result in cellular damage. The overall mechanism for drug-induced liver damage is still poorly

Table 2 Common Causes of Idiosyncratic DILI

Antiinfectives
Amoxicillin–clavulanate, Azithromycin, Ciprofloxacin, Doxycyline, Flucloxacillin, Isoniazid, Levofloxacin, Minocycline, Nitrofurantoin, Sulfamethoxazole–trimethoprim, Terbinafine
Others
Atorvastatin, Azathioprine, Diclofenac, Infliximab, Phenytoin, Propylthiouracil, Valproic acid

Based on data from the following sources: Bjornsson, E. S., Bergmann, O. M., Bjornsson, H. K., Kvaran, R. B., & Olafsson, S. (2013). Incidence, presentation, and outcomes in patients with drug-induced liver injury in the general population of Iceland. *Gastroenterology, 144*, 1419–1425, 1425 e1411–1413; Chalasani, N., Bonkovsky, H. L., Fontana, R., Lee, W., Stolz, A., Talwalkar, J., et al. (2015). Features and outcomes of 899 patients with drug-induced liver injury: The DILIN prospective study. *Gastroenterology, 148*, 1340–1352.e1347; Shin, J., Hunt, C. M., Suzuki, A., Papay, J. I., Beach, K. J., & Cheetham, T. C. (2013). Characterizing phenotypes and outcomes of drug-associated liver injury using electronic medical record data. *Pharmacoepidemiology and Drug Safety, 22*, 190–198; Suzuki, A., Andrade, R. J., Bjornsson, E., Lucena, M. I., Lee, W. M., Yuen, N. A., et al. (2010). Drugs associated with hepatotoxicity and their reporting frequency of liver adverse events in VigiBase: Unified list based on international collaborative work. *Drug Safety, 33*, 503–522.

understood. This is due, at least in part, to the complex phenotype which is quite drug dependent. Typically, a hepatotoxic drug will cause one or more of the following phenotypes: hepatocyte necrosis, hepatitis where inflammation occurs, cholestasis with normal flow of bile through the bile duct impaired, or steatosis where lipid accumulates. Idiosyncratic DILI generally involves hepatitis and/or cholestasis (Verma & Kaplowitz, 2009) and on this basis is most easily divided into three types: hepatocellular, cholestatic, and mixed. Importantly, up to 13% of patients suffering hepatocellular DILI may progress to acute liver failure. Drug-induced cholestasis is rarely fatal but may result occasionally in chronic liver disease.

3.1.2.2 HLA Associations in DILI

For DILI, the first reports linking HLA with susceptibility to this reaction involved the general anesthetic halothane, which was used widely until the 1980s but was an important cause of idiosyncratic DILI. This association, which was reported before HLA genes were well understood, involved an increased risk of DILI in those positive for the HLA class II serotype DR2 (Otsuka et al., 1985). More recently, HLA associations with DILI have been studied directly by genotyping. Initially this involved direct HLA genotyping but recently GWAS have been performed on DILI cohorts and a number of these have shown associations with the MHC region. A relatively large number of different associations with specific HLA class I and II alleles for DILI due to particular drugs have been reported as summarized in Table 3. A number of conclusions can be made from these data. In particular, though certain drugs are generally associated with a particular DILI phenotype, e.g., flucloxacillin most frequently gives rise to a cholestatic or mixed phenotype, HLA associations extend across all three common DILI phenotypes. Some associations with the same HLA allele are seen for several structurally unrelated drugs; for example, carrying the class II allele *DRB1*15:01* is a risk factor for DILI due to both amoxicillin–clavulanate and lumiracoxib, and the class I allele *A*33:01* is a risk factor for DILI relating to both terbinafine and ticlopidine in addition to a number of other unrelated drugs (Nicoletti et al., 2017). Effect sizes in HLA associations vary depending on the drug with odds ratios for risk of DILI of between 2 and 80 reported. The strongest HLA association reported to date with DILI is for reactions due to the antimicrobial flucloxacillin, which is used in some countries to treat staphylococcal infections. A highly significant association with the HLA class I allele *B*57:01* was detected for flucloxacillin DILI with an odds ratio of approximately 80 (Daly et al., 2009). As discussed earlier, this allele has been

Table 3 HLA Alleles Associated With Idiosyncratic DILI

Compound	No. of Cases	HLA Allele	Predominant DILI Phenotype	Odds Ratio (95% CI) and *P* Value	References
Flucloxacillin	51	*B*57:01*	Cholestatic/mixed	80.6 (22.8–284.9), $P=9\times10^{-19}$	Daly et al. (2009)
Amoxicillin–clavulanic acid	201	*A*02:01* *DRB1*15:01-DQB1*06:02*	Cholestatic/mixed	2.3 (1.8–2.9), $P=1.8\times10^{-10}$ 2.8 (2.1–3.8), $P=3.5\times10^{-11}$	Lucena et al. (2011)
Lumiracoxib	41	*DRB1*15:01-DQB1*06:02*	Hepatocellular	5.0 (3.6–7.0), $P=6.8\times10^{-25}$	Singer et al. (2010)
Lapatinib	35	*DRB1*07:01-DQA1*02:01*	Hepatocellular	2.9 (1.3–6.6), $P=0.007$	Spraggs et al. (2011)
Ximelagatran	74	*DRB1*07:01-DQA1*02:01*	Hepatocellular	4.4 (2.2–8.9), $P=6\times10^{-6}$	Kindmark et al. (2008)
Ticlopidine	22	*A*33:03*	Cholestatic/mixed	13.0 (4.4–38.6), $P=1.2\times10^{-5}$	Hirata et al. (2008)
	5	*A*33:01*		163.1(16.2–1642), $P=0.00002$	Nicoletti et al. (2017)
Terbinafine	14	*A*33:01*	Cholestatic/mixed	40.5 (12.5–131.4), $P=6.7\times10^{-10}$	Nicoletti et al. (2017)
Minocycline	25	*B*35:02*	Hepatocellular	29.6 (7.8–89.8), $P=2.57\times10^{-8}$	Urban et al. (2017)
Flupirtine	6	*DRB1*16:01-DQB1*05:02*	Hepatocellular	18.7 (2.5–140.5), $P=0.002$	Nicoletti et al. (2016)
*Anti-HIV/anti-TB combination	46	*B*57:02, B*57:03*	Cholestatic/mixed	30.08 (3.44–263.11), $P=0.002$	Petros et al. (2017)
Pazopanib	24	*B*57:01*	Hepatocellular	2.1 (1.3–3.60), $P=0.0058$	Xu et al. (2016)

*African population. All other data are from White European populations.

shown previously to be a strong risk factor for hypersensitivity reactions to abacavir (see Section 3.1.1), but this reaction generally does not involve the liver. Two alleles closely related to *B*57:01*, *B*57:02*, and **57:03* are risk factors for development of DILI relating to exposure to both anti-HIV and anti-TB drugs (Petros et al., 2017); this finding relates to an African population where the two observed HLA risk alleles are more common than *B*57:01*. It is not known whether *B*57:01* is also a risk factor for this type of DILI. However, an association between raised transaminase enzyme levels following treatment with the anticancer drug pazopanib and *B*57:01* has also been reported in a mainly European population, suggesting this association might not be unique to flucloxacillin DILI. The odds ratio for development of pazopanib toxicity is much lower than that seen for flucloxacillin DILI, however. Another example of differences between ethnic groups relates to ticlopidine DILI where *A*33:03* was found to be a risk factor in a Japanese population (Hirata et al., 2008). This allele is rarer in Europeans than the related *A*33:01*, which was later shown to also be a risk factor for this form of DILI (Nicoletti et al., 2017).

The observed HLA associations are interesting but even for flucloxacillin DILI, only 1 in every 500–1000 patients carrying the risk allele *B*57:01* develop the reaction when given the drug. This means additional risk factors contribute to risk and these may include factors such as age and gender on the basis of epidemiological data (Devereaux, Crawford, Purcell, Powell, & Roeser, 1995; Russmann, Kaye, Jick, & Jick, 2005; Wing et al., 2017).

The underlying mechanism involved in the flucloxacillin DILI reaction also appears to be slightly different to the mechanism reported for abacavir hypersensitivity (Monshi et al., 2013; Wuillemin et al., 2013). There is some evidence that flucloxacillin binds covalently to proteins prior to triggering a T-cell response (Monshi et al., 2013), though a second study using a different approach suggests that covalent binding is not essential (Wuillemin et al., 2013). For DILI due to amoxicillin–clavulanate, evidence for T-cell responses involving both amoxicillin and clavulanate has been obtained (Kim et al., 2015) but in the case of lapatinib DILI, no evidence of drug-specific activation of T-cells was obtained in a study of five patients either using the parent drug or several metabolites (Faulkner, Meng, Naisbitt, Spraggs, & Park, 2016). A recent report on minocycline DILI suggests that direct binding of minocycline to the *HLA-B*35:02* protein may occur (Nicoletti et al., 2017), but this is based entirely on molecular modeling and did not involve T-cell stimulation by the drug.

3.1.3 Other HLA Associations With ADRs

Hypersensitivity reactions, severe cutaneous reactions, and DILI are currently the best studied ADRs in terms of HLA associations. There is also increasing evidence, mainly obtained using GWAS approaches, that additional ADRs show HLA associations. As summarized in Table 4, drug-induced agranulocytosis is the best-studied additional example. Drug-specific HLA associations in relation to clozapine, thionamide antithyroid drugs, and sulfasalazine have now been demonstrated. HLA genotype also appears to be a predictor of susceptibility to a rare form of myositis induced by statins which has autoimmune features (circulating antibodies to 3-hydroxy-3-methylglutaryl coenzyme A reductase) and to thiopurine-induced pancreatitis. There is no information to date on the underlying mechanisms, but they are likely to show similarities to those demonstrated for drug-induced hypersensitivity, cutaneous, and liver reactions.

3.2 Non-HLA Genetic Risk Factors for ADRs

In addition to HLA genes, a number of other genetic risk factors for idiosyncratic ADRs have been identified, though few of these have been well replicated. Type B ADRs are often considered to be concentration independent but genetic factors that affect drug concentration also make a contribution to susceptibility to some ADRs. Other genetic risk factors investigated include polymorphisms affecting the innate immune system and proteins protecting the cell against oxidative stress. Cardiotoxicity reactions are somewhat different to other forms of ADR in that polymorphisms in cardiac ion channels are important genetic risk factors. This section will consider non-HLA risk factors for both DILI and cardiotoxicity. These factors are different with no obvious overlap so will be considered in separate sections.

3.2.1 Non-HLA Genetic Risk Factors in DILI

In general, progress to date in identifying non-HLA genetic risk factors for DILI has been very limited. There are examples of drugs that are common causes of DILI such as diclofenac, isoniazid, and statins where data from GWAS analysis suggest HLA genotype is not a risk factor (Nicoletti et al., 2017; Urban et al., 2012). With respect to genes relevant to drug disposition, a recent review has considered their relevance as DILI risk factors in detail (Daly, 2017), but concluded that only a small number of the associations reported appear likely to be genuine and that almost all still require replication in larger numbers of cases, ideally using approaches such as GWAS. The most widely studied association with a non-HLA gene to date for DILI

Table 4 HLA Associations With Other ADRs

ADR	Compound	Population	HLA Allele	Odds Ratio (95% CI) and *P* Value	References
Agranulocytosis	Clozapine	White European	*DQB1 amino acid (Q126)	0.19 (0.12–0.29), $P=4.7\times10^{-14}$	Goldstein et al. (2014)
			*B amino acid (T158)	3.3 (2.3–4.9), $P=6.4\times10^{-10}$	
Agranulocytosis	Thionamides (methimazole, carbimazole, or propylthiouracil)	Chinese	*B*38:02*	265.5 (27.9–2528), $P=2.5\times10^{-14}$	Cheung et al. (2016)
		Swedish	*B*27:05*	7.30 (3.81–13.96), $P=1.91\times10^{-9}$	Hallberg et al. (2016)
Agranulocytosis	Sulfasalazine	Swedish	*B*08:01*	2.25 (1.02–4.97), $P=0.0439$	Wadelius et al. (2017)
			*A*31:01*	4.81 (1.52–15.26), $P=0.0077$	
Myositis	Statin	White European and African-American	*DRB1*11:01*	11.7 (4.0–35.3), $P=4.1\times10^{-7}$	Mammen et al. (2012)
Pancreatitis	Thiopurine	White European	*DRB1*07:01*	2.55 (2.01–3.23), $P=1\times10^{-14}$	Heap et al. (2014)

*Association shown for particular amino acids in HLA-B and HLA-DQB1 may involve several alleles.

is *N*-acetyltransferase 2 (*NAT2*) for isoniazid-related DILI. The enzyme encoded by this gene has a clear role in isoniazid metabolism and the polymorphisms investigated as DILI risk factors show well-established functional significance. As discussed recently (Daly, 2017), the possible *NAT2* association remains problematic for several reasons. In particular, most studies to date have been on mild DILI where genetic factors may be less important. The complexity of treatment regimens for tuberculosis with several potentially hepatotoxic drugs used together makes it challenging to ensure that all DILI cases included in a study are due to isoniazid. The failure to confirm the *NAT2* association in GWAS is a particular limitation, though studies performed up to the present may not be adequately powered to detect small effects (Nicoletti et al., 2017; Urban et al., 2012).

Some progress in detecting non-HLA genetic risk factors for DILI has been reported recently in the largest GWAS to date which involved 862 cases relating to a large number of causative prescribed drugs (Nicoletti et al., 2017). This study excluded cases of DILI due to the two most common causative drugs amoxicillin–clavulanate and flucloxacillin in an attempt to improve coverage of rarer causative drugs. In addition to the HLA signal for *A*33:01* discussed earlier, a genome-wide significant signal in an intergenic region of chromosome 2 was detected together with a signal on chromosome 4 in the *LRBA* gene for hepatocellular cases only (Nicoletti et al., 2017). When individual drug classes were investigated separately, a signal on chromosome 18, also in an intergenic region, for statin-related cases was seen. Attempts to replicate these signals in additional DILI cases have to date been unsuccessful which indicates the genome-wide significance could have been detected by chance only. The fact that the chromosome 2 and 4 signals relate to a number of different drug causes makes them particularly interesting but also more difficult to replicate as finding similar cases for replication purposes is quite challenging.

It remains possible that genes relevant to hepatic function more generally, to protection against oxidative stress, or the innate immune response could be risk factors for DILI. In general, oxidative stress genes in DILI, especially those affecting mitochondrial function, have been the best investigated of these three gene classes with some borderline significant findings reported in candidate gene studies (Boelsterli & Lee, 2014; Nanashima et al., 2012; Suzuki et al., 2010). In addition and also on the basis of candidate gene studies, polymorphisms in the immune-related genes *PTPN22* and *STAT4* may be more general DILI risk factors, but these findings need to be followed up in additional cases (Urban et al., 2011, 2012).

Non-HLA-associated DILI may still involve an immune response. Though several GWAS failed to detect any HLA association for DILI relating to isoniazid or other antituberculosis medications (Nicoletti et al., 2017; Urban et al., 2011), there is some evidence that T-cell responses may contribute to this form of DILI (Usui et al., 2017, 2016) and also that autoantibodies to isoniazid are produced in isoniazid DILI (Metushi, Sanders, Lee, & Uetrecht, 2014). Diclofenac DILI is also not HLA associated and, though less extensively studied in vitro than the isoniazid-related disease, has also been shown to be associated with autoantibody formation (Aithal et al., 2004).

It is also possible that in some cases the drug or a metabolite may have a direct toxic effect within the liver in a manner similar to that occurring during acetaminophen overdose (Kaplowitz, 2005). Direct effects of the drug on a variety of organelles including mitochondria may occur resulting in cellular apoptosis or necrosis, and there have been a variety of studies using both cellular and animal models in relation to DILI (Boelsterli & Lee, 2014). Genetic studies have not yet confirmed the importance of such mechanisms in human DILI. Another toxicity mechanism may involve accumulation of bile acids within hepatocytes at toxic levels due to inhibition of ABC transporters by the hepatotoxic drug resulting in apoptosis or necrosis (Woolbright et al., 2015). There is some evidence that an ABCC2 variant may be a risk factor for diclofenac DILI (Daly et al., 2007), but this has not been confirmed independently and, as discussed elsewhere (Daly, 2017), polymorphisms in ABC transporters do not generally appear to be important risk factors for DILI.

3.2.2 Drug-Induced Cardiotoxicity

Drug-induced cardiotoxicity is the most common reason for a drug's license to be withdrawn from the market (Daly, 2013). Manifestations of cardiotoxicity include increased arrhythmogenicity and risk of sudden cardiac death with prolonged QT interval and cardiomyocyte toxicity leading to heart failure. The QT interval is the time taken for the ventricles of the heart to depolarize, then repolarize. It is easily measured on an electrocardiogram and is closely monitored in clinical trials and when relevant in clinical practice. When the QT interval is prolonged, there is a significantly increased risk of developing arrhythmias. This can include torsades de pointes (TdP), a dangerous polymorphic ventricular tachycardia which can degenerate into ventricular fibrillation and sudden death (Fig. 2). Various risk factors increase the risk of developing a prolonged QT interval,

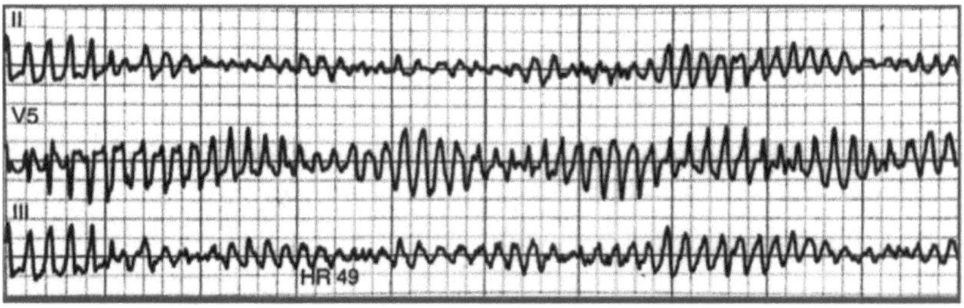

Fig. 2 Electrocardiogram traces showing profiles observed during a torsades de pointes episode. The traces shown are for a single individual and show the signals obtained by three different electrodes, i.e., II, V5, and III.

such as hypokalemia, hypomagnesaemia, female sex, bradycardia, heart failure, ischemic heart disease, and certain drugs (Kannankeril, Roden, & Darbar, 2010; Niemeijer, van den Berg, Eijgelsheim, Rijnbeek, & Stricker, 2015). There are many drugs that prolong the QT interval, some of which are in widespread use. The proton pump inhibitors omeprazole and lansoprazole are examples, which were dispensed over 50 million times in England in 2014 (NHS, 2015). On balance, drugs that prolong the QT interval are often prescribed as the risk-balance ratio of the drug favors the use of the drug. However, this is far from ideal. Various resources are available to health professionals that list drugs known to prolong the QT interval, including "crediblemeds.org" (Combined list of drugs that prolong QT and/or cause torsades de pointes (TDP), 2017). In addition to these factors, genetic predisposition also contributes to prolonged QT interval and the risk of sudden cardiac death.

There is no convincing data that the QT interval itself varies significantly dependent on ethnicity. However, the prevalence of certain polymorphisms that are associated with a prolonged QT interval varies with ethnicity (Niemeijer et al., 2015). In terms of the QT interval response following administration of drugs, there is limited evidence on interethnic differences. One study using quinidine suggested that British people are more susceptible to QT prolongation than Nigerian people (Olatunde & Evans, 1982). However, another trial found that Afro-Caribbean people carried the higher risk compared with Hispanic people in prolonging the QT interval following suspected poisoning (Manini, Stimmel, & Vlahov, 2014).

Research into congenital long QT syndrome (cLQTS) has established the involvement of various ion channels. Long QT syndrome 1 (LQT1) and LQT2 are responsible for the vast majority of confirmed cases of cLQTS. These both encode for cardiac potassium channels, such as the human

Ether-a-go-go-Related Gene channel. Around 15% of cLQTS cases are due to LQT3, where a polymorphism in *SCN5A* causes a defect in sodium channels (Niemeijer et al., 2015).

Drug-induced long QT syndrome (diLQTS) usually affects voltage-gated potassium channels, albeit via a different mechanism. This is thought to be secondary to disrupted protein channeling that reduces the number of functioning ion channels (Kannankeril et al., 2010). Nishio et al. (2009) found that D85N, a *KCNE1* polymorphism that encodes for voltage-gated potassium channels was present more frequently in subjects with prolonged QT intervals (Nishio et al., 2009). A separate high density candidate gene approach also found that D85N correlated with diLQTS with an odds ratio of 9 (Aberg et al., 2012). NOS1AP has also been implicated in diLQTS. This is a nitric oxide synthase-activating protein that regulates intracellular calcium levels. In a prospective study of over 7500 participants, a variant of *NOS1AP* (rs10494366) was shown to significantly potentiate (Niemeijer et al., 2015) the QT prolonging effects of Verapamil (van Noord et al., 2009). A GWAS looking at nearly half a million SNPs in over 700 patients taking antipsychotics again found that *NOS1AP* was implicated, but that another gene, *NUBPL* was also implicated in diLQTS (Aberg et al., 2012). Other studies have failed to find significant associations. A GWAS analysis of 216 cases of diLQTS that precipitated TdP, using 771 controls, found no significant link to any SNP (Aberg et al., 2012).

Doxorubicin, an anthracycline used in the treatment of various malignancies has been associated with the development of arrhythmias and congestive cardiac failure. It has various mechanisms of action, including inhibition of topoisomerase 2. However, there are also other pathways that are less well understood that are implicated in cardiotoxicity. Schneider et al. (2017) performed a GWAS on over 3000 patients on a phase III breast cancer trial, identifying 11 SNPs with potential (P value $<10^{-5}$) to increase congestive heart failure risk. One of the top SNPs, rs28714259, was validated in two separate cohorts being associated with heart failure in one cohort and reduced left ventricular ejection fraction in another cohort (Schneider et al., 2017). This SNP is located in the binding site for the glucocorticoid receptor protein (Rosenbloom et al., 2013). Mice with deficient glucocorticoid receptors have been shown to have disorganized myofibrils, impaired contraction, and overall impaired cardiac function (Rog-Zielinska et al., 2013). Furthermore, work undertaken by a Canadian group has identified variants in *RARG*, *SLC22A17*, and *SLC22A7*, as being associated with anthracycline-induced cardiotoxicity in children

(Aminkeng et al., 2015). The lack of agreement between the different studies may be related to differences in phenotype used to classify patients as suffering from cardiotoxicity.

In summary, although there is some evidence of genetic factors predisposing to drug-induced cardiotoxicity as discussed earlier, these are not used in clinical practice to assess risk at present.

4. CURRENT EXAMPLES OF GENETIC TESTING TO PREVENT ADRs

Genetic testing relating to both type A and type B ADRs has been implemented clinically though overall the number of implemented examples remains small. For a type A reaction, a recommendation that patients have their TPMT status determined prior to thiopurine drug prescription has been made in a number of countries. As reviewed recently (Lennard, 2014), this can be done either by measuring enzyme levels in red blood cells or by genotyping. Normally, individuals who are found to lack TPMT activity will not be prescribed thioguanines as immunosuppressants. However, for leukemia patients, a decreased dose is prescribed (approximately 20-fold less than normal) with close monitoring during treatment (Relling et al., 2011). Approximately 10% of Europeans are heterozygous; genotyping is needed to identify these individuals accurately but measuring TPMT enzyme levels is a reasonable predictor. It is recommended that heterozygotes can still be prescribed thiopurines but that doses of 30%–70% of normal should be used initially combined with monitoring of full blood counts; the dose can then be titrated upward over time (Meggitt, Anstey, Mohd Mustapa, Reynolds, & Wakelin, 2011; Relling et al., 2011).

With increasing knowledge of specific HLA associations with type B ADRs, genetic testing has been used to prevent significant morbidity and mortality in certain populations. For abacavir, *HLA-B*57:01* screening is now recommended by the US Food and Drug Administration, the EMA, and many other drug regulatory agencies worldwide (MHRA, 2017). This prospective screening has been highly effective reducing the incidence of abacavir hypersensitivity from over 5% to less than 1%. Although the prevalence of *HLA-B*57:01* is lower in Africans than in Europeans, prospective screening has still been shown to be effective.

For carbamazepine skin reactions, the ethnic variation seen for *HLA-B*15:02* as a risk factor led to drug label changes which mandate testing for *HLA-B*15:02* in some populations only. Despite the evidence of the effectiveness of *HLA-B*15:02* genetic testing for carbamazepine-induced SJS (Chen et al., 2011), its use in Hong Kong provides a salutary lesson of the difficulties in implementing genetic testing despite acceptance of the test by regulators. Though the Hong Kong government agreed to pay for genetic testing and included it in guidelines, clinicians avoided the use of carbamazepine and switched patients over to lamotrigine and phenytoin. The net result was that SJS due to phenytoin or lamotrigine increased, and the overall incidence of SJS did not change over the years after introduction of *HLA-B*15:02* genetic testing (Alfirevic & Pirmohamed, 2017; Bernal, Lee, Wendon, Larsen, & Williams, 2015; Plumpton et al., 2017).

Despite the relatively large number of reported HLA associations with DILI, the positive predictive values are all considered too low to currently justify introduction of screening.

5. FUTURE PROSPECTS

Due to the relative rarity of severe type B ADRs, pharmacogenetic research has often suffered from low sample sizes. Future research requires increased collaborations between research groups in different countries, facilitating identification of ADRs of moderate significance or those affecting small cohorts. Collaborations should also be utilized to standardize phenotyping, as a poor phenotype is likely to lead to an inadequate genotypic association. To this end, the International Serious Adverse Event Consortium, a collaboration between academia, regulatory agencies, and industry (https://www.saeconsortium.org/), facilitated the phenotype standardization project, which looked to standardize phenotypic definitions for ADRs involving DILI, drug-induced TdP, and drug-induced skin injury (Pirmohamed, Aithal, Behr, Daly, & Roden, 2011). Information standardized includes terminology, diagnostic criteria, severity, and chronicity which should assist in advancing the field and facilitate further genetic studies.

As genotyping technology continues its rapid development, and demand increases, the costs of genome sequencing will likely to continue its rapid descent. As we move to the next generation of whole genome sequencing, it may become easier to identify rarer gene variants that may further explain the interindividual variability and novel pathways involved in drug responses and ADRs. However, large patient sample sizes are going to be needed to identify rare mutations predisposing to ADRs.

As we see a shift in drug development further toward personalized medicines, with over 30% of drugs in development (Lybecker, 2016) being biologicals, and this is likely to increase further, another aspect that will need consideration is how drug development can be streamlined to more easily identify subsets of patients that are more likely to be treatment responsive. There already exists interregulatory body differences in the amount of genetic information disclosed to patients in PILs/SmPCs. Increased harmonization between regulatory authorities in the genetic knowledge included in drug labels will be important for the future.

Car insurance companies often claim to provide cheaper cover for those who install telematics systems that monitor their driving. Although they are not mandatory, they are becoming increasingly common and eventually may become the norm. Legislation and regulatory safeguards are imperative to prevent a similar trend of insurance and financial institutions demanding genetic information as part of their health insurance quotations. If genetic testing may have financial, insurance, or other implications, patients require counseling and to be given the opportunity to make an informed decision. This will require increased training and support of medical healthcare professionals.

Patient education is a significant issue in clinical medicine. With complex pharmacogenetics, this issue becomes more challenging, and significant time and effort will need to be expended to provide them with informed decision-making. Reassurance will need to be given that information will not be shared unnecessarily with third parties, including financial or insurance institutes. Education and engagement of medical health professionals are also important. With new testing, healthcare professionals will need to keep up to date with the changing field of pharmacogenetic testing and how to interpret the results, especially if point-of-care testing is to be performed at the bedside.

Personalized medicine can improve outcomes and reduce harm from ADRs. However, through its nature, it also generates inequality. This inequality is an ethical concern and is present at an interindividual and an interstate level. Care is required to ensure safeguards and recommendations such as the WHO essential medicines list, which already contains drugs such as trastuzumab (WHO, 2015), are reproduced in pharmacogenetics to minimize health and pharmacogenetic inequality.

6. CONCLUSION

ADRs are an important cause of morbidity and mortality. Genetic factors are important in predisposing to many ADRs, irrespective of whether they are categorized as type A or type B. The overall contribution of genetics will vary according to drug and ADR, and should be one of the components taken into account in predicting and preventing ADRs. Although we currently prospectively genotype for particular ADRs prior to drug prescription, it is likely that this will become more preemptive in the future as more and more people undergo whole genome sequencing.

CONFLICT OF INTEREST

The authors have no conflicts of interest to declare.

REFERENCES

Aberg, K., Adkins, D. E., Liu, Y., McClay, J. L., Bukszar, J., Jia, P., et al. (2012). Genome-wide association study of antipsychotic-induced QTc interval prolongation. *The Pharmacogenomics Journal, 12*, 165–172.

Aithal, G. P., Ramsay, L., Daly, A. K., Sonchit, N., Leathart, J. B., Alexander, G., et al. (2004). Hepatic adducts, circulating antibodies, and cytokine polymorphisms in patients with diclofenac hepatotoxicity. *Hepatology, 39*, 1430–1440.

Alfirevic, A., & Pirmohamed, M. (2017). Genomics of adverse drug reactions. *Trends in Pharmacological Sciences, 38*, 100–109.

Alomar, M. J. (2014). Factors affecting the development of adverse drug reactions. *Saudi Pharmaceutical Journal, 22*, 83–94.

Aminkeng, F., Bhavsar, A. P., Visscher, H., Rassekh, S. R., Li, Y., Lee, J. W., et al. (2015). A coding variant in RARG confers susceptibility to anthracycline-induced cardiotoxicity in childhood cancer. *Nature Genetics, 47*, 1079–1084.

Anderson, J. L., Horne, B. D., Stevens, S. M., Grove, A. S., Barton, S., Nicholas, Z. P., et al. (2007). Randomized trial of genotype-guided versus standard warfarin dosing in patients initiating oral anticoagulation. *Circulation, 116*, 2563–2570.

Bernal, W., Lee, W. M., Wendon, J., Larsen, F. S., & Williams, R. (2015). Acute liver failure: A curable disease by 2024? *Journal of Hepatology, 62*, S112–120.

Bernal, W., & Wendon, J. (2013). Acute liver failure. *The New England Journal of Medicine, 369*, 2525–2534.

Bjornsson, E. S., Bergmann, O. M., Bjornsson, H. K., Kvaran, R. B., & Olafsson, S. (2013). Incidence, presentation, and outcomes in patients with drug-induced liver injury in the general population of Iceland. *Gastroenterology, 144*, 1419–1425. 1425 e1411–1413; quiz e1419–1420.

Boelsterli, U. A., & Lee, K. K. (2014). Mechanisms of isoniazid-induced idiosyncratic liver injury: Emerging role of mitochondrial stress. *Journal of Gastroenterology and Hepatology, 29*, 678–687.

Borzelleca, J. F. (2000). Paracelsus: Herald of modern toxicology. *Toxicological Sciences, 53*, 2–4.

Buranova, D. D. (2015). The value of Avicenna's heritage in development of modern integrative medicine in Uzbekistan. *Journal of International Medical Research, 4*, 220–224.

Burmester, J. K., Berg, R. L., Yale, S. H., Rottscheit, C. M., Glurich, I. E., Schmelzer, J. R., et al. (2011). A randomized controlled trial of genotype-based Coumadin initiation. *Genetics in Medicine, 13*, 509–518.

Bush, W. S., & Moore, J. H. (2012). Chapter 11: Genome-wide association studies. *PLoS Computational Biology, 8*, e1002822.

Caraco, Y., Blotnick, S., & Muszkat, M. (2008). CYP2C9 genotype-guided warfarin prescribing enhances the efficacy and safety of anticoagulation: A prospective randomized controlled study. *Clinical Pharmacology and Therapeutics*, *83*, 460–470.

Carr, D. F., Chaponda, M., Jorgensen, A. L., Castro, E. C., van Oosterhout, J. J., Khoo, S. H., et al. (2013). Association of human leukocyte antigen alleles and nevirapine hypersensitivity in a Malawian HIV-infected population. *Clinical Infectious Diseases*, *56*, 1330–1339.

Cascorbi, I. (2011). P-glycoprotein: Tissue distribution, substrates, and functional consequences of genetic variations. *Handbook of Experimental Pharmacology*, *201*, 261–283.

Caudle, K. E., Rettie, A. E., Whirl-Carrillo, M., Smith, L. H., Mintzer, S., Lee, M. T., et al. (2014). Clinical pharmacogenetics implementation consortium guidelines for CYP2C9 and HLA-B genotypes and phenytoin dosing. *Clinical Pharmacology and Therapeutics*, *96*, 542–548.

Chen, P., Lin, J. J., Lu, C. S., Ong, C. T., Hsieh, P. F., Yang, C. C., et al. (2011). Carbamazepine-induced toxic effects and HLA-B*1502 screening in Taiwan. *The New England Journal of Medicine*, *364*, 1126–1133.

Cheung, Y. K., Cheng, S. H., Chan, E. J., Lo, S. V., Ng, M. H., & Kwan, P. (2013). HLA-B alleles associated with severe cutaneous reactions to antiepileptic drugs in Han Chinese. *Epilepsia*, *54*, 1307–1314.

Cheung, C. L., Sing, C. W., Tang, C. S., Cheng, V. K., Pirmohamed, M., Choi, C. H., et al. (2016). HLA-B*38:02:01 predicts carbimazole/methimazole-induced agranulocytosis. *Clinical Pharmacology and Therapeutics*, *99*, 555–561.

Chung, W. H., Chang, W. C., Lee, Y. S., Wu, Y. Y., Yang, C. H., Ho, H. C., et al. (2014). Genetic variants associated with phenytoin-related severe cutaneous adverse reactions. *JAMA*, *312*, 525–534.

Chung, W.-H., Hung, S.-I., Hong, H.-S., Hsih, M.-S., Yang, L.-C., Ho, H.-C., et al. (2004). A marker for Stevens–Johnson syndrome. *Nature*, *428*, 486.

Combined list of drugs that prolong QT and/or cause torsades de pointes (TDP). (2017). https://crediblemeds.org/new-drug-list/. Accessed 25 January 2018.

Crews, K. R., Gaedigk, A., Dunnenberger, H. M., Leeder, J. S., Klein, T. E., Caudle, K. E., et al. (2014). Clinical pharmacogenetics implementation consortium guidelines for cytochrome P450 2D6 genotype and codeine therapy: 2014 Update. *Clinical Pharmacology and Therapeutics*, *95*, 376–382.

Daly, A. K. (2013). Pharmacogenomics of adverse drug reactions. *Genome Medicine*, *5*, 5.

Daly, A. K. (2017). Are polymorphisms in genes relevant to drug disposition predictors of susceptibility to drug-induced liver injury? *Pharmaceutical Research*, *34*, 1564–1569.

Daly, A. K., Aithal, G. P., Leathart, J. B., Swainsbury, R. A., Dang, T. S., & Day, C. P. (2007). Genetic susceptibility to diclofenac-induced hepatotoxicity: Contribution of UGT2B7, CYP2C8, and ABCC2 genotypes. *Gastroenterology*, *132*, 272–281.

Daly, A. K., Donaldson, P. T., Bhatnagar, P., Shen, Y., Pe'er, I., Floratos, A., et al. (2009). HLA-B*5701 genotype is a major determinant of drug-induced liver injury due to flucloxacillin. *Nature Genetics*, *41*, 816–819.

Dean, L. (2017). Amitriptyline therapy and CYP2D6 and CYP2C19 genotype. In V. Pratt, H. Mc Leod, & L. Dean (Eds.), *Medical Genetics Summaries*. Bethesda (MD): National Center for Biotechnology Information.

Devereaux, B. M., Crawford, D. H., Purcell, P., Powell, L. W., & Roeser, H. P. (1995). Flucloxacillin associated cholestatic hepatitis. An Australian and Swedish epidemic? *European Journal of Clinical Pharmacology*, *49*, 81–85.

Devi, K., George, S., Criton, S., Suja, V., & Sridevi, P. K. (2005). Carbamazepine—The commonest cause of toxic epidermal necrolysis and Stevens–Johnson syndrome: A study of 7 years. *Indian Journal of Dermatology, Venereology and Leprology*, *71*, 325–328.

Dickens, D., Owen, A., Alfirevic, A., & Pirmohamed, M. (2013). ABCB1 single nucleotide polymorphisms (1236C > T, 2677G > T, and 3435C > T) do not affect transport activity of human P-glycoprotein. *Pharmacogenetics and Genomics*, *23*, 314–323.

Edwards, I. R., & Aronson, J. K. (2000). Adverse drug reactions: Definitions, diagnosis, and management. *The Lancet*, *356*, 1255–1259.

Ehmann, F., Caneva, L., Prasad, K., Paulmichl, M., Maliepaard, M., Llerena, A., et al. (2015). Pharmacogenomic information in drug labels: European medicines agency perspective. *The Pharmacogenomics Journal*, *15*, 201–210.

Epstein, R. S., Moyer, T. P., Aubert, R. E., DJ, O. K., Xia, F., Verbrugge, R. R., et al. (2010). Warfarin genotyping reduces hospitalization rates results from the MM-WES (Medco-Mayo warfarin effectiveness study). *Journal of the American College of Cardiology*, *55*, 2804–2812.

Faulkner, L., Meng, X., Naisbitt, D. J., Spraggs, C. F., & Park, B. K. (2016). No evidence for drug-specific activation of circulating T cells from patients with HLA-DRB1*07:01-restricted Lapatinib-induced liver injury. *Chemical Research in Toxicology*, *29*, 2111–2113.

Gage, B. F., Bass, A. R., Lin, H., Woller, S. C., Stevens, S. M., Al-Hammadi, N., et al. (2017). Effect of genotype-guided warfarin dosing on clinical events and anticoagulation control among patients undergoing hip or knee arthroplasty: The GIFT randomized clinical trial. *JAMA*, *318*, 1115–1124.

Goldstein, J. I., Jarskog, L. F., Hilliard, C., Alfirevic, A., Duncan, L., Fourches, D., et al. (2014). Clozapine-induced agranulocytosis is associated with rare HLA-DQB1 and HLA-B alleles. *Nature Communications*, *5*, 4757.

Guideline on summary of product characteristics (SmPC). (2009). *European commission enterprise and industry directorate-general*. European Commission. https://ec.europa.eu/health/sites/health/files/files/eudralex/vol-2/c/smpc_guideline_rev2_en.pdf. Accessed 25 January 2018.

Hallberg, P., Eriksson, N., Ibanez, L., Bondon-Guitton, E., Kreutz, R., Carvajal, A., et al. (2016). Genetic variants associated with antithyroid drug-induced agranulocytosis: A genome-wide association study in a European population. *The Lancet Diabetes and Endocrinology*, *4*, 507–516.

Harr, T., & French, L. E. (2010). Toxic epidermal necrolysis and Stevens–Johnson syndrome. *Orphanet Journal of Rare Diseases*, *5*, 39.

Heap, G. A., Weedon, M. N., Bewshea, C. M., Singh, A., Chen, M., Satchwell, J. B., et al. (2014). HLA-DQA1-HLA-DRB1 variants confer susceptibility to pancreatitis induced by thiopurine immunosuppressants. *Nature Genetics*, *46*, 1131–1134.

Henney, J. E. (2000). Withdrawal of troglitazone and cisapride. *JAMA*, *283*, 2228.

Hirata, K., Takagi, H., Yamamoto, M., Matsumoto, T., Nishiya, T., Mori, K., et al. (2008). Ticlopidine-induced hepatotoxicity is associated with specific human leukocyte antigen genomic subtypes in Japanese patients: A preliminary case-control study. *The Pharmacogenomics Journal*, *8*, 29–33.

Hoffmeyer, S., Burk, O., von Richter, O., Arnold, H. P., Brockmoller, J., Johne, A., et al. (2000). Functional polymorphisms of the human multidrug-resistance gene: Multiple sequence variations and correlation of one allele with P-glycoprotein expression and activity in vivo. *Proceedings of the National Academy of Sciences of the United States of America, Early Edition*, *97*, 3473–3478.

Hughes, D. A., Vilar, F. J., Ward, C. C., Alfirevic, A., Park, B. K., & Pirmohamed, M. (2004). Cost-effectiveness analysis of HLA B*5701 genotyping in preventing abacavir hypersensitivity. *Pharmacogenetics*, *14*, 335–342.

Hung, S. I., Chung, W. H., Liou, L. B., Chu, C. C., Lin, M., Huang, H. P., et al. (2005). HLA-B*5801 allele as a genetic marker for severe cutaneous adverse reactions caused by allopurinol. *Proceedings of the National Academy of Sciences of the United States of America*, *102*, 4134–4139.

Hung, S. I., Chung, W. H., Liu, Z. S., Chen, C. H., Hsih, M. S., Hui, R. C., et al. (2010). Common risk allele in aromatic antiepileptic-drug induced Stevens–Johnson syndrome and toxic epidermal necrolysis in Han Chinese. *Pharmacogenomics*, *11*, 349–356.

Ikeda, H., Takahashi, Y., Yamazaki, E., Fujiwara, T., Kaniwa, N., Saito, Y., et al. (2010). HLA class I markers in Japanese patients with carbamazepine-induced cutaneous adverse reactions. *Epilepsia*, *51*, 297–300.

Illing, P. T., Vivian, J. P., Dudek, N. L., Kostenko, L., Chen, Z., Bharadwaj, M., et al. (2012). Immune self-reactivity triggered by drug-modified HLA-peptide repertoire. *Nature*, *486*, 554–558.

Ingelman-Sundberg, M., Oscarson, M., & McLellan, R. A. (1999). Polymorphic human cytochrome P450 enzymes: An opportunity for individualized drug treatment. *Trends in Pharmacological Sciences*, *20*, 342–349.

Ionescu, C., & Caira, M. R. (2005). *Drug metabolism: Current concepts*. The Netherlands: Springer.

Johansson, I., & Ingelman-Sundberg, M. (2008). CNVs of human genes and their implication in pharmacogenetics. *Cytogenetic and Genome Research*, *123*, 195–204.

Johnson, J. A., Gong, L., Whirl-Carrillo, M., Gage, B. F., Scott, S. A., Stein, C. M., et al. (2011). Clinical pharmacogenetics implementation consortium guidelines for CYP2C9 and VKORC1 genotypes and warfarin dosing. *Clinical Pharmacology and Therapeutics*, *90*, 625–629.

Jorgensen, A. L., FitzGerald, R. J., Oyee, J., Pirmohamed, M., & Williamson, P. R. (2012). Influence of CYP2C9 and VKORC1 on patient response to warfarin: A systematic review and meta-analysis. *PLOS one*, *7*, e44064.

Kang, H. R., Jee, Y. K., Kim, Y. S., Lee, C. H., Jung, J. W., Kim, S. H., et al. (2011). Positive and negative associations of HLA class I alleles with allopurinol-induced SCARs in Koreans. *Pharmacogenetics and Genomics*, *21*, 303–307.

Kaniwa, N., Saito, Y., Aihara, M., Matsunaga, K., Tohkin, M., Kurose, K., et al. (2008). HLA-B locus in Japanese patients with anti-epileptics and allopurinol-related Stevens–Johnson syndrome and toxic epidermal necrolysis. *Pharmacogenomics*, *9*, 1617–1622.

Kaniwa, N., Saito, Y., Aihara, M., Matsunaga, K., Tohkin, M., Kurose, K., et al. (2010). HLA-B*1511 is a risk factor for carbamazepine-induced Stevens–Johnson syndrome and toxic epidermal necrolysis in Japanese patients. *Epilepsia*, *51*, 2461–2465.

Kaniwa, N., Sugiyama, E., Saito, Y., Kurose, K., Maekawa, K., Hasegawa, R., et al. (2013). Specific HLA types are associated with antiepileptic drug-induced Stevens–Johnson syndrome and toxic epidermal necrolysis in Japanese subjects. *Pharmacogenomics*, *14*, 1821–1831.

Kannankeril, P., Roden, D. M., & Darbar, D. (2010). Drug-induced long QT syndrome. *Pharmacological Reviews*, *62*, 760–781.

Kaplowitz, N. (2005). Idiosyncratic drug hepatotoxicity. *Nature Reviews. Drug Discovery*, *4*, 489–499.

Katara, P., & Kuntal, H. (2016). TPMT polymorphism: When shield becomes weakness. *Interdisciplinary Sciences*, *8*, 150–155.

Kim, S. H., Kim, M., Lee, K. W., Kim, S. H., Kang, H. R., Park, H. W., et al. (2010). HLA-B*5901 is strongly associated with methazolamide-induced Stevens–Johnson syndrome/toxic epidermal necrolysis. *Pharmacogenomics*, *11*, 879–884.

Kim, S. H., Saide, K., Farrell, J., Faulkner, L., Tailor, A., Ogese, M., et al. (2015). Characterization of amoxicillin- and clavulanic acid-specific T cells in patients with amoxicillin-clavulanate-induced liver injury. *Hepatology*, *62*, 887–899.

Kimmel, S. E., French, B., Kasner, S. E., Johnson, J. A., Anderson, J. L., Gage, B. F., et al. (2013). A pharmacogenetic versus a clinical algorithm for warfarin dosing. *The New England Journal of Medicine*, *369*, 2283–2293.

Kindmark, A., Jawaid, A., Harbron, C. G., Barratt, B. J., Bengtsson, O. F., Andersson, T. B., et al. (2008). Genome-wide pharmacogenetic investigation of a hepatic adverse event without clinical signs of immunopathology suggests an underlying immune pathogenesis. *The Pharmaceutical Journal, 8*, 186–195.

Klein, T. E., Altman, R. B., Eriksson, N., Gage, B. F., Kimmel, S. E., Lee, M. T., et al. (2009). Estimation of the warfarin dose with clinical and pharmacogenetic data. *The New England Journal of Medicine, 360*, 753–764.

Ko, T.-M., Tsai, C.-Y., Chen, S.-Y., Chen, K.-S., Yu, K.-H., Chu, C.-S., et al. (2015). Use of HLA-B*58:01 genotyping to prevent allopurinol induced severe cutaneous adverse reactions in Taiwan: National prospective cohort study. *British Medical Journal, 351*, h4848.

Kongpan, T., Mahasirimongkol, S., Konyoung, P., Kanjanawart, S., Chumworathayi, P., Wichukchinda, N., et al. (2015). Candidate HLA genes for prediction of co-trimoxazole-induced severe cutaneous reactions. *Pharmacogenetics and Genomics, 25*, 402–411.

Kwon, J. M., & Goate, A. M. (2000). The candidate gene approach. *Alcohol Research & Health, 24*, 164–168.

Lennard, L. (1992). The clinical pharmacology of 6-mercaptopurine. *European Journal of Clinical Pharmacology, 43*, 329–339.

Lennard, L. (2014). Implementation of TPMT testing. *British Journal of Clinical Pharmacology, 77*, 704–714.

Lonjou, C., Borot, N., Sekula, P., Ledger, N., Thomas, L., Halevy, S., et al. (2008). A European study of HLA-B in Stevens–Johnson syndrome and toxic epidermal necrolysis related to five high-risk drugs. *Pharmacogenetics and Genomics, 18*, 99–107.

Lucena, M. I., Molokhia, M., Shen, Y., Urban, T. J., Aithal, G. P., Andrade, R. J., et al. (2011). Susceptibility to amoxicillin-clavulanate-induced liver injury is influenced by multiple HLA class I and II alleles. *Gastroenterology, 141*, 338–347.

Lybecker, K. M. (2016). *The biologics revolution in the production of drugs*. Fraser Institute.

Madadi, P., Amstutz, U., Rieder, M., Ito, S., Fung, V., Hwang, S., et al. (2013). Clinical practice guideline: CYP2D6 genotyping for safe and efficacious codeine therapy. *Journal of Population Therapeutics and Clinical Pharmacology, 20*, e369–396.

Mallal, S., Nolan, D., Witt, C., Masel, G., Martin, A. M., Moore, C., et al. (2002). Association between presence of HLA-B*5701, HLA-DR7, and HLA-DQ3 and hypersensitivity to HIV-1 reverse-transcriptase inhibitor abacavir. *Lancet, 359*, 727–732.

Mallal, S., Phillips, E., Carosi, G., Molina, J. M., Workman, C., Tomazic, J., et al. (2008). HLA-B*5701 screening for hypersensitivity to abacavir. *The New England Journal of Medicine, 358*, 568–579.

Mammen, A. L., Gaudet, D., Brisson, D., Christopher-Stine, L., Lloyd, T. E., Leffell, M. S., et al. (2012). Increased frequency of DRB1*11:01 in anti-hydroxymethylglutaryl-coenzyme a reductase-associated autoimmune myopathy. *Arthritis Care and Research, 64*, 1233–1237.

Manini, A. F., Stimmel, B., & Vlahov, D. (2014). Racial susceptibility for QT prolongation in acute drug overdoses. *Journal of Electrocardiology, 47*, 244–250.

McCormack, M., Alfirevic, A., Bourgeois, S., Farrell, J. J., Kasperavičiūtė, D., Carrington, M., et al. (2011). HLA-A*3101 and carbamazepine-induced hypersensitivity reactions in Europeans. *The New England Journal of Medicine, 364*, 1134–1143.

McMillin, G. A., Melis, R., Wilson, A., Strong, M. B., Wanner, N. A., Vinik, R. G., et al. (2010). Gene-based warfarin dosing compared with standard of care practices in an orthopedic surgery population: A prospective, parallel cohort study. *Therapeutic Drug Monitoring, 32*, 338–345.

Meggitt, S. J., Anstey, A. V., Mohd Mustapa, M. F., Reynolds, N. J., & Wakelin, S. (2011). British Association of Dermatologists' guidelines for the safe and effective prescribing of azathioprine 2011. *The British Journal of Dermatology, 165*, 711–734.

Meletis, J., & Konstantopoulos, K. (2010). The beliefs, myths, and reality surrounding the word hema (blood) from homer to the present. *Anemia*, *2010*, 857657.

Metushi, I. G., Sanders, C., Lee, W. M., & Uetrecht, J. (2014). Detection of anti-isoniazid and anti-cytochrome P450 antibodies in patients with isoniazid-induced liver failure. *Hepatology*, *59*, 1084–1093.

Meyer, U. A. (2000). Pharmacogenetics and adverse drug reactions. *The Lancet*, *356*, 1667–1671.

MHRA (2013) Codeine for analgesia: Restricted use in children because of reports of morphine toxicity In: mhra.gov.uk. https://www.gov.uk/drug-safety-update/codeine-for-analgesia-restricted-use-in-children-because-of-reports-of-morphine-toxicity Accessed 25/01/2018, UK Government.

MHRA. (2016). *Summary of product characteristics*. UK Government. http://www.mhra.gov.uk/home/groups/spcpil/documents/spcpil/con1502428749713.pdf.

MHRA (2017) Abacavir/lamivudine. In: mhra.gov.uk. http://www.mhra.gov.uk/spc-pil/?prodName=ABACAVIR/LAMIVUDINE SANDOZ 600 MG/300 MG FILM-COATED TABLETS&subsName=ABACAVIR HYDROCHLORIDE&pageID=SecondLevel.

Monshi, M. M., Faulkner, L., Gibson, A., Jenkins, R. E., Farrell, J., Earnshaw, C. J., et al. (2013). Human leukocyte antigen (HLA)-B*57:01-restricted activation of drug-specific T cells provides the immunological basis for flucloxacillin-induced liver injury. *Hepatology*, *57*, 727–739.

Moosavi, J. (2009). The place of Avicenna in the history of medicine. *Avicenna Journal of Medical Biotechnology*, *1*, 3–8.

Moriyama, T., Nishii, R., Perez-Andreu, V., Yang, W., Klussmann, F. A., Zhao, X., et al. (2016). NUDT15 polymorphisms alter thiopurine metabolism and hematopoietic toxicity. *Nature Genetics*, *48*, 367–373.

Nanashima, K., Mawatari, T., Tahara, N., Higuchi, N., Nakaura, A., Inamine, T., et al. (2012). Genetic variants in antioxidant pathway: Risk factors for hepatotoxicity in tuberculosis patients. *Tuberculosis (Edinburgh, Scotland)*, *92*, 253–259.

Narayan, H., Thomas, S. H., Eddleston, M., Dear, J. W., Sandilands, E., & Bateman, D. N. (2015). Disproportionate effect on child admissions of the change in medicines and healthcare products regulatory agency guidance for management of paracetamol poisoning: An analysis of hospital admissions for paracetamol overdose in England and Scotland. *British Journal of Clinical Pharmacology*, *80*, 1458–1463.

NHS. (2015). *Prescriptions dispensed in the community, statistics for England—2004–2014. In NHS DIgital.* UK Government. http://digital.nhs.uk/catalogue/PUB17644.

Nicoletti, P., Aithal, G. P., Bjornsson, E. S., Andrade, R. J., Sawle, A., Arrese, M., et al. (2017). Association of liver injury from specific drugs, or groups of drugs, with polymorphisms in HLA and other genes in a genome-wide association study. *Gastroenterology*, *152*, 1078–1089.

Nicoletti, P., Werk, A. N., Sawle, A., Shen, Y., Urban, T. J., Coulthard, S. A., et al. (2016). HLA-DRB1*16: 01-DQB1*05: 02 is a novel genetic risk factor for flupirtine-induced liver injury. *Pharmacogenetics and Genomics*, *26*, 218–224.

Niemeijer, M. N., van den Berg, M. E., Eijgelsheim, M., Rijnbeek, P. R., & Stricker, B. H. (2015). Pharmacogenetics of drug-induced QT interval prolongation: An update. *Drug Safety*, *38*, 855–867.

Nishio, Y., Makiyama, T., Itoh, H., Sakaguchi, T., Ohno, S., Gong, Y. Z., et al. (2009). D85N, a KCNE1 polymorphism, is a disease-causing gene variant in long QT syndrome. *Journal of the American College of Cardiology*, *54*, 812–819.

Norcross, M. A., Luo, S., Lu, L., Boyne, M. T., Gomarteli, M., Rennels, A. D., et al. (2012). Abacavir induces loading of novel self-peptides into HLA-B*57: 01: An autoimmune model for HLA-associated drug hypersensitivity. *AIDS*, *26*, F21–F29.

Olatunde, A., & Evans, P. D. A. (1982). Blood quinidine levels and cardiac effects in white British and Nigerian subjects. *British Journal of Clinical Pharmacology, 14*, 513–518.

Ostrov, D. A., Grant, B. J., Pompeu, Y. A., Sidney, J., Harndahl, M., Southwood, S., et al. (2012). Drug hypersensitivity caused by alteration of the MHC-presented self-peptide repertoire. *Proceedings of the National Academy of Sciences of the United States of America, 109*, 9959–9964.

Otsuka, S., Yamamoto, M., Kasuya, S., Ohtomo, H., Yamamoto, Y., Yoshida, T. O., et al. (1985). HLA antigens in patients with unexplained hepatitis following halothane anesthesia. *Acta Anaesthesiologica Scandinavica, 29*, 497–501.

Ozeki, T., Mushiroda, T., Yowang, A., Takahashi, A., Kubo, M., Shirakata, Y., et al. (2011). Genome-wide association study identifies HLA-A*3101 allele as a genetic risk factor for carbamazepine-induced cutaneous adverse drug reactions in Japanese population. *Human Molecular Genetics, 20*, 1034–1041.

Patnala, R., Clements, J., & Batra, J. (2013). Candidate gene association studies: A comprehensive guide to useful in silicotools. *BMC Genetics, 14*, 39.

Petros, Z., Kishikawa, J., Makonnen, E., Yimer, G., Habtewold, A., & Aklillu, E. (2017). HLA-B*57 allele is associated with concomitant anti-tuberculosis and antiretroviral drugs induced liver toxicity in Ethiopians. *Frontiers in Pharmacology, 8*, 90.

Pirmohamed, M. (2001). Pharmacogenetics and pharmacogenomics. *British Journal of Clinical Pharmacology, 52*, 345–347.

Pirmohamed, M. (2011). Pharmacogenetics: Past, present and future. *Drug Discovery Today, 16*, 852–861.

Pirmohamed, M. (2014). Personalized pharmacogenomics: Predicting efficacy and adverse drug reactions. *Annual Review of Genomics and Human Genetics, 15*, 349–370.

Pirmohamed, M., Aithal, G. P., Behr, E., Daly, A., & Roden, D. (2011). The phenotype standardization project: Improving pharmacogenetic studies of serious adverse drug reactions. *Clinical Pharmacology and Therapeutics, 89*, 784–785.

Pirmohamed, M., Burnside, G., Eriksson, N., Jorgensen, A. L., Toh, C. H., Nicholson, T., et al. (2013). A randomized trial of genotype-guided dosing of warfarin. *The New England Journal of Medicine, 369*, 2294–2303.

Pirmohamed, M., James, S., Meakin, S., Green, C., Scott, A. K., Walley, T. J., et al. (2004). Adverse drug reactions as cause of admission to hospital: Prospective analysis of 18 820 patients. *British Medical Journal, 329*, 15–19.

Pirmohamed, M., Kamali, F., Daly, A. K., & Wadelius, M. (2015). Oral anticoagulation: A critique of recent advances and controversies. *Trends in Pharmacological Sciences, 36*, 153–163.

Plumpton, C. O., Alfirevic, A., Pirmohamed, M., & Hughes, D. A. (2017). Cost effectiveness analysis of HLA-B*58:01 genotyping prior to initiation of allopurinol for gout. *Rheumatology (Oxford), 56*, 1729–1739.

Relling, M. V., Gardner, E. E., Sandborn, W. J., Schmiegelow, K., Pui, C. H., Yee, S. W., et al. (2011). Clinical pharmacogenetics implementation consortium guidelines for thiopurine methyltransferase genotype and thiopurine dosing. *Clinical Pharmacology and Therapeutics, 89*, 387–391.

Rog-Zielinska, E. A., Thomson, A., Kenyon, C. J., Brownstein, D. G., Moran, C. M., Szumska, D., et al. (2013). Glucocorticoid receptor is required for foetal heart maturation. *Human Molecular Genetics, 22*, 3269–3282.

Rosenbloom, K. R., Sloan, C. A., Malladi, V. S., Dreszer, T. R., Learned, K., Kirkup, V. M., et al. (2013). ENCODE data in the UCSC genome browser: Year 5 update. *Nucleic Acids Research, 41*, D56–D63.

Routledge, P. (1998). 150 Years of pharmacovigilance. *Lancet, 351*, 1200–1201.

Russmann, S., Kaye, J. A., Jick, S. S., & Jick, H. (2005). Risk of cholestatic liver disease associated with flucloxacillin and flucloxacillin prescribing habits in the UK: Cohort study using data from the UK general practice research database. *British Journal of Clinical Pharmacology, 60*, 76–82.

Schneider, B. P., Shen, F., Gardner, L., Radovich, M., Li, L., Miller, K. D., et al. (2017). Genome-wide association study for anthracycline-induced congestive heart failure. *Clinical Cancer Research*, *23*, 43–51.

Shah, R. R., & Shah, D. R. (2013). Response to the comments from Drs Shimazawa and Ikeda. *British Journal of Clinical Pharmacology*, *75*, 1368–1369.

Shimazawa, R., & Ikeda, M. (2013). Differences in pharmacogenomic biomarker information in package inserts from the United States, the United Kingdom and Japan. *Journal of Clinical Pharmacy and Therapeutics*, *38*, 468–475.

Singer, J. B., Lewitzky, S., Leroy, E., Yang, F., Zhao, X., Klickstein, L., et al. (2010). A genome-wide study identifies HLA alleles associated with lumiracoxib-related liver injury. *Nature Genetics*, *42*, 711–714.

Spraggs, C. F., Budde, L. R., Briley, L. P., Bing, N., Cox, C. J., King, K. S., et al. (2011). HLA-DQA1*02:01 is a major risk factor for Lapatinib-induced hepatotoxicity in women with advanced breast cancer. *Journal of Clinical Oncology*, *29*, 667–673.

Susce, M. T., Murray-Carmichael, E., & de Leon, J. (2006). Response to hydrocodone, codeine and oxycodone in a CYP2D6 poor metabolizer. *Progress in Neuro-Psychopharmacology and Biological Psychiatry*, *30*, 1356–1358.

Suzuki, A., Andrade, R. J., Bjornsson, E., Lucena, M. I., Lee, W. M., Yuen, N. A., et al. (2010). Drugs associated with hepatotoxicity and their reporting frequency of liver adverse events in VigiBase: Unified list based on international collaborative work. *Drug Safety*, *33*, 503–522.

Tassaneeyakul, W., Jantararoungtong, T., Chen, P., Lin, P. Y., Tiamkao, S., Khunarkornsiri, U., et al. (2009). Strong association between HLA-B*5801 and allopurinol-induced Stevens–Johnson syndrome and toxic epidermal necrolysis in a Thai population. *Pharmacogenetics and Genomics*, *19*, 704–709.

Tempark, T., Satapornpong, P., Rerknimitr, P., Nakkam, N., Saksit, N., Wattanakrai, P., et al. (2017). Dapsone-induced severe cutaneous adverse drug reactions are strongly linked with HLA-B*13:01 allele in the Thai population. *Pharmacogenetics and Genomics*, *27*, 429–437.

Tong, H. Y., Medrano, N., Borobia, A. M., Martinez, A. M., Martin, J., Ruiz, J. A., et al. (2015). Hepatotoxicity induced by acute and chronic paracetamol overdose in adults. Where do we stand? *Regulatory Toxicology and Pharmacology*, *72*, 370–378.

Urban, T. J., Nicoletti, P., Chalasani, N., Serrano, J., Stolz, A., Daly, A. K., et al. (2017). Minocycline hepatotoxicity: Clinical characterization and identification of HLA-B *35:02 as a risk factor. *Journal of Hepatology*, *67*, 137–144.

Urban, T., Shen, Y. F., Chalasani, N. P., Fontana, R. J., Rochon, J., Stolz, A., et al. (2011). A genome-wide association study identifies potential susceptibility loci for hepatotoxicity due to various drugs. *Gastroenterology*, *140*, S886.

Urban, T. J., Shen, Y., Stolz, A., Chalasani, N., Fontana, R. J., Rochon, J., et al. (2012). Limited contribution of common genetic variants to risk for liver injury due to a variety of drugs. *Pharmacogenetics and Genomics*, *22*, 784–795.

Usui, T., Meng, X., Saide, K., Farrell, J., Thomson, P., Whitaker, P., et al. (2017). From the cover: Characterization of isoniazid-specific T-cell clones in patients with anti-tuberculosis drug-related liver and skin injury. *Toxicological Sciences*, *155*, 420–431.

Usui, T., Whitaker, P., Meng, X., Watson, J., Antoine, D. J., French, N. S., et al. (2016). Detection of drug-responsive T-lymphocytes in a case of fatal antituberculosis drug-related liver injury. *Chemical Research in Toxicology*, *29*, 1793–1795.

van Noord, C., Aarnoudse, A. J., Eijgelsheim, M., Sturkenboom, M. C., Straus, S. M., Hofman, A., et al. (2009). Calcium channel blockers, NOS1AP, and heart-rate-corrected QT prolongation. *Pharmacogenetics and Genomics*, *19*, 260–266.

Verma, S., & Kaplowitz, N. (2009). Diagnosis, management and prevention of drug-induced liver injury. *Gut*, *58*, 1555–1564.

Vogel, F. (1959). Moderne probleme der humangenetik. *Ergebnisse der Innere Medizinische und Kinderheilkunde*, *12*, 52–62.

Wadelius, M., Eriksson, N., Kreutz, R., Bondon-Guitton, E., Ibanez, L., Carvajal, A., et al. (2017). Sulfasalazine-induced agranulocytosis is associated with the human leukocyte antigen locus. *Clinical Pharmacology and Therapeutics*, (Epub ahead of print).

Wadelius, M., & Pirmohamed, M. (2007). Pharmacogenetics of warfarin: Current status and future challenges. *The Pharmacogenomics Journal*, 7, 99–111.

WHO. (2009). *WHO*. http://www.who.int/medicines/areas/coordination/English_Glossary.pdf. Accessed October 2017.

WHO. (2015). *19th WHO model list of essential medicines (April 2015) essential medicines and health products*. WHO.

Wilke, R. A., Lin, D. W., Roden, D. M., Watkins, P. B., Flockhart, D., Zineh, I., et al. (2007). Identifying genetic risk factors for serious adverse drug reactions: Current progress and challenges. *Nature Reviews. Drug Discovery*, *6*, 904–916.

Wing, K., Bhaskaran, K., Pealing, L., Root, A., Smeeth, L., van Staa, T. P., et al. (2017). Quantification of the risk of liver injury associated with flucloxacillin: A UK population-based cohort study. *The Journal of Antimicrobial Chemotherapy*, *72*, 2636–2646.

Woolbright, B. L., Dorko, K., Antoine, D. J., Clarke, J. I., Gholami, P., Li, F., et al. (2015). Bile acid-induced necrosis in primary human hepatocytes and in patients with obstructive cholestasis. *Toxicology and Applied Pharmacology*, *283*, 168–177.

Wuillemin, N., Adam, J., Fontana, S., Krahenbuhl, S., Pichler, W. J., & Yerly, D. (2013). HLA haplotype determines hapten or p-i T cell reactivity to flucloxacillin. *Journal of Immunology*, *190*, 4956–4964.

Xu, C. F., Johnson, T., Wang, X., Carpenter, C., Graves, A. P., Warren, L., et al. (2016). HLA-B*57:01 confers susceptibility to Pazopanib-associated liver injury in patients with Cancer. *Clinical Cancer Research*, *22*, 1371–1377.

Yang, J., Chen, Y., Li, X., Wei, X., Chen, X., Zhang, L., et al. (2013). Influence of CYP2C9 and VKORC1 genotypes on the risk of hemorrhagic complications in warfarin-treated patients: A systematic review and meta-analysis. *International Journal of Cardiology*, *168*, 4234–4243.

Yip, V. L., Alfirevic, A., & Pirmohamed, M. (2015). Genetics of immune-mediated adverse drug reactions: A comprehensive and clinical review. *Clinical Reviews in Allergy and Immunology*, *48*, 165–175.

Zanger, U. M., & Schwab, M. (2013). Cytochrome P450 enzymes in drug metabolism: Regulation of gene expression, enzyme activities, and impact of genetic variation. *Pharmacology & Therapeutics*, *138*, 103–141.

CHAPTER EIGHT

Pharmacogenetics: Applications to Pediatric Patients

Tiphaine Adam de Beaumais[*,2], **Evelyne Jacqz-Aigrain**[*,†,‡,1]
[*]Department of Paediatric Pharmacology and Pharmacogenetics, Robert Debré Hospital, APHP, Paris, France
[†]University Paris Diderot Sorbonne Paris Cité, Paris, France
[‡]Clinical Investigation Center CIC1426, INSERM, Paris, France
[1]Corresponding author: e-mail address: evelyne.jacqz-aigrain@aphp.fr

Contents

1. Introduction 192
2. Developmental Pharmacology and Pharmacogenetics 192
3. Clinical Applications 194
   3.1 Pharmacogenetics of Acute Lymphoblastic Leukemia in Pediatric Patients 194
   3.2 Codeine and Tramadol in Children 198
   3.3 Pharmacogenetics and Adverse Drugs Reactions 200
4. Conclusion 206
References 208

Abstract

Individual genomic differences may affect drug disposition and effects of many drugs, and identification of biomarkers are crucial to personalize dosage and optimize response. In children, developmental changes associated with growth and maturation translate into different relationships between genotype and phenotype and different responses to treatment compared to adults. This review aims to summarize some developmental aspects of pharmacogenetics, based on practical examples.

ABBREVIATIONS

6-MMPN 6-methylmercaptopurine nucleotides metabolites
6-MP 6-mercaptopurine
6-TGN 6-thioguanine active metabolites
ALL acute lymphoblastic leukemia
COMT cathecol-*O*-methytransferase
CYP cytochrome
ITPA inosine triphosphate pyrophosphatase
NUDT15 Nudix (nucleoside diphosphate-linked moiety X)-type motif 15

[2] Current address: Precision Cancer Medicine Team, Gustave Roussy, Villejuif, France.

Advances in Pharmacology, Volume 83
ISSN 1054-3589
https://doi.org/10.1016/bs.apha.2018.04.006

PG	pharmacogenetic(s)
SNP	single-nucleotide polymorphism
TKI	tyrosine kinase inhibitor
TPMT	thiopurine *S*-methyltransferase

1. INTRODUCTION

The pediatric population is characterized by progressive developmental changes linked to growth and maturation of organs and functions. In particular, the pharmacogenetic (PG) expression of genes controlling the different pathways evolved in drug-metabolizing enzymes; transporters and targets change over time. Most PG biomarkers are identified in adult populations but the impacts of ontogeny and variability linked to the disease, drug associations, or environmental factors limit their therapeutic use by simple extrapolation from adults to children. Only studies evaluating the interactions between PG, ontogeny, and pediatric specificities allow validation of PG biomarkers in pediatric patients of different age groups for implementation to personalize treatments.

2. DEVELOPMENTAL PHARMACOLOGY AND PHARMACOGENETICS

Age plays a central role in the variability of drug disposition and effects among patients treated with standard dosage schedules (Allegaert, Mian, & van den Anker, 2017; Allegaert et al., 2008; Kearns et al., 2003; Leeder & Meibohm, 2016). In addition to age-dependent growth and maturation, PG variants are identified in most key metabolizing enzymes and transporters (Ahmed, Zhou, Zhou, & Chen, 2016). In pediatrics, the PG challenge is to understand and analyze the impact of growth/maturation on differences in genotype/phenotype correlations between adults and children (Leeder, 2009).

At birth, all physiological systems and functions are immature. They develop gradually but irregularly with growth, rapidly in the newborn, more slowly until adolescence, with modifications of body composition, integumentary development, changes in gastrointestinal function, ontogeny of metabolism enzymes and transporters, and maturation of renal function. After oral administration, the extent of drug absorption depends on many developmental changes occurring in physical and biological barriers; gastric acid secretion, gastric emptying, intestinal motility, and effective surface of absorption are reduced in neonates and develop in older infants and children, thus affecting bioavailability. Drug distribution depends on size and age-related modifications of body composition. Both phase 1 and phase 2 metabolisms are highly dependent on the patient's age. Phase I metabolism is essentially carried out by the cytochrome P-450 (CYP) enzyme system. Hepatic drug-metabolizing enzymes can be categorized into three classes based on developmental trajectories, as reviewed by Hines (2013) and illustrated by the developmental changes of CYP3A subfamily members: class 1: CYP3A7 is the fetal form of CYP3A expressed at the higher level before birth, and decreases rapidly after birth but remains detected at low levels in the adult liver; class 2: CYP3A5 is polymorphic and highly variable during all stages of maturation; class 3: CYP3A4 increases rapidly after birth. Additional pathways involve carboxylesterases (Hines, Simpson, & McCarver, 2016).

Detailed impacts of ontogeny on pharmacogenetically controlled activities were studied for most metabolic pathways, including CYP2C8 (Naraharisetti et al., 2010), CYP2C19 (Zhao, Leroux, Biran, & Jacqz-Aigrain, 2018), CYP2D6 (Blake et al., 2007; Jacqz-Aigrain, Funck-Brentano, & Cresteil, 1993), and CYP3A4 (Kearns et al., 2003). Pathway-dependent maturation is also reported for phase 2 enzymes, and along with the impact of PG variations has been reported in almost all UGT family members (De Wildt, Kearns, Leeder, & Van den Anker, 1999; Krekels, Danhof, Tibboel, & Knibbe, 2012; Miners, McKinnon, & Mackenzie, 2002; Vanhaesebrouck, Verbesselt, & van den Anker, 2009).

Maturation of elimination through the renal route is faster, with immaturity of glomerular filtration, tubular secretion, and reabsorption affecting the elimination of renal-cleared drugs in the first years of life.

The ontogeny of drug transporters and drug targets is also important in drug disposition and effects. Although numerous studies reported PG variants, data on ontogeny and its impact on growth are limited (Brouwer, Aleksunes, Brandys, Giacoia, Knipp, Lukacova, 2015; Mooij et al., 2016).

Altogether, these data demonstrate that the different genes are expressed in an independent manner during growth and maturation (Stevens et al., 2013), with different ontogenic profiles, resulting in pharmacokinetic and pharmacodynamic differences between adults and pediatric patients, and between the different age groups from neonates to adolescents. Clearly, extrapolation of adult data to pediatric patients may not be straightforward.

Drug dosage and treatment personalized to children require the taking into account of age, organ maturation status, disease, and expression of PG polymorphisms (Ahmed et al., 2016; Leeder, Kearns, Spielberg, & van den Anker, 2010; Maagdenberg et al., 2016).

3. CLINICAL APPLICATIONS

Among all polymorphisms studied in adults, some do not translate into major differences in response between children and adults (e.g., antiretrovirals (Mattevi & Tagliari, 2017; Tozzi, 2010) and deferiprone (Limenta, Jirasomprasert, Tankanitlert, et al., 2008)), while genetic variations lead more frequently to differences in response in children and adults, as reported for antidepressants (Blazquez, Mas, Plana, Lafuente, & Lázaro, 2012; Elie, de Beaumais, Fakhoury, & Jacqz-Aigrain, 2011), antitumor agents (Mlakar, Huezo-Diaz, Satyanarayana Uppugunduri, Krajinovic, & Ansari, 2016), and immunosuppressant and antiinflammatory drugs (Elie et al., 2011). Some polymorphisms were discovered and evaluated in adults prior to their being studied in pediatric populations: VKORC1/CYP2C9 and warfarin (Biss et al., 2012; Hamberg & Wadelius, 2014; Tang et al., 2017; Vear et al., 2014; Zhang et al., 2017) or CYP2C19—clopidogrel interactions (Simon et al., 2009).

The following examples were selected as they are of importance in pediatrics.

3.1 Pharmacogenetics of Acute Lymphoblastic Leukemia in Pediatric Patients

Acute lymphoblastic leukemia (ALL) is the most common cancer in childhood. Therapeutic protocols are complex, but the disease is now curable in at least 90% of patients. This provides a model to analyze all research trials—environmental, genetic, and PG—to personalize treatment and improve survival (Hunger & Mullighan, 2015).

Several genetic factors associated with favorable or poor outcomes are identified and considered when selecting intensification treatment along with early response to treatment, after the initial remission therapy (Hunger & Mullighan, 2015; Maxwell & Cole, 2017). When remission is obtained, treatment aims at prevention of relapse during the consolidation and maintenance phases. Current efforts focus on analyzing all factors that will allow treatment optimization by (1) devising molecular-based therapy for the subsets of ALL that are most resistant to current therapy, and (2) identifying the patient's characteristics that influence drug disposition and side effects (Bertholee, Maring, & Van Kuilenburg, 2017).

3.1.1 Pharmacogenetics of 6-Mercaptopurine

Single-nucleotide polymorphism (SNP) in enzymes metabolizing 6-mercaptopurine (6-MP) metabolism have been well established (e.g., thiopurine *S*-methyltransferase (TPMT) and inosine triphosphate pyrophosphatase (ITPA)).

6-MP is a prodrug metabolized by multiple enzymatic steps of the purine salvage pathway to 6-thioguanine active metabolites (6-TGN) incorporated into DNA and 6-methylmercaptopurine nucleotides metabolites (6-MMPN) (Fig. 1). The genetic polymorphisms of TPMT influence the balance between 6-TGN and 6-MMPN and both the efficacy and side

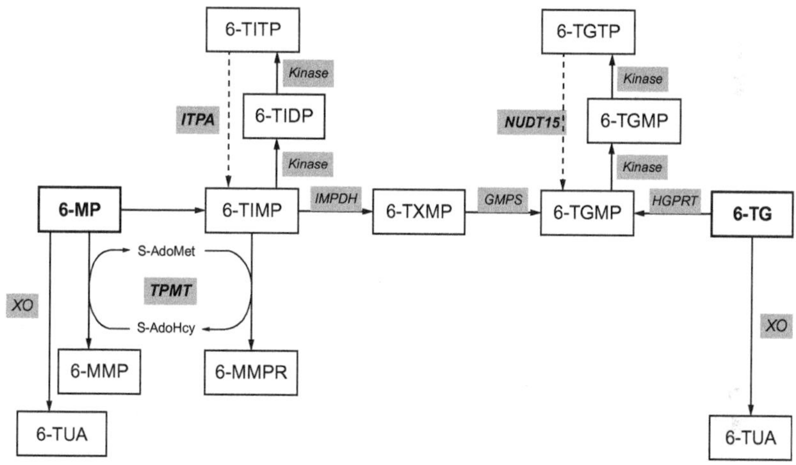

Fig. 1 Simplified scheme of 6-mercaptopurine metabolism. Compounds: *6-MP*, 6-mercaptopurine; *6-TG*, 6-thioguanine; *6-MMP*, 6-methylmercaptopurine; *6-TUA*, 6-thiouric acid; *6-MMPR*, 6-methylmercaptopurine ribonucleotides; *6-TIMP*, 6-thioinosine monophosphate; *6-TIDP*, 6-thioinosine diphosphate; *6-TITP*, 6-thioinosine triphosphate; *6-TXMP*, 6-thioxanthosine monophosphate; *6-TGMP*, 6-thioguanine monophosphate; *6-TGDP*, 6-thioguanine diphosphate; *6-TGTP*, 6-thioguanine triphosphate; *A-AdoHcy*, *S*-adenosyl-L-homocysteine; *S-adoMet*, *S*-adenosyl-L-methionine; Enzymes: *IMPDH*, inosine monophosphate dehydrogenase; *GMPS*, guanosine monophosphate synthetase; *HGPRT*, hypoxanthine-guanine phosphoribosyltransferase; *ITPA*, inosine triphosphate pyrophosphatase; *NUDT15*, Nudix type 15-nucleoside diphosphate-linked moiety X-type motif 15; *XO*, xanthine oxidase; *TPMT*, thiopurine *S*-methyltransferase.

effects of 6-MP, with a high risk of myelosuppression in homozygous TPMT-deficient patients (Adam de Beaumais & Jacqz-Aigrain, 2012; Fakhoury, de Beaumais, Médard, & Jacqz-Aigrain, 2010; McLeod, Krynetski, Relling, & Evans, 2000). Over 95% of TPMT deficiency is attributed to variants located in exons 5 (*2: 238G>C), 7 (*3B: 460G>A), and 10 (*3C: 719A>G), and 7+10 (*3A: 460G>A, 719A>G). Genotyping children receiving 6-MP treated for leukemia or Crohn's disease for TPMT polymorphism helps in dosage adaptation of 6-MP (Relling et al., 2013).

During exposure to thiopurines, and in addition to TPMT polymorphism, variants on ITPA and Nudix (nucleoside diphosphate-linked moiety X)-type motif 15 (NUDT15) are associated with variability in response to 6-MP and hematopoietic and hepatic toxicities (Moriyama et al., 2017; Singh, Bhatia, Khera, & Trehan, 2017).

ITPA hydrolyzes deaminated purine nucleoside triphosphates. One variant (94C>A; Pro32Thr) results in reduced activity in heterozygous patients (Sumi et al., 2002). When analyzed simultaneously, both TPMT and ITPA genotypes influence 6-MP metabolism and hepatotoxicity (Adam de Beaumais et al., 2011).

NUDT15 encodes a nucleoside diphosphatase that dephosphorylates the 6-thioguanine diphosphate (TdGTP) and triphosphate (TGTP), preventing their incorporation into DNA. NUDT15 variants with reduced enzyme activity are liable to lead to accumulation of active 6-MP metabolites in cells and hence increased rate of toxicity. NUDT15 415 C>T is also strongly associated with myelosuppression as initially reported by Yang in Asian ALL children (Yang et al., 2014): patients with TT genotype were highly sensitive to MP and tolerated only 8.3% of the standard dose of 6-MP.

Both TPMT and NUDT15 polymorphisms contribute to 6-MP sensitivity. TPMT testing is already recommended for thiopurine dosage adaptation and is currently performed for 6-MP dosage adaptation in ALL patients (Relling et al., 2013).

Recommendations for additional PG testing will need to take into account important ethnic differences: the frequencies of TPMT SNPs vary widely when Asians cohorts are compared to European cohorts (3% vs 10%–15%). NUDT15 variants are frequent in Asians but exceptional in Europeans and absent in Africans (Zgheib et al., 2017). The implications of transporters and potential additional polymorphisms will also need to be considered (Rubin, Marable, & Huang, 2017; Tanaka et al., 2018).

3.1.2 Pharmacogenetics of Methotrexate

Methotrexate (MTX) is an antifolate with antikeulemic effects, acting by inhibition of the folate pathway. MTX enters cells by the active transporter reduced folate carrier (RFC1 or SLCO19A1), and acts through accumulation of long-chain active MTX polyglutamates. MTX interferes with the folate–homocysteine cycle, inhibiting the pharmacogenetically controlled dihydrofolate reductase (DHFR), thymidylate synthase (TYMS), and 5,10-methylenetetrahydrofolate reductase (MTHFR). Corresponding gene variants affect MTX intracellular metabolism, while polymorphism of the transporter SLCO1B1 expressed in the liver is associated with variability in MTX clearance. This results in resistance or severe toxicity to MTX (Ishikawa, 2012; Mishra et al., 2007; Ramsey et al., 2013; Trevino et al., 2009).

In addition, metabolic interactions between 6-MP and MTX are well documented but their therapeutic impact remains to be investigated (Adam de Beaumais & Jacqz-Aigrain, 2012). All of these polymorphisms were studied by candidate gene approaches and were not clearly associated with response to an individual drug, except for TPMT.

3.1.3 Tyrosine Kinases Inhibitors and Personalized ALL Treatment in Children

Imatinib (Glivec®) is a potent tyrosine kinase inhibitor (TKI) of the fusion gene product BCR-ABL (Philadelphia gene rearrangement, Ph+), indicated in adult and pediatric Ph+ leukemic patients. It greatly improved the outcome of Ph_ALL children when added to the treatment of ALL (Schultz et al., 2014). In addition to inhibition of this target, success requires sufficient exposure. Recent studies have shown the impact of PG biomarkers on pharmacokinetics and monitoring is recommended.

Although outcomes for children with ALL improved, 10%–20% of them relapse, with acquired resistance to reinduction chemotherapy. In such a context, new biological subgroups such as "Ph-like ALL" are now characterized by gene rearrangements affecting pathways involving different kinase and cytokine receptor activation, making them potential targets for specific therapies (Reshmi et al., 2017; Roberts et al., 2017, 2014; Tasian, Loh, & Hunger, 2017).

A limited number of clinical trials, listed in the clinical trials.gov database, are ongoing to evaluate different TKI (imatinib, dasatinib, or nilotinib) in "Ph-like" childhood ALL (Loh et al., 2015; Santiago, Vairy, Sinnett, Krajinovic, & Bittencourt, 2017; Suttorp, Bornhäuser, Metzler, Millot, & Schleyer, 2017).

3.1.4 Immunotherapy

Immunotherapy is an extremely promising therapeutic option in cancer, including in pediatric patients experiencing multiple relapses (Foster & Maude, 2018; Raffaella et al., 2017; Schalper, 2016). Very preliminary data are available in children with relapsed B-ALL, but clinical trials with blinatumomab, inotuzumab, or CART cells are ongoing in North America and Europe (Franca et al., 2017; Pierro, Hogan, Bhatla, & Carroll, 2017; Rytting, Triche, Thomas, O'Brien, & Kartajian, 2017; von Stackelberg et al., 2016).

PG variability is the key issue in the treatment of childhood ALL. In addition to biomarkers of drug pharmacokinetics and disposition, biomarkers of drug pharmacodynamics characterizing disease phenotype are promising tools to treat or even prevent high-risk relapses.

3.2 Codeine and Tramadol in Children

Codeine is an analgesic drug, partly inactivated by glucuronidation (UGT2B7) and demethylation (CYP3A4) and metabolized to active morphine (CYP2D6): the analgesic and side effects of codeine depend on the relative activity of these different pathways (Fig. 2A). Accordingly, administration of codeine does not provide the expected level of analgesia in CYP2D6 poor metabolizers (PM, 5%–10% of Caucasian subjects). Extensive metabolizers (EM, ~70% of Caucasians) (Hicks, Swen, & Gaedigk, 2014) produce morphine, the proportion of which corresponds to about 10% of the codeine dose. Ultrarapid metabolizers (UM, about 1%–10% of the Caucasians) develop an accentuated codeine effect, through a high production of morphine, and individuals are at risk of severe poisoning with respiratory depression when receiving standard dosages. During ontogeny, CYP2D6 gene expression and activity are extremely low at birth and gradually increase to reach their final level in adolescents (Blake et al., 2007; Leeder & Kearns, 1997).

Severe poisonings and deaths have been reported with codeine use in children and neonates from breastfeeding mothers. Koren et al. described the tragic case of an infant who developed lethargy and decrease in milk intake while being breastfed by his mother who was treated by codeine and paracetamol at standard doses for postpartum pain. The toxicological analysis revealed that the mother was an ultrarapid CYP2D6 metabolizer, with very high morphine blood and milk levels (Koren, Cairns, Chitayat, Gaedigk, & Leeder, 2006). Additional cases confirmed that codeine not

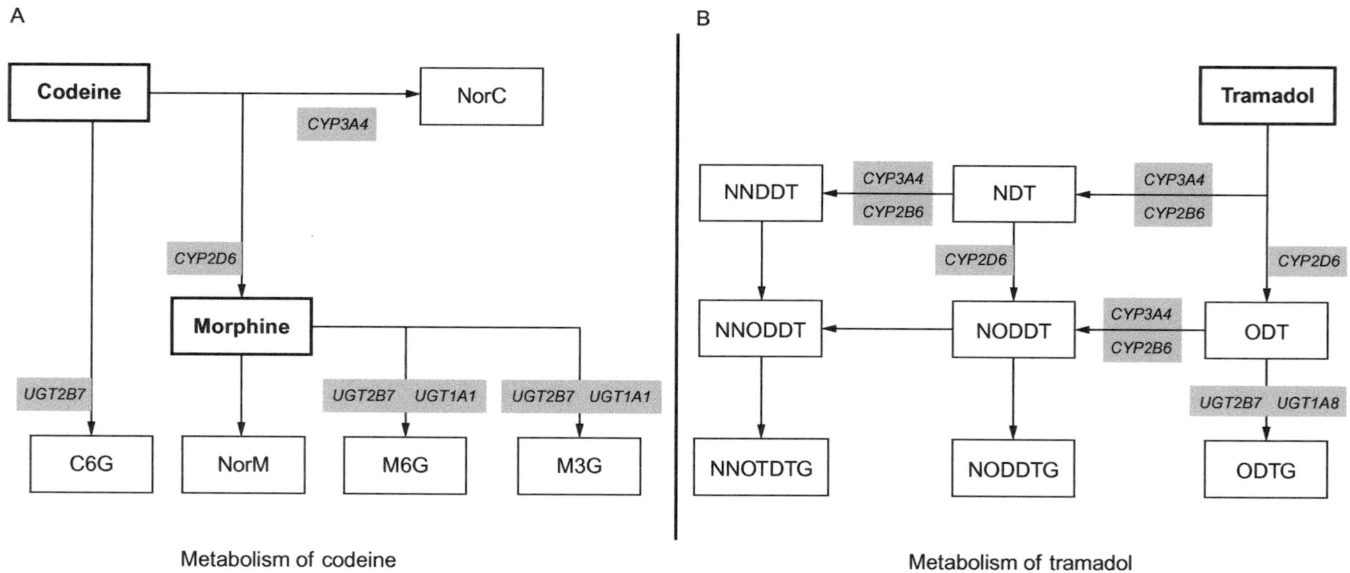

Fig. 2 Simplified scheme of codeine and tramadol metabolisms. (A) Metabolism of codeine. Compounds: *NorC*, norcodeine; *C6G*, codeine-6-glucuronide; *NorM*, normorphine; *M3G*, morphine-3-glucuronide; *M6G*, morphine-6-glucuronide. Enzymes: *Cytochrome (CYP)*: CYP2D6, CYP3A4, *Glucuronosyltransferase (UGT)*: UGT1A1, UGT2B7. (B) Metabolism of tramadol. Compounds: *ODT*, *O*-desmethyltramadol; *ODTG*, *O*-desmethyltramadol glucuronide; *NDT*, *N*-desmethyltramadol; *NODDT*, *N,O*-didesmethyltramadol; *NODDTG*, *N,O*-didesmethyltramadol glucuronides; *NNDDT*, *N,N*-didesmethytramadol; *NNODDT*, *N,N,O*-tridesmethytramadol; *NNOTDTG*, *N,N-O*-trimethyltramadol. Enzymes: *Cytochrome (CYP)*: CYP2B6, CYP3A4, *Glucuronosyltransferase (UGT)*: UGT2B7. *Panel (A): Adapted from PharmKB: https://www.pharmgkb.org/pathway/PA146123006. Panel (B): Adapted from PharmKB: https://www.pharmgkb.org/pathway/PA165946349.*

be prescribed for breastfeeding mothers (Lazaryan, Shasha-Zigelman, Dagan, & Berkovitch, 2015). In older children, life-threatening respiratory depression, anoxic brain injuries, and even death occurred under appropriate weight-based doses of codeine for postoperative pain, primarily following tonsillectomy (Prows et al., 2014; Racoosin, Roberson, Pacanowski, & Nielsen, 2013). The adverse event reports submitted to the FDA (Food and Drug Administration) from January 1969 to May 2015 identified 64 cases of serious breathing problems, including 24 deaths, with codeine-containing medicines in children younger than 18 years (FDA Drug Safety Communication, 2017).

Tramadol is also a weak opioid agonist with a CYP2D6-dependent metabolism and active metabolite (Fig. 2B). It is mainly used in children for postoperative pain and also associated with a few cases of respiratory depression (Hassanian-Moghaddam, Farnaghi, & Rahimi, 2015; Schnabel, Reichl, Meyer-Frießem, Zahn, & Pogatzki-Zahn, 2015).

Both the FDA and EMA (European Medical Agency) issued warnings regarding the use of codeine and tramadol during breastfeeding and to treat pain in children and adolescents (Table 1). However, whether similar restrictions should apply to both drugs remains a matter of large debate (Jin, 2017; Palmer, Anderson, Linscott, Paech, & Allegaert, 2018; Rodieux et al., 2018).

In the neonatal period, the first cost-effectiveness analysis of maternal CYP2D6 genetic testing to guide treatment for postpartum pain was recently published (Moretti et al., 2017). In children, additional studies are required to optimize the use of opioids, as limited data are available on efficacy and adverse events in both cancer and noncancer pediatric pain (Cooper et al., 2017; Wiffen et al., 2017). In the absence of emergency and prior to surgery, systematic genotyping might be discussed, weighted against the real positive analgesic effect of codeine (Chidambaran, Sadhasivam, & Mahmoud, 2017).

3.3 Pharmacogenetics and Adverse Drugs Reactions

3.3.1 Safety of Anticancer Drugs in Children

Many PG studies in the field of childhood cancer have focused on treatment toxicity. Selected examples will be detailed later, illustrating that studies reporting association between PG biomarkers and toxic events may be difficult to replicate.

Table 1 Summary of EMA and FDA Publications for Codeine and Tramadol Use in Children and During Breastfeeding

Issue	Drug	EMA	FDA	Comment
CYP2D6	Codeine	Codeine is contraindicated in CYP2D6 ultrarapid metabolizers, but genetic testing is not required	The prescribing physician is alerted to the risk of codeine toxicity in CYP2D6 ultrarapid metabolizers, as mentioned in the black box warning and the warning and precautions sections, but genetic testing prior to therapy is not required (2)	Both agencies agree on the risk of toxicity in CYP2D6 ultrarapid metabolizers. They also agree that genetic testing prior to administration is not required. However, the management of this risk differs in that in the European Union, being an ultrarapid metabolizer is a contraindication and in the United States, although the risk in ultrarapid metabolizers is mentioned, it is not a contraindication (1,2)
	Tramadol	The EMA is currently updating the tramadol label with a warning on the risk of tramadol toxicity in ultrarapid CYP2D6 metabolizers	The prescribing physician is alerted to the risk of tramadol toxicity in CYP2D6 ultrarapid metabolizers, in the black box warning and the warning and precautions section, but genetic testing prior to therapy is not required (2, 4, 5)	Both agencies agree on the risk of tramadol toxicity in ultrarapid CYP2D6 metabolizers. While the FDA has already included the relevant information in the label, the EMA is currently in the process of updating the tramadol label based on the recommendations made by the PRAC. The FDA cites a case report by Orliaguet et al. on a child with an ultrarapid CYP2D6 metabolism suffering from respiratory depression following the administration of tramadol. The FDA provides information in their reports and the product label on the risk of tramadol toxicity in ultrarapid CYP2D6 metabolizers (2–5)

Continued

Table 1 Summary of EMA and FDA Publications for Codeine and Tramadol Use in Children and During Breastfeeding—cont'd

Issue	Drug	EMA	FDA	Comment
Pain in children	Codeine	Indicated for children >12 years if other analgesics have not been effective Contraindicated in all children for postoperative pain management following tonsillectomy/ adenoidectomy for sleep apnea (6, 7)	Contraindicated in children <12 years Contraindicated in children ≥12 to <18 years following surgery for tonsillectomy and/or adenoidectomy	EMA and FDA agree on not using codeine for pain relief in all children <12 years Some variability exists in the EMA's and FDA's assessment for children aged ≥12 to <18 years: The EMA considers that codeine could be given, if other analgesics have not been effective, and that it could be given in children who had a tonsillectomy and/or adenoidectomy for any other reason than obstructive sleep apnea The FDA does not make a difference between a tonsillectomy/adenoidectomy for obstructive sleep apnea or for any other reason (2, 6, 7)
	Tramadol	Tramadol is not recommended in children <12 years The EMA is currently updating the label warning about the risk of life-threatening adverse events if tramadol is used postoperatively and in children with compromised respiratory function (3)	Contraindicated in children <12 years Contraindicated in children >12 to <18 years following surgery for tonsillectomy and/or adenoidectomy (2)	Tramadol risk communication for children differs between the FDA and the EMA While tramadol is not recommended in the European Union for children under 12 years of age, it is contraindicated for this age group in the United States. Similarly, for children aged 12–18 years the FDA has contraindicated the use of tramadol following surgery for tonsillectomy/adenoidectomy, while the EMA is in the process of updating the label with a general warning relating to its use following surgery in children and a more specific warning of the use in children with compromised respiratory function (2, 3)

Cough	Codeine	Codeine is not recommended for the treatment of cough in children (0–18 years) (1)	Codeine is not recommended for the treatment of cough in children (0–18 years) (2)	Both agencies agree that codeine should not be used in children (0–18 years) for the treatment of cough (1, 2)
	Tramadol	Not applicable	Not applicable	Not applicable—cough is not an indication
Diarrhea	Codeine	Codeine is not recommended for the treatment of diarrhea in children (0–18 years). No reference is provided on the EMEA website or in the label for this information	Not applicable (diarrhea is not an indication in the United States)	In the European Union, single-ingredient codeine is not recommended for the treatment of diarrhea in children (0–18 years) Diarrhea is not an indication in the United States, thus any use of codeine for treatment of diarrhea is considered off-label. No reference is provided on the MEA website or in the label for this information
	Tramadol	Not applicable	Not applicable	Not applicable—diarrhea is not an indication
Breastfeeding	Codeine	The EMA has contraindicated breast feeding for all codeine-containing products regardless of the indication (1)	The FDA warns against use during breastfeeding (2)	Both agencies advise against the use of codeine containing drugs in breastfeeding women. However, the risk management differs: in the European Union breastfeeding is a contraindication, while in the United States it is only included in the warnings and precautions section (1, 2)

Continued

Table 1 Summary of EMA and FDA Publications for Codeine and Tramadol Use in Children and During Breastfeeding—cont'd

Issue	Drug	EMA	FDA	Comment
	Tramadol	The EMA is currently updating the label providing information on the risks during breastfeeding in the corresponding breastfeeding section of the label (3)	The FDA warns against use during breastfeeding (2)	The EMA provides information in the section on lactation and considers that a single dose of tramadol is not harmful The FDA advises against the use of tramadol during breastfeeding (2,3)

EMA, European Medical Agency; *FDA*, Food and Drug Administration.

References

1. European Medicines Agency. Assessment report of the Pharmacovigilance Risk Assessment Committee (PRAC): Codeine containing medicinal products for the treatment of cough and/or cold in paediatric patients. EMA/235820/2015, March 12, 2015. URL: http://www.ema.europa.eu/docs/en_GB/document_library/Referrals_document/Codeine_cough_or_cold_in_children/Recommendation_provided_by_Pharmacovigilance_Risk_Assessment_Committee/WC500186522.pdf, accessed March 27, 2018.
2. Food and Drug Administration. Background document pediatric advisory committee meeting, September 11, 2017: Benefit/risk assessment of prescription opioid antitussive products for treatment of cough in pediatric patients. URL: https://www.fda.gov/downloads/AdvisoryCommittees/CommitteesMeetingMaterials/PediatricAdvisoryCommittee/UCM573222.pdf, accessed March 26, 2018.
3. European Medicines Agency. Tramadol—Scientific conclusions and grounds for the variation to the terms of the Marketing Authorisation(s), 2018. URL: http://www.ema.europa.eu/docs/en_GB/document_library/Periodic_safety_update_single_assessment/2018/03/WC500245268.pdf, accessed March 28, 2018.
4. Food and Drug Administration. FDA evaluating the risks of using the pain medicine tramadol in children aged 17 and younger, September 21, 2015. URL: https://www.fda.gov/downloads/Drugs/DrugSafety/UCM463471.pdf, accessed March 28, 2018.
5. Orliaguet, G., Hamza, J., Couloigner, V., Denoyelle, F., Loriot, M.A., Broly, F., & Garabedian, E.N. (2015). A case of respiratory depression in a child with ultrarapid CYP2D6 metabolism after tramadol. *Pediatrics*, *135*, e753–e755.
6. European Medicines Agency. Restrictions on use of codeine for pain relief in children—CMDh endorses PRAC recommendation, June 28, 2013. URL: http://www.ema.europa.eu/docs/en_GB/document_library/Referrals_document/Codeine_containing_medicinal_products/Position_provided_by_CMDh/WC500144850.pdf, accessed March 28, 2018.
7. European Medicines Agency. Assessment report of the Pharmacovigilance Risk Assessment Committee (PRAC): Assessment report for codeine-containing medicinal products indicated in the management of pain in children, June 24, 2013; EMA/441891/2013. URL: http://www.ema.europa.eu/docs/en_GB/document_library/Referrals_document/Codeine_containing_medicinal_products/Recommendation_provided_by_Pharmacovigilance_Risk_Assessment_Committee/WC500147065.pdf, accessed March 28, 2018.

Cisplatin

Patients, both adults and children, treated with cisplatin for solid tumors have a high risk of developing irreversible hearing loss. The first pediatric study identified TPMT and cathecol-*O*-methytransferase (COMT) variants as PG markers in a cohort of 54 children treated in oncology units, with a replication cohort of 112 children (Pussegoda et al., 2013; Ross et al., 2009). Additional replication studies were conducted in different pediatric cohorts, with less significant or contradictory results (Hagleitner et al., 2014; Lanvers-Kaminsky et al., 2014; Yang et al., 2013). Very recently, a wild type and *3A TPMT variant was transfected into murine ear cell lines and cells exposed to cisplatin, showing that cisplatin toxicity was higher in *3A expressing cells. The underlying mechanism may involve diminished detoxification of cisplatin reactive metabolite and abnormal "low utilization" of *S*-adenosyl-methionine. Such a mechanism of ototoxicity remains under discussion and would need to be confirmed, but this study provides an additional argument for the involvement of TPMT (Bhavsar et al., 2017; Lanvers-Kaminsky et al., 2014). Additional risk variants were identified in transporters (ABCC3, LRP2), conjugaison enzymes (UGTs), or deafness genes (GJB2, SLC26A4, mitochondrial DNA polymorphisms). For now, genotyping children exposed to cisplatin for TPMT might help early diagnosis and management in high-risk patients. However, even this is a matter of debate (Lee et al., 2016).

Anthracyclines (Aminkeng et al., 2016, 2017; Lenneman & Sawyer, 2016) and *vincristine* (Lopez-Lopez et al., 2016; van de Velde et al., 2017) are also known to be responsible for severe ADRs, particularly cardiotoxicity, with a major impact on quality of life in survivors.

3.3.2 Additional Safety Issues in Children

Valproate administration is associated with severe and even fatal hepatotoxicity. Developmental and genetic factors may potentially interact, explaining higher risk in young patients under the age of 6, compared to older children and adults (Star, Edwards, & Choonara, 2014).

Regarding *statins* (Niemi, 2010), the *SLCO1B1* gene encodes the OATP1B1 hepatic uptake transporter, showed to play a role in statin disposition. Only one variant of *SLCO1B1* coding for OATP1B1 has been linked to statin myopathy in a genome-wide association study. Although multifactorial, the risk for muscular toxicity, associated with higher simvastatin concentrations, increases in adult carriers of a variant of SLCO1B1 (rs4149056) (Ramsey et al., 2014). However, the effects of this variant differ markedly depending on the statin in question. Additional genes were tested as potential contributors to variability in the response and safety of statins with contradictory results in adults (Maxwell et al., 2017). As indications of statins are limited in children, the only data in pediatric patients on simvastatin disposition were published very recently, showing that simvastatin and simvastatin acid systemic exposure was highly variable in children and adolescents (8–20 years old), and that the impact of the *SLCO1B1* genotype was more pronounced. Additional studies are required to confirm these data, in the light of the possible impact of ontogeny (Wagner & Leeder, 2012).

Human leukocyte antigen (*HLA*) polymorphisms have been identified as high-risk factors of immunologic-mediated ADRs (Fricke-Galindo, LLerena, & Lopez-Lopez, 2017). Association between HLA-B*58:01 and ADRs induced by *allopurinol* is rare, occurring mainly in patients with Asian ancestry but also reported in a limited number of studies in Caucasians.

Carbamazepine is commonly prescribed in children for the treatment of seizures, and in HLA-B*1502 carriers may induce life-threatening reactions of the skin, such as Stevens–Johnson syndrome or toxic epidermal necrolysis, initially reported in a Han Chinese case (Wang et al., 2017). Patients who carry the HLA-B*5701 allele are at high risk of hypersensitivity reaction/lactic acidosis and severe hepatomegaly in response to *abacavir*.

Additional PG associations were reported with *antiretroviral drugs*: CYP2B6 alleles and *efavirenz*, and UGT1A1 alleles and *atazanavir*-associated hyperbilirubinemia. Screening for the HLA-B*1502 or *5701 alleles before treatment initiation is justified in patients from high-risk populations.

4. CONCLUSION

Advances in PG offer significant potential for improving individual patient management. However, the continuum of research in PG is complex, ranging from the discovery of genes to clinical trials, and therefore translation of research findings into clinical practice is slow. More than 50 years have elapsed since the description of the first PG polymorphism and more than 10 years since the complete sequencing of the human genome. Although the value of individual genetic information in medical care has been demonstrated, it is recommended only for a limited number of drugs and patients (Farfan et al., 2014; Green et al., 2015; Nava et al., 2018).

When involved in PG, pediatricians and pediatric pharmacologists have to face many challenges to validate and use developmental PG information in pediatric care, including the following:

(1) Increase knowledge of all developmental aspects of drug metabolism and elimination including ontogeny of transporters and the mechanisms underlying the different developmental trajectories, in order to understand the differences between adults, children, and neonates, between ethnicities, and between diseases (Leeder & Meibohm, 2016).

(2) Integrate PG into clinical trials. These studies are almost exclusively conducted in adults and are lacking in children. The challenge is to develop and use methodologies for "appropriate integration" of pharmacogenetic data, along with other biological markers, to quantify and explain variability in drug response. Accordingly, advanced molecular biology techniques should be incorporated in pediatric drug evaluation early, and include appropriate follow-up to demonstrate the benefit of individualized drug therapy based on genetic testing on clinical outcomes. In the long term, this will increase the likelihood of treatment success and decrease adverse drug reactions, thus reducing the cost of health care (Lauschke, Milani, & Ingelman-Sundberg, 2017).

(3) Develop consensus based on the level of evidence required to implement specific genetic testing in children. Because of the known barriers to pediatric trials, randomized trials evaluating drug effects based on genotyped patients are not feasible, and it is therefore not surprising that there is a real lack of available data to catalyze changes in clinical practice (Piana et al., 2012) and that the implementation of genotype-guided therapy for children remains limited (Aka et al., 2017). In this context, the Clinical Pharmacogenetics Implementation Consortium (CPIC®) is working to issue expertly approved guidelines for a translation from genetics to therapeutics in order to use genetic tests when important for the patient and guide the choice of treatment.

(4) Respect ethical issues related to pediatric PG testing. Written informed consent from both parents is mandatory, as is making detailed information about the drug and biomarkers understandable for families. For children and adolescents, who are requested to give assent, the issue is also complex, as it relies on their capacities to understand the implications of PG testing, including identifying PG variants unrelated to any current or planned therapies but predisposing them to adult disease (Schiavone et al., 2017; Zhang, Bruce, Hayde, & Rieder, 2014). In this context, pediatricians have a central role to ensure the strict respect of regulatory and ethical requirements and good clinical practices and guidance at the European and international levels (ICH Expert Working Group, 2017; Maliepaard et al., 2013).

(5) Develop training in developmental pharmacology and molecular genetics, and increase PG expertise. Recent US surveys revealed that pediatricians feel insufficiently educated and trained in the corresponding fields, and that drugs even with high PG variability are prescribed without determining a patient's genotype. Beyond the lack of knowledge/training, interpreting the results of PG analysis remains a challenge for clinicians, given the "multivariate" and "multigenic" nature of most drug effects with contribution of physiological and pathological factors, particularly in pediatric patients (Daly, 2014; Zhang et al., 2014).

(6) Evaluate the economic benefits of PG testing. Reducing inadequate therapeutic responses will in turn reduce the important societal and financial cost associated with lack of efficacy, adverse events, hospitalization, sequelae, and even death. In children, it will also reduce the potential impact on growth, organ maturation, and neurological development. The technological advances that reduce the cost of genetic testing are rapid, while progress allowing the validation of polygenic models with ontogenic variables will be much slower.

CONFLICT OF INTEREST

The authors have no conflicts of interest to declare.

REFERENCES

Adam de Beaumais, T., Fakhoury, M., Medard, Y., Azougagh, S., Zhang, D., Yakouben, K., et al. (2011). Determinants of mercaptopurine toxicity in paediatric acute lymphoblastic leukemia maintenance therapy. *British Journal of Clinical Pharmacology*, *71*(4), 575–584. https://doi.org/10.1111/j.1365-2125.2010.03867.x.

Adam de Beaumais, T., & Jacqz-Aigrain, E. (2012). Pharmacogenetic determinants of mercaptopurine disposition in children with acute lymphoblastic leukemia. *European Journal of Clinical Pharmacology*, *68*, 1233–1242.

Ahmed, S., Zhou, Z., Zhou, J., & Chen, S. Q. (2016). Pharmacogenomics of drug metabolizing enzymes and transporters: Relevance to precision medicine. *Genomics, Proteomics & Bioinformatics*, *14*, 298–313. https://doi.org/10.1016/j.gpb.2016.03.008 [Epub 2016 Oct 8].

Aka, I., Bernal, C. J., Carroll, R., Maxwell-Horn, A., Oshikoya, K. A., & Van Driest, S. L. (2017). Clinical pharmacogenetics of cytochrome P450-associated drugs in children. *Journal of Personalized Medicine*, 7, 1–20. pii: E14. https://doi.org/10.3390/jpm7040014.

Allegaert, K., Verbesselt, R., Naulaers, G., Van den Anker, J. N., Rayyan, M., Debeer, A., et al. (2008). Developmental pharmacology: Neonates are not just small adults. *Acta Clinica Belgica*, *63*, 16–24.

Allegaert, K., Mian, P., & van den Anker, J. N. (2017). Developmental pharmacokinetics in neonates: Maturational changes and beyond. *Current Pharmaceutical Design*, *23*, 5769–5778. https://doi.org/10.2174/1381612823666170926121124.

Aminkeng, F., Ross, C. J. D., Rassekh, S. R., Rieder, M. J., Bhavsar, A. P., Sanatani, S., et al. (2016). Recommendations for genetic testing to reduce the incidence of anthracycline-induced cardiotoxicity. *British Journal of Clinical Pharmacology, 82,* 683–695.

Aminkeng, F., Ross, C. J. D., Rassekh, S. R., Rieder, M. J., Bhavsar, A. P., Sanatani, S., et al. (2017). Pharmacogenetic screening for anthracycline-induced cardiotoxicity in childhood cancer. Letter to the Editor. *British Journal of Clinical Pharmacology, 83*(5), 1143–1145.

Bhavsar, A. P., Gunaretnam, E. P., Li, Y., Hasbullah, J. S., Carleton, B. C., & Ross, C. J. D. (2017). Pharmacogenetic variants in TPMT alter cellular responses to cisplatin in inner ear cell lines. *PLoS One, 12*(4), 1–10. e0175711. https://doi.org/10.1371/journal.pone.0175711. eCollection 2017.

Biss, T. T., Avery, P. J., Brandão, L. R., Chalmers, E. A., Williams, M. D., Grainger, J. D., et al. (2012). VKORC1 and CYP2C9 genotype and patient characteristics explain a large proportion of the variability in warfarin dose requirement among children. *Blood, 119,* 868–873. https://doi.org/10.1182/blood-2011-08-372722 [Epub 2011 Oct 18].

Blake, M. J., Gaedigk, A., Pearce, R. E., Bomgaars, L. R., Christensen, M. L., Stowe, C., et al. (2007). Ontogeny of dextromethorphan O- and N-demethylation in the first year of life. *Clinical Pharmacology and Therapeutics, 81,* 510–516.

Blazquez, A., Mas, S., Plana, M. T., Lafuente, A., & Lázaro, L. (2012). Fluoxetine pharmacogenetics in child and adult populations. *European Child & Adolescent Psychiatry, 21*(11), 599–610. https://doi.org/10.1007/s00787-012-0305-6 [Epub 2012 Jul 12].

Brouwer, K. L., Aleksunes, L. M., Brandys, B., Giacoia, G. P., Knipp, G., Lukacova, V., et al. (2015). Human ontogeny of drug transporters: Review and recommendations of the pediatric transporter working group. *Clinical Pharmacology and Therapeutics, 98,* 266–287. https://doi.org/10.1002/cpt.176.

Chidambaran, V., Sadhasivam, S., & Mahmoud, M. (2017). Codeine and opioid metabolism: Implications and alternatives for pediatric pain management. *Current Opinion in Anaesthesiology, 30,* 349–356.

Cooper, T. E., Fisher, E., Gray, A. L., Krane, E., Sethna, N., van Thilburg, M. A., et al. (2017). Opioids for chronic non-cancer pain in children and adolescents. *The Cochrane Database of Systematic Reviews,* 7, CD012538.

Bertholee, D., Maring, J. G., & Van Kuilenburg, A. B. (2017). Genotypes affecting the pharmacokinetics of anticancer drugs. *Clinical Pharmacokinetics, 56*(4), 317–337.

Daly, A. K. (2014). Is there a need to teach pharmacogenetics? *Clinical Pharmacology and Therapeutics, 95*(3), 245–247. https://doi.org/10.1038/clpt.2013.184.

De Wildt, S. N., Kearns, G. L., Leeder, J. S., & Van den Anker, J. N. (1999). Glucuronidation in humans. Pharmacogenetic and developmental aspects. *Clinical Pharmacokinetics, 36,* 439–452.

Elie, V., de Beaumais, T., Fakhoury, M., & Jacqz-Aigrain, E. (2011). Pharmacogenetics and individualized therapy in children: Immunosuppressants, antidepressants, anticancer and anti-inflammatory drugs. *Pharmacogenomics, 12,* 827–843.

Fakhoury, M., de Beaumais, T., Médard, Y., & Jacqz-Aigrain, E. (2010). Therapeutic drug monitoring of 6-thioguanine nucleotides in paediatric acute lymphoblastic leukaemia: Interest and limits. *Thérapie, 65,* 187–193.

Farfan, M. J., Salas, C., Canales, C., Silva, F., Villarroel, M., Kopp, K., et al. (2014). Prevalence of TPMT and ITPA gene polymorphisms and effect on mercaptopurine dosage in Chilean children with acute lymphoblastic leukemia. *BMC Cancer 14,* 299. https://doi.org/10.1186/1471-2407-14-299.

Foster, J. B., & Maude, S. L. (2018). New developments in immunotherapy for pediatric leukemia. *Current Opinion in Pediatrics, 30*(1), 25–29.

FDA Drug Safety Communication. (2017). *Safety announcement, US Food and Drug Administration, US Department of Health and Human Services.* available at https://www.fda.gov/Drugs/DrugSafety/ucm549679.htm.

Franca, R., Favretto, D., Granzotto, M., Decorti, G., Rabusin, M., & Stocco, G. (2017). Epratuzumab and blinatumomab as therapeutic antibodies for treatment of pediatric acute lymphoblastic leukemia: Current status and future perspectives. *Current Medicinal Chemistry, 24*(11), 1050–1065. https://doi.org/10.2174/0929867324666170113105733.

Fricke-Galindo, I., LLerena, A., & Lopez-Lopez, M. (2017). An update on HLA alleles associated with adverse drug reactions. *Drug Metabolism and Personalized Therapy, 32*, 73–87.

Green, D. J., Mummaneni, P., Kim, I. W., Oh, J. M., Pacanowski, M., & Burckaert, G. J. (2015). Pharmacogenomic information in FDA-approved drug labels: Application to paediatric patients. *Clinical Pharmacology and Therapeutics, 99*(6), 622–632.

Hagleitner, M. M., Coenen, M. J., Patino-Garcia, A., de Bont, E. S., Gonzales-Neira, A., Vos, H. L., et al. (2014). Influence of genetic variants in TMPT and COMT associated woith cisplatin induced hearing loss in patients with cancer: Two new cohort and meta-analysis reveal significant heterogeneity between cohorts. *PLoS One, 9*, e115869.

Hamberg, A. K., & Wadelius, M. (2014). Pharmacogenetics-based warfarin dosing in children. *Pharmacogenomics, 15*(3), 361–374. https://doi.org/10.2217/pgs.14.8.

Hassanian-Moghaddam, H., Farnaghi, F., & Rahimi, M. (2015). Tramadol overdose and apnea in hospitalized children, a review of 20 cases. *Research in Pharmaceutical Sciences, 10*(6), 544–552.

Hicks, J. K., Swen, J. J., & Gaedigk, A. (2014). Challenges in CYP2D6 phenotype assignment from genotype data: A critical assessment and call for standardization. *Current Drug Metabolism, 15*, 218–232.

Hines, R. N., Simpson, P. M., & McCarver, D. G. (2016). Age-dependent human hepatic carboxylesterase 1 (CES1) and carboxylesterase 2 (CES2) postnatal ontogeny. *Drug Metabolism and Disposition, 44*, 959–966. https://doi.org/10.1124/dmd.115.068957 [Epub 2016 Jan 29].

Hines, R. N. (2013). Developmental expression of drug metabolizing enzymes: Impact on disposition in neonates and young children. *International Journal of Pharmaceutics, 16*, 3–7.

Hunger, S. P., & Mullighan, C. G. (2015). Acute lymphoblastic leukemia in children. *The New England Journal of Medicine, 373*, 1541–1552.

ICH Expert Working Group. (2017). *ICH E18 Guideline on genomic sampling and management of genomic data, International Council for Harmonisation of Technical Requirements for Pharmaceuticals for Human Use.* Geneva, Switzerland: ICH Secretariat, available at http://www.ich.org/ichnews.

Ishikawa, T. (2012). Genetic variants in the human SLCO1B1 gene and individual variations in methotrexate clearance. *Pharmacogenomics, 13*, 993–994. https://doi.org/10.2217/pgs.12.74.

Jacqz-Aigrain, E., Funck-Brentano, C., & Cresteil, T. (1993). CYP2D6- and CYP3A-dependent metabolism of dextromethorphan in humans. *Pharmacogenetics, 3*, 197–204.

Jin, J. (2017). Risks of codeine and tramadol in children. *JAMA, 318*(15), 1514. https://doi.org/10.1001/jama.2017.13534.

Kearns, G. L., Abdel-Rahman, S. M., Alander, S. W., Blowey, D. L., Leeder, J. S., & Kauffman, R. E. (2003). Developmental pharmacology—Drug disposition, action, and therapy in infants and children. *The New England Journal of Medicine, 18*, 1157–1167.

Kearns, G. L., Robinson, P. K., Wilson, J. T., Wilson-Costello, D., Knight, G. R., Ward, R. M., et al. (2003). Pediatric pharmacology research unit network. Cisapride disposition in neonates and infants: In vivo reflection of cytochrome P450 3A4 ontogeny. *Clinical Pharmacology and Therapeutics, 74*, 312–325.

Koren, G., Cairns, J., Chitayat, D., Gaedigk, A., & Leeder, S. J. (2006). Pharmacogenetics of morphine poisoning in a breastfed neonate of a codeine-prescribed mother. *Lancet (London, England), 368*, 704.

Krekels, E. H., Danhof, M., Tibboel, D., & Knibbe, C. A. (2012). Ontogeny of hepatic glucuronidation; methods and results. *Current Drug Metabolism*, *13*, 728–743.

Lanvers-Kaminsky, C., Malath, I., Deuster, D., Ciarimboli, G., Boos, J., & Am Zehnhoff-Dinnesen, A. G. (2014). Evaluation of pharmacogenetic markers to predict the risk of cisplatin-induced ototoxicity. *Clinical Pharmacology and Therapeutics*, *96*(2), 156–157. https://doi.org/10.1038/clpt.2014.67. Epub 2014 Mar 18.

Lauschke, V. M., Milani, L., & Ingelman-Sundberg, M. (2017). Pharmacogenomic biomarkers for improved drug therapy-recent progress and future developments. *The AAPS Journal*, *20*(1), 4. https://doi.org/10.1208/s12248-017-0161-x.77. PG techniques a mettre en fin.

Lazaryan, M., Shasha-Zigelman, C., Dagan, Z., & Berkovitch, M. (2015). Codeine should not be prescribed for breastfeeding mothers or children under the age of 12. *Acta Paediatrica*, *104*, 550–556.

Lee, J. W., Pussegoda, K., Rassekh, S. R., Monzon, J. G., Liu, G., Hwang, S., et al.Clinical Recommendations Group, (2016). Clinical practice recommendations for the management and prevention of cisplatin-induced hearing loss using pharmacogenetic markers. *Therapeutic Drug Monitoring*, *38*(4), 423–431. https://doi.org/10.1097/FTD.0000000000000298.

Leeder, J. S., & Kearns, G. L. (1997). Pharmacogenetics in pediatrics. Implications for practice. *Pediatric Clinics of North America*, *44*, 55–77.

Leeder, J. S. (2009). Developmental pharmacogenetics: A general paradigm for application to neonatal pharmacology and toxicology. *Clinical Pharmacology and Therapeutics*, *86*, 678–682. https://doi.org/10.1038/clpt.2009.195. Epub 2009 Oct 28.

Leeder, J. S., Kearns, G. L., Spielberg, S. P., & van den Anker, J. (2010). Understanding the relative roles of pharmacogenetics and ontogeny in paediatric drug development and regulatory sciences. *Journal of Clinical Pharmacology*, *50*, 1377–1387.

Leeder, J. S., & Meibohm, B. (2016). Challenges and opportunities for increasing the knowledge base related to drug biotransformation and pharmacokinetics during growth and development. *Drug Metabolism and Disposition*, *44*(7), 916–923. https://doi.org/10.1124/dmd.116.071159.

Lenneman, C. G., & Sawyer, D. B. (2016). Cardio-oncology: An update on cardiotoxicity of cancer related treatment. *Circulation Research*, *118*, 1008–1020.

Limenta, L. M., Jirasomprasert, T., Tankanitlert, J., et al. (2008). UGT1A6 genotype-related pharmacokinetics of deferiprone (L1) in healthy volunteers. *British Journal of Clinical Pharmacology*, *65*, 908–916.

Loh, M. L., Tasian, S. K., Rabin, K. R., Brown, P., Magoon, D., Reid, J. M., et al. (2015). A phase 1 dosing study of ruxolitinib in children with relapsed or refractory solid tumors, leukemias, or myeloproliferative neoplasms: A children's oncology group phase 1 consortium study (ADVL1011). *Pediatric Blood & Cancer*, *62*, 1717–1724. https://doi.org/10.1002/pbc.25575. Epub 2015 May 13.

Lopez-Lopez, E., Gutierrez-Camino, A., Astigarraga, I., Navajas, A., Echebarria-Barona, A., Garcia-Miguel, P., et al. (2016). Vincristine pharmacokinetic pathway and neurotoxicity during early phases of treatment in paediatric acute lymphoblastic leukemia. *Pharmacogenomics*, *17*, 731–741.

Maagdenberg, H., Vijverberg, S. J., Bierings, M. B., Carleton, B. C., Arets, H. G., de Boer, A., et al. (2016). Pharmacogenomics in pediatric patients: Towards personalized medicine. *Paediatric Drugs*, *18*, 251–260. https://doi.org/10.1007/s40272-016-0176-2.

Maliepaard, M., Nofziger, C., Papaluca, M., Zineh, I., Uyama, Y., Prasad, K., et al. (2013). Pharmacogenetics in the evaluation of new drugs: A multiregional regulatory perspective. *Nature Reviews. Drug Discovery*, *12*, 103–115.

Mattevi, V. S., & Tagliari, C. F. (2017). Pharmacogenetic considerations in the treatment of HIV. *Pharmacogenomics*, *18*, 85–98.

Maxwell, R. R., & Cole, P. D. (2017). Pharmacogenetic predictors of treatment-related toxicity among children with acute lymphoblastic leukemia. *Current Hematologic Malignancy Reports*, *12*, 176–186.

Maxwell, W. D., Ramsey, L. B., Johnson, S. G., Moore, K. G., Shtutman, M., Schoonover, J. H., et al. (2017). Impact of pharmacogenetics on efficacy and safety of statin therapy for dyslipidemia. *Pharmacotherapy*, *37*(9), 1172–1190. https://doi.org/10.1002/phar.1981. Epub 2017 Aug 23.

McLeod, H. L., Krynetski, E. Y., Relling, M. V., & Evans, W. E. (2000). Genetic polymorphism of thiopurine methyltransferase and its clinical relevance for childhood acute lymphoblastic leukemia. *Leukemia*, *14*, 567–572.

Miners, J. O., McKinnon, R. A., & Mackenzie, P. I. (2002). Genetic polymorphisms of UDP glucuronosyltransferases and their functional significance. *Toxicology*, *181*, 453–456.

Mishra, P. J., Humeniuk, R., Mishra, P. J., Longo-Sorbello, G. S., Barnerjee, D., & Bertino, J. R. (2007). A miR-24 microRNA binding site polymorphism in dihydrofolate gene reductase gene leads to methotrexate resistance. *Proceedings of the National Academy of Sciences of the United States of America*, *104*, 13513–13518.

Mlakar, V., Huezo-Diaz Curtis, P., Satyanarayana Uppugunduri, C. R., Krajinovic, M., & Ansari, M. (2016). Pharmacogenomics in pediatric oncology: Review of gene-drug associations for clinical use. *International Journal of Molecular Sciences*, *17*(9), 1502–1536. pii: E1502. https://doi.org/10.3390/ijms17091502.

Mooij, M. G., van de Steeg, E., van Rosmalen, J., Windster, J. D., de Koning, B. A., Vaes, W. H., et al. (2016). Proteomic analysis of the developmental trajectory of human hepatic membrane transporter proteins in the first three months of life. *Drug Metabolism and Disposition: The Biological Fate of Chemicals*, *55*, 507–524. https://doi.org/10.1007/s40262-015-0328-5. Review.

Moretti, M. E., Lato, D. F., Berger, H., Koren, G., Ito, S., & Ungar, W. J. (2017). A cost-effectiveness analysis of maternal CYP2D6 genetic testing to guide treatment for postpartum pain and avert infant adverse events. *The Pharmacogenomics Journal*. https://doi.org/10.1038/tpj.2017.33. Epub ahead of print.

Moriyama, T., Yang, Y. L., Nishii, R., Ariffin, H., Liu, C., Lin, T. N., et al. (2017). Novel variants in NUDT15 and thiopurine intolerance in children with acute lymphoblastic leukemia from diverse ancestry. *Blood*, *130*, 1209–1212.

Naraharisetti, S. B., Lin, Y. S., Rieder, M. J., Marciante, K. D., Psaty, B. M., Thummel, K. E., et al. (2010). Human liver expression of CYP2C8: Gender, age, and genotype effects. *Drug Metabolism and Disposition*, *38*, 889–893. https://doi.org/10.1124/dmd.109.031542. Epub 2010 Feb 26.

Nava, T., Kassir, N., Rezgui, M. A., Uppugunduri, C. R., Huezo-Diaz Curtis, P., & Duval, M. (2018). Incorporation of GSTA1 genetic variations into a population pharmacokinetic model for IV busulfan in paediatric hematopoietic stem cell transplantation. *British Journal of Clinical Pharmacology*. https://doi.org/10.1111/bcp.13566. Epub ahead of print.

Niemi, M. (2010). Transporter pharmacogenetics and statin toxicity. *Clinical Pharmacology and Therapeutics*, *87*, 130–133.

Palmer, G. M., Anderson, B. J., Linscott, D. K., Paech, M. J., & Allegaert, K. (2018). Tramadol, breast feeding and safety in the newborn. *Archives of Disease in Childhood*. https://doi.org/10.1136/archdischild-2017-313786. pii: archdischild, 313786. Epub ahead of publication.

Piana, C., Surh, L., Furst-Recktenwald, S., Iolascon, A., Jacqz-Aigrain, E. M., Jonker, I., et al. (2012). Integration of pharmacogenetics and pharmacogenomics in drug development: Implications for regulatory and medical decision making in pediatric diseases. *Journal of Clinical Pharmacology*, *52*, 704–716.

Pierro, J., Hogan, L. E., Bhatla, T., & Carroll, W. L. (2017). New targeted therapies for relapsed pediatric acute lymphoblastic leukemia. *Expert Review of Anticancer Therapy, 17*(8), 725–736. https://doi.org/10.1080/14737140.2017.1347507. Epub 2017 Jul 5.

Prows, C. A., Zhang, X., Huth, M. M., Zhang, K., Saldaña, S. N., Daraiseh, N. M., et al. (2014). Codeine-related adverse drug reactions in children following tonsillectomy: A prospective study. *The Laryngoscope, 124*, 1242–1250.

Pussegoda, K., Ross, C. J., Visscher, H., Yazdanpanah, M., Brooks, B., Rassekh, S. R., et al. (2013). Replication of TPMT and ABCC3 genetic variants associated with cisplatin-induced hearing loss in children. *Clinical Pharmacology and Therapeutics, 94*, 243–251.

Racoosin, J. A., Roberson, D. W., Pacanowski, M. A., & Nielsen, D. R. (2013). New evidence about an old drug—Risk with codeine after adenotonsillectomy. *The New England Journal of Medicine, 368*, 2155–2157.

Raffaella, F., Kuzelicki, N. K., Sorio, C., Toffoletti, E., Montecchini, O., Poropat, A., et al. (2017). Targeting kinase-activating genetic lesions to improve therapy of pediatric acute lymphoblastic leukemia. *Current Medicinal Chemistry,* 27 [Epub ahead of print]66.

Ramsey, L. B., Johnson, S. G., Caudle, K. E., Haidar, C. E., Voora, D., Wilke, R. A., et al. (2014). The clinical pharmacogenetics implementation consortium guideline for SLCO1B1 and simvastatin-induced myopathy: 2014 Update. *Clinical Pharmacology and Therapeutics, 96*(4), 423–428. https://doi.org/10.1038/clpt.2014.125. Epub 2014 Jun 11.

Ramsey, L. B., Panetta, J. C., Smith, C., Yang, W., Fan, Y., & Winick, N. J. (2013). Genome-wide study of methotrexate clearance replicates SLCO1B1. *Blood, 121*(6), 898–904. https://doi.org/10.1182/blood-2012-08-452839. Epub 2012 Dec 11.

Relling, M. V., Gardner, E. E., Sandborn, W. J., Schmiegelow, K., Pui, C.-H., Yee, S. W., et al. (2013). Clinical pharmacogenetics implementation consortium guidelines for thiopurine methyltransferase genotype and thiopurine dosing: 2013 Update. *Clinical Pharmacology and Therapeutics, 93*, 324–325.

Reshmi, S. C., Harvey, R. C., Roberts, K. G., Stonerock, E., Smith, A., Jenkins, H., et al. (2017). Targetable kinase gene fusions in high-risk B-ALL: A study from the Children's Oncology Group. *Blood, 129*(25), 3352–3361. 22. https://doi.org/10.1182/blood-2016-12-758979. Epub 2017 Apr 13.

Roberts, K. G., Li, Y., Payne-Turner, D., Harvey, R. C., Yang, Y. L., Pei, D., et al. (2014). Tragetable kinase-activating lesions in Ph-lie acute leukemia. *The New England Journal of Medicine, 371*, 1005–1015.

Roberts, K. G., Gu, Z., Payne-Turner, D., McCastlain, K., Harvey, R. C., Chen, I. M., et al. (2017). High frequency and poor outcome of Philadelphia chromosome-like acute lymphoblastic leukemia in adults. *Journal of Clinical Oncology, 35*(4), 394–401. https://doi.org/10.1200/JCO.2016.69.0073. Epub 2016 Nov 21.

Rodieux, F., Vutskits, L., Posfay-Barbe, K. M., Habre, W., Piguet, V., Desmeules, J. A., et al. (2018). When the safe alternative is not that safe: Tramadol prescribing in children. *Frontiers in Pharmacology, 9*, 148.

Ross, C. J., Katzov-Eckert, H., Dube, M. P., Brooks, B., Rassekh, S. R., Barhdadi, A., et al. (2009). Genetic variants in TPMT and COMT are associated with hearing loss in children receiving cisplatin chemotherapy. *Nature Genetics, 41*, 1345–1349.

Rubin, S., Marable, M., & Huang, R. S. (2017). The promise of pharmacogenomics in reducing toxicity during acute lymphoblastic leukemia maintenance therapy. *Genomics, Proteomics & Bioinformatics, 15*(2), 82–93.

Rytting, M., Triche, L., Thomas, D., O'Brien, S., & Kartajian, H. (2017). Initial experience with CMC-544 (inotuzumab ozogamicin) in pediatric patients wit remapsed-B cell acute lymphoblastic leukemia. *Expert Review of Anticancer Therapy, 17*, 725–736. https://doi.org/10.1080/14737140.2017.1347507. Epub 2017 Jul 5.

Santiago, R., Vairy, S., Sinnett, D., Krajinovic, M., & Bittencourt, H. (2017). Novel therapy for childhood acute lymphoblastic leukemia. *Expert Opinion on Pharmacotherapy*, *18*, 1081–1099.

Schalper, K. (2016). Basic overview of current immunotherapy approaches in cancer. *American Society of Clinical Oncology Educational Book. American Society of Clinical Oncology. Meeting*, *35*, 298–308. https://doi.org/10.14694/EDBK_156572.

Schiavone, S., Neri, M., Pomara, C., Riezzo, I., Trabace, L., & Turillazzi, E. (2017). Personalized medicine in the paediatric population: The balance between pharmacogeetics progress and bioethics. *Current Pharmaceutical Biotechnology*, *18*(3), 253–262. https://doi.org/10.2174/1389201018666170207130236.

Schnabel, A., Reichl, S. U., Meyer-Frießem, C., Zahn, P. K., & Pogatzki-Zahn, E. (2015). Tramadol for postoperative pain treatment in children. *The Cochrane Database of Systematic Reviews*, *18*(3), CD009574. https://doi.org/10.1002/14651858.CD009574.pub2.

Schultz, K. R., Carroll, A., Heerema, N. A., Bowman, W. P., Aledo, A., Slayton, W. B., et al. (2014). Long-term follow-up of imatinib in pediatric Philadelphia chromosome-positive acute lymphoblastic leukemia: Children's oncology group study. *Leukemia*, *28*, 1467–1471.

Simon, T., Verstuyft, C., Mary-Krause, M., Quteineh, L., Drouet, E., Méneveau, N., et al. (2009). Genetic determinants of response to clopidogrel and cardiovascular events. *The New England Journal of Medicine*, *360*, 363–375.

Singh, M., Bhatia, P., Khera, S., & Trehan, A. (2017). Emerging role of NUDT15 polymorphisms in 6-mercaptopurine metabolism and dose related toxicity in acute lymphoblastic leukaemia. *Leukemia Research*, *62*, 17–22.

Star, K., Edwards, I. R., & Choonara, I. (2014). Valproic acid and fatalities in children: A review of individual case safety reports in VigiBase. *PLoS One*, *9*, e108970.

Stevens, A., Hanson, D., Whamore, A., Destenaves, B., Chatelin, P., & Clayton, P. (2013). Human growth is associated with distinct patterns of gene expression in evolutionary conserved networks. *BMC Genomics*, *14*, 547. https://doi.org/10.1186/1471-2164-14-547.

Sumi, S., Marinaki, A. M., Arenas, M., Fairbanks, L., Shobowale-Bakre, M., Rees, D. C., et al. (2002). Genetic basis of inosine triphosphate pyrophosphohydrolase deficiency. *Human Genetics*, *111*(4–5), 360–367. Epub 2002 Aug 15.

Suttorp, M., Bornhäuser, M., Metzler, M., Millot, F., & Schleyer, E. (2017). Pharmacology and pharmacokinetics of imatinib in pediatric patients. *Expert Review of Clinical Pharmacology*, *11*(3), 219–231. https://doi.org/10.1080/17512433.2018.1398644.

Tanaka, Y., Nakadate, H., Kondoh, K., Nakamura, K., Koh, K., & Manabe, A. (2018). Interaction between NUDT15 and ABCC4 variants enhances intolerability of 6-mercaptopurine in Japanese patients with childhood acute lymphoblastic leukemia. *The Pharmacogenomics Journal*, *18*(2), 275–280. https://doi.org/10.1038/tpj.2017.12. Epub 2017 Apr 18.

Tang, W., Shi, Q. P., Ding, F., Yu, M. L., Hua, J., & Wang, Y. X. (2017). Impact of VKORC1 gene polymorphisms on warfarin maintenance dosage: A novel systematic review and meta-analysis of 53 studies. *International Journal of Clinical Pharmacology and Therapeutics*, *55*(4), 304–321. https://doi.org/10.5414/CP202833.

Tasian, S. K., Loh, M. L., & Hunger, S. P. (2017). Philadelphia chromosome-like acute lymphoblastic leukemia. *Blood*, *130*(19), 2064–2072. https://doi.org/10.1182/blood-2017-06-743252. Epub 2017 Oct 2.

Tozzi, V. (2010). Pharmacogenetics of antiretrovirals. *Antiviral Research*, *85*, 190–200.

Trevino, L. R., Shimasaki, N., Yang, W., Panetta, J. C., Cheng, C., Pei, D., et al. (2009). Germilne genetic variation in an organic anion transporter polypeptide associated with methotrexate pharmacokinetics and clinical effects. *Journal of Clinical Oncology*, *27*, 5972–5978.

van de Velde, M. E., Kaspers, G. L., Abbink, F. C. H., Wilhelm, A. J., Ket, J. C. F., & van den Berg, M. H. (2017). Vincristine-induced peripheral neuropathy in children with cancer: A systematic review. *Critical Reviews in Oncology/Hematology, 114*, 114–130.

Vanhaesebrouck, S., Verbesselt, R., & van den Anker, J. N. (2009). In vivo glucuronidation activity of drugs in neonates: Extensive interindividual variability despite their young age. *Therapeutic Drug Monitoring, 31*, 411–415.

Vear, S. I., Ayers, G. D., Van Driest, S. L., Sidonio, R. F., Stein, C. M., & Ho, R. H. (2014). The impact of age and CYP2C9 and VKORC1 variants on stable warfarin dose in the paediatric population. *British Journal of Haematology, 165*(6), 832–835. https://doi.org/10.1111/bjh.12817. Epub 2014 Mar 6.

von Stackelberg, A., Locatelli, F., Zugmaier, G., Handgretinger, R., Trippett, T. M., Rizzari, C., et al. (2016). Phase I/phase II study of blinatumomab in Pediatric patients with relapsed/refractory actue lymphoblastic leukemia. *Journal of Clinical Oncology, 43*, 4381–4389.

Wagner, J., & Leeder, J. S. (2012). Pediatric pharmacogenomics: A systematic assessment of ontogeny and genetic variation to guide the design of statin studies in children. *Pediatric Clinics of North America, 59*(5), 1017–1037. https://doi.org/10.1016/j.pcl.2012.07.008. Epub 2012 Aug 22.

Wang, Q., Sun, S., Xie, M., Zhao, K., Li, X., & Zhao, Z. (2017). Association between the HLA-B alleles and carbamazepine-induced SJS/TEN: A meta-analysis. *Epilepsy Research, 135*, 19–28.

Wiffen, P. J., Cooper, T. E., Anderson, A. K., Gray, A. L., Grégoire, M. C., et al. (2017). Opioids for cancer-related pain in children and adolescents. *Cochrane Database of Systematic Reviews* (7), CD012564. https://doi.org/10.1002/14651858.CD012564.pub2.

Yang, S. K., Hong, M., Baek, J., Choi, H., Zhao, W., Jung, Y., et al. (2014). A common missense variant in NUDT15 confers susceptibility to thiopurine-induced leukopenia. *Nature Genetics, 46*(9), 1017–1020. https://doi.org/10.1038/ng.3060. Epub 2014 Aug 10.

Yang, J. J., Lim, J. Y., Huang, J., Bass, J., Wu, J., Wang, C., et al. (2013). The role of inherited TPMT and COMT genetic variation in cysplatin induced ototoxicity in children with cancer. *Clinical Pharmacology and Therapeutics, 94*, 252–259.

Zhang, S. C., Bruce, C., Hayde, M., & Rieder, M. (2014). Public perceptions of pharmacogenomics. *Pediatrics, 133*, e1258.

Zhang, J., Tian, L., Huang, J., Huang, S., Chai, T., & Shen, J. (2017). Cytochrome P450 2C9 gene polymorphism and warfarin maintenance dosage in pediatric patients: A systematic review and meta-analysis. *Cardiovascular Therapeutics, 35*, 26–32. https://doi.org/10.1111/1755-5922.12230.

Zhao, W., Leroux, S., Biran, V., & Jacqz-Aigrain, E. (2018). Developmental pharmacogenetics of CYP2C19 in neonates and young infants: Omeprazole as a probe drug. *British Journal of Clinical Pharmacology, 84*(5), 997–1005. https://doi.org/10.1111/bcp.13526. Epub 2018 Mar 9.

Zgheib, N. K., Akika, R., Mahfouz, R., Aridi, C. A., Ghanem, K. M., Saab, R., et al. (2017). NUDT15 and TPMT genetic polymorphisms are related to 6-mercaptopurine intolerance in children treated for acute lymphoblastic leukemia at the Children's Cancer Center of Lebanon. *Pediatric Blood & Cancer, 64*(1), 146–150. https://doi.org/10.1002/pbc.26189. Epub 2016 Aug 31.

SECTION IV

Pharmacogenetics in Therapy

CHAPTER NINE

Implementation of Pharmacogenomics in Everyday Clinical Settings

Paul C.D. Bank, Jesse J. Swen, Henk-Jan Guchelaar[1]
Department of Clinical Pharmacy & Toxicology, Leiden University Medical Center, Leiden, The Netherlands
[1]Corresponding author: e-mail address: h.j.guchelaar@lumc.nl

Contents

1. Introduction 220
2. Players in the Field 220
3. Challenges for Implementation of PGx 223
   3.1 Selecting Clinically Relevant Pharmacogenes 223
   3.2 Providing Data on Diagnostic Criteria of PGx Testing 231
   3.3 Guidelines Directing the Clinical Use of PGx Test Results 232
   3.4 Providing Scientific Evidence for Improvement in Patient Care by PGx Testing 233
   3.5 Providing Information on Cost-Effectiveness and Cost-Consequences of PGx Testing 236
   3.6 Improving Acceptance of PGx Testing 237
4. Conclusion 239
Acknowledgments 239
References 240

Abstract

Currently, germline pharmacogenomics (PGx) is successfully implemented within certain specialties in clinical care. With the integration of PGx in pharmacotherapy multiple stakeholders are involved, which are identified in this chapter. Clinically relevant pharmacogenes with their related PGx test are discussed, along with diagnostic test criteria to guide clinicians and policy makers in PGx test selection. The chapter further reviews the similarities and the differences between the guidelines of the Dutch Pharmacogenetics Working Group and the Clinical Pharmacogenetics Implementation Consortium which both support healthcare professionals in understanding PGx test results and help guiding pharmacotherapy by providing evidence-based dosing recommendations. Finally, clinical studies which provide scientific evidence and information on cost-effectiveness supporting clinical implementation of PGx in clinical care are discussed along with the remaining barriers for adoption of PGx testing by healthcare professionals.

Advances in Pharmacology, Volume 83
ISSN 1054-3589
https://doi.org/10.1016/bs.apha.2018.04.003

1. INTRODUCTION

In the last decade pharmacogenomics (PGx) has made the transition from a field within clinical pharmacology research to an integral part of pharmacotherapy. Barriers obstructing the integration of PGx in clinical care included a lack of clinical grade tests, a lack of evidence-based guidelines providing interpretation and therapeutic recommendations, and a lack of integration into the workflow of healthcare professionals (Swen et al., 2007). Currently, many of these barriers have been successfully addressed. Multiple genotyping tests suitable for clinical use have been developed. Consortia such as the Dutch Pharmacogenetics Working Group (DPWG) and the Clinical Pharmacogenetics Implementation Consortium (CPIC) both have provided widely acclaimed guidelines (Relling & Klein, 2011; Swen et al., 2011, 2008). Clinical decision support (CDS) integrating electronic medication surveillance based on genotype into the workflow has become available on institutional or national level (O'Donnell et al., 2012, 2014; Swen et al., 2011, 2008; Van Driest et al., 2014). For several PGx genes large studies have provided evidence that information on germline variants in single genes can lead to more effective or safer therapy. The first part of this review identifies the parties that play a role in the widespread implementation of PGx in clinical care. The second part covers various topics regarding current implementation of PGx in clinical practice, including: clinically relevant tests; diagnostic criteria; guidelines containing evidence-based therapeutic recommendations; multiple implementation programs; and barriers still hindering the full and widespread integration of PGx in clinical care.

2. PLAYERS IN THE FIELD

On the road to widespread integration of PGx into clinical care multiple parties play a role in PGx becoming a part of routine practice. These roles include making decisions to adopt PGx testing, enforcing research on genetic biomarkers, providing the materials for clinical laboratories to test patients, or reviewing available evidence to provide healthcare professionals the tools to optimize pharmacotherapy. Different stakeholders can be involved in the implementation process including the biotechnology industry, governments, clinicians, healthcare insurers, and patients.

Research institutions and the analytical industry are developing new methods for detection of genetic variants. Although this technology is mostly developed to detect mutations responsible for genetic diseases, clinical laboratories can optimize the developed assays to detect relevant (germline) PGx variants. In licensed medicine, information on PGx markers in drug labels increasingly will lead to ordering a PGx test before the use of the drug. However, the pharmaceutical industry still is somewhat divided regarding the concept of personalized medicine and as long as development of "one-size-fits-all" drugs is an aim, pharmaceutical companies will probably consider the need for PGx markers as a disadvantage. Currently, PGx is mainly used by the pharmaceutical industry as a manner to salvage drugs that do not appear effective or safe in clinical trials. Erlotinib is an example of a drug that in the initial phase appeared not to show the expected results in terms of overall survival in phase II and III studies, whereas a small subgroup performed exceptionally well. Further research revealed specific mutations in the EGFR receptor that could explain the gain in survival (Rosell et al., 2009). Although mandatory genetic testing before prescribing is mainly seen in combination with somatic mutations, genetic testing for germline variants is required before starting certain treatments, such as eliglustat which requires *CYP2D6* testing with an FDA-cleared test. For the actionable phenotype "poor metabolizer" the dosage has to be halved, while for the phenotype "ultra-rapid metabolizer" this therapy is not recommended as it might not achieve adequate levels of concentrations of eliglustat (FDA Approvals of Brand-Name Prescription Drugs in 2014, 2015). However, patents have expired for many drugs with gene interactions and producers of generic drugs are not interested in advancing the research in (germline) biomarkers for the drugs in their portfolio. For multiple gene–drug pairs the regulators had to step in and issue boxed warnings to enforce healthcare professionals to take gene-pairs interactions into account when prescribing (e.g., *CYP2C19* and clopidogrel and *CYP2C9*/*VKORC1* and warfarin). Additionally, because of the efforts of EMA and FDA policy innovative pharmaceutical companies are enforced to investigate the influence of PGx variants. As an outcome, the FDA reported an increase in the number of registered drugs with information on genetic biomarkers in corporate in drug labels (Whirl-Carrillo et al., 2012). Similarly, in 2015 Ehmann et al. showed an increased uptake of information on PGx biomarkers in drug labels of drugs registered in the European Union in the last decades (Ehmann et al., 2015).

Based on information from drug labels and guidelines, healthcare professionals are expected to adjust pharmacotherapy if the genotype of the patient is known and is actionable. However, currently the clinically relevant genotypes are not known for the majority of the patients. Since no solid evidence is available which supports the use of upfront panel-based (or preemptive) genotyping, the use of PGx is restricted mainly to single-gene testing mostly performed retrospectively in order to explain a lack of efficacy or adverse reactions. Many physicians and pharmacists are not yet fully aware of the potential of PGx notwithstanding the fact that in the last decades clinical research has generated data on the existence and frequencies of genetic variants in a variety of pharmacogenes. In addition, several multidisciplinary initiatives of healthcare professionals and researchers have translated the effects of aberrant phenotypes into widely acclaimed clinical guidelines providing therapeutic recommendations (Relling & Klein, 2011; Swen et al., 2011, 2008).

Obviously, patients play an important role in the uptake of PGx in clinical care. Relative to secondary care, in primary care patients have a large impact on the decisions that are made concerning pharmacotherapy. Using a survey Haga et al. showed that the majority of patients are positive toward PGx as this diagnostic in the eyes of the surveyed patients can lead toward selecting the right drug by healthcare professionals and ultimately to safer and more effective pharmacotherapy. However, concerns whether third parties can access the results of a PGx test result or the fear that PGx results can be used for nefarious reasons by employers or healthcare insurance are reasons to reject a PGx test (O'Daniel et al., 2010).

Finally, one of the players with a large influence in primary care regarding implementation of PGx testing are health insurers. This stakeholder determines whether costs of PGx and other laboratory test used in primary care are reimbursed, whereas in secondary care laboratory test are usually part of integral treatment plans that are reimbursed. Lack of coverage of PGx testing by insurance companies is an important demotivator in patients' uptake of PGx testing. Haga et al. have shown that 81% of patient in their study are likely to decline if the test was not reimbursed (O'Daniel et al., 2010). Additionally, the current (lack of) policy regarding coverage of PGx testing is also a major reason why the adoption of PGx testing among healthcare professionals is low. In a recent survey 14.0% of the pharmacists indicate that uncertainty regarding the reimbursement is a reason for not having ordered or recommended a PGx test in the previous 6 months (Bank, Swen, & Guchelaar, 2017b).

3. CHALLENGES FOR IMPLEMENTATION OF PGx

In the process of widespread implementation of PGx in clinical care several challenges still play a role. These hurdles include the answers to the question which pharmacogenes should be incorporated in routine care and which known variants in the gene should be tested for. The decision on whether genetic testing for a pharmacogene is implemented is dependent on several aspects including the diagnostic criteria of the assays, available therapeutic recommendations for patients with an aberrant phenotype and evidence whether PGx testing improves patient care. Additionally, in certain healthcare settings data on cost-effectiveness and cost-consequences also can play a role. These topics will be covered in the next sections.

3.1 Selecting Clinically Relevant Pharmacogenes

Regarding the above-mentioned challenges, the first question to be asked is which pharmacogenes are clinically relevant and should be tested. The answer can partially be found in the guidelines of the CPIC and the DPWG. Although the guidelines created by both consortia are written on the premise that the genotype of the patient is already known, and the guidelines do not provide a recommendation who to test, the consortia have already selected gene–drug pairs with a clinically relevant impact on outcome of pharmacotherapy. Testing for genetic variants in genes other than described in these guidelines can be considered to be of very limited clinical use. The selection of pharmacogenes discussed below is based on the pharmacogenes most frequently determined in the Netherlands.

One of the examples of a clinically relevant pharmacogene where genetic variation results in a difference in specific treatment outcomes is *CYP2D6*, a gene that metabolizes 20%–25% of the drugs that have gained market approval (Owen, Sangkuhl, Klein, & Altman, 2009). It was described in one of the first reports of hereditary influence on drug metabolism (Eichelbaum, Spannbrucker, Steincke, & Dengler, 1979; Mahgoub, Idle, Dring, Lancaster, & Smith, 1977). Currently, more than 100 variants (including single nucleotide polymorphisms, insertions, and deletions) resulting in 113 possible combinations of genetic variations (haplotypes) have been described in literature. Furthermore, reports have shown that the entire gene can be deleted or duplicated [http://www.cypalleles.ki.se/] (Sim & Ingelman-Sundberg, 2006). In the last decade multiple commercial platforms have been developed to genotype *CYP2D6*.

In addition to *CYP2D6* the CPIC and DPWG guidelines have described many more clinically relevant pharmacogenes including *CYP2C9*, *CYP2C19*, *CYP3A5*, *DPYD*, *TPMT*, and *VKORC1* (for the associated drugs with these genes see Table 1). For these pharmacogenes research has shown that the number of common genetic variants that have a well-known clinical relevant impact on the function of the protein are much lower and range from one in case of *VKORC1* to four for *DPYD*. As a result, for the limited number of variants per gene it is relatively simple to design and validate assays based on methodologies such as Taqman, pyrosequencing, or high-resolution melting. An important aspect with home-brew assays is quality assurance of the assay by means of the use of multiple techniques, controls using plasmids or reference samples from the Coriell Institute for Medical Research and participation in proficiency testing (Pratt et al., 2010; van der Straaten, Swen, Baak-Pablo, & Guchelaar, 2008).

3.1.1 *CYP2D6*

One commercial test to genotype *CYP2D6* was the Roche Amplichip (Hoffmann-La Roche, Basel, Switzerland) which was one of the first genetic tests to receive FDA approval. The assay was based on the Affymetrix Genechip platform (Affymetrix, Santa Clara, CA) (Roche Diagnostics, 2005) and allowed for testing of 2 variant alleles of *CYP2C19* and 32 variant alleles of *CYP2D6* including deletion (*5) and duplication of the gene. At the time it was on the market it was considered the gold standard in *CYP2C19* and *CYP2D6* genotyping in clinical practice. A disadvantage of the platform, partly a result of the FDA approval, was that sometimes analyses resulted in a no-call (Gaedigk, Garcia-Ribera, Jeong, Shin, & Hernandez-Sanchez, 2014; Gaedigk, Hernandez, Garcia-Solaesa, Sanchez, & Isidoro-Garcia, 2011; Gaedigk, Riffel, et al., 2014). Additionally, problems with the calling of the *CYP2D6**41* by the Amplichip have been reported in literature (Bank, Swen, Guchelaar, & van der Straaten, 2015; Dodgen et al., 2013; Pratt et al., 2010). The miscalling of the *41 by the Amplichip can be explained by the manner that is used to call this allele by this platform. It uses a combination of the detected presence of 1661G > C, 2850C > T, and 4180G > C SNPs and the absence of the −1584C > G SNP. Platforms that have been developed at a later stage using oligonucleotide markers for SNP detection call the *41 allele solely based on the 2988G > A SNP (Bank et al., 2015; Roche Diagnostics, 2005). After the discovery of the 2988G > A SNP in 2004 (after the development of the Roche Amplichip) the definition of the *41 changed as The Human Cytochrome P450 Allele Nomenclature Committee decided

Table 1 Overview of the Guidelines of the CPIC and the DPWG

Gene	Drugs
COMT	Methylphenidate[a]
CYP1A2	Clozapine[a], olanzapine[a]
CYP2B6	Efavirenz[a]
CYP2C9	Acenocoumarol[a], phenprocoumon[a], phenytoin, glibenclamide[a], gliclazide[a], glimepiride[a], tolbutamide[a], warfarin
CYP2C19	Amitriptyline, citalopram, clomipramine, clopidogrel, desipramine[b], doxepin, escitalopram, esomeprazole[a], fluvoxamine[a], imipramine, lansoprazole[a], mirtazapine[a] moclobemide[a], omeprazole[a], pantoprazole[a], prasugrel[a], rabeprazole[a], sertraline, ticagrelor[a], trimipramine[b], voriconazole
CYP2D6	Amiodaron[a], amitriptyline, aripiprazole[a], atenolol[a], atomoxetine[a], bisoprolol[a], carvedilol[a], citalopram[a], clomipramine, clonidine[a], clozapine[a], codeine, desipramine[b], disopyramide[a], doxepin, duloxetine[a], eliglustat[a], escitalopram[a], flecainide[a], fluphenazine[a], fluoxetine[a], flupentixol[a], fluvoxamine, gefitinib[a], haloperidol[a], imipramine, quinidine[a], methylphenidate[a], metoprolol[a], mirtazapine†, nortriptyline, olanzapine[a], ondansetron[b], oxycodone[a], paroxetine, pimozide[a], propafenone[a], quetiapine[a], risperidone[a] sertraline[a], sotalol[a], tamoxifen, tramadol[a], trimipramine[b], tropisetron[b], venlafaxine[a], zuclopenthixol[a]
CYP3A4	Quetiapine[a]
CYP3A5	Tacrolimus
CFTR	Ivacaftor[b]
CYP4F2	Warfarin[b]
DPYD	Capecitabine, 5-fluorouracil, tegafur
G6PD	Rasburicase[b]
Factor V Leiden	Oral contraceptives containing estrogen derivatives[a]
HLA-A and HLA-B	Abacavir, allopurinol, carbamazepine, flucloxacillin[a], phenytoin[b], ribavirin[a]
IFNL3	Peginterferon alfa-2a[b], peginterferon alfa-2b[b], ribavirin[b]
MTHFR	Methotrexate[a]
SLCO1B1	Atorvastatin[a], simvastatin
TPMT	Azathioprine, 6-mercaptopurine, thioguanine
UGT1A1	Atazanavir[b], irinotecan[a]
VKORC1	Warfarin, phenprocoumon[a], acenocoumarol[a]

[a]DPWG only.
[b]CPIC only.

the 2988G>A SNP was indicative of the *41 allele (Raimundo et al., 2004; Sim & Ingelman-Sundberg, 2006; Toscano et al., 2006). As a result of the FDA approval, this new SNP could not be (directly) incorporated into the platform resulting in erroneous calling of the *41. Despite this known problem the assay was still recommended for genotyping *CYP2D6* until Roche discontinued the platform in 2016, partly because the assay was not used frequently in clinical practice because of its high costs. At the moment xTag 2D6 assay by Luminex (Luminex Molecular Diagnostics, Austin, TX) which uses the Luminex® 100/200™ platform is one of the CYP2D6 assays most frequently used in the clinic. The third version of the assay currently on the market detects 16 variant alleles of the *CYP2D6* gene. In this assay two separate multiplex long-range PCRs are carried out followed by a process of multiplex allele-specific primer extension.

The downside to the assays described above is that the required platforms are relatively expensive. The major disadvantage of using commercial assays is the limited number of variant alleles which can be detected. Based on the total number of variants in *CYP2D6* one can deduce that using assays that can detect from 11 up to 32 variant alleles do not cover all known genetic variants in the *CYP2D6* gene and patients might be designated an incorrect genetic predicted phenotype based on a *1 auto call by the platform (Sim & Ingelman-Sundberg, 2006). A solution for this problem is sequencing of *CYP2D6* to read all nucleotides and compare it to a reference gene. In 2013 Dodgen et al. described a platform that combines *CYP2D6* long-range PCR with multiple rounds of Sanger sequencing per sample. The long-range PCR was used for an amplicon used in Sanger sequencing as well as products to identify deletion and duplication of the gene (Dodgen et al., 2013; Gaedigk et al., 2007). Attempts have been made by analyzing the *CYP2D6* gene directly in a single sequencing reaction using second-generation sequencing; however, due to the existence of the pseudogenes *CYP2D7* and *CYP2D8* and the homology with other CYP450 genes this has proven difficult. Buermans et al. have circumvented this problem by using a long-range PCR in combination with the Pacific Biosciences RSII which allows for reliable full-length sequencing of *CYP2D6*. As a result of the full-length read complete phasing of the sequencing data is possible resulting in calling of complete haplotype across the entire *CYP2D6* gene which includes up- and downstream regions, introns, and exons (Buermans et al., 2017). Although sequencing is considered an improvement upon genotyping assays, as all the genetic variants in the gene are uncovered, in a clinical setting this could present a problem. With sequencing new genetic variants within the

CYP2D6 gene will be found of unknown functionality and unknown influence on the function of the metabolizing enzyme. Attempts have been made to quantify the effects of new genetic variants on the metabolizing capacity of enzymes using in silico prediction (Fukuyoshi et al., 2016). However, with different settings of the analyses concordance for predicted effects of newly found variants has been low (McCarthy et al., 2014). In the case of implementing next-generation sequencing in a clinical setting the discovery of novel uncharacterized variants in the *CYP2D6* gene could present a challenge. A solution for this problem would be to limit the results of the sequencing analysis to known mutations that are fully characterized. In conclusion, despite the complexity of *CYP2D6* multiple commercial assays are available for a broad coverage of genetic variants in this gene. Furthermore, research will likely lead to novel techniques which in the future can be used in the clinic for a more detailed analysis of this pharmacogene.

3.1.2 *CYP2C9+VKORC1*

The *CYP2C9* gene will mostly be tested in combination with *VKORC1* to guide dosing of coumarins or explain adverse reactions to vitamin K antagonists. Testing for *CYP2C9*2* and **3* along with the −1639G>A mutation in the promotor of *VKORC1* appears to be sufficient in patients of non-African ancestry to adjust the maintenance dose of coumarins or to determine the starting dose in case the INR is measured routinely at follow-up. In case of patients of African descent, the additional variants of **5*, **6*, **8*, and **11* appear relevant as a reduction of 15%–30% of the maintenance dose is required if patients are carriers of these alleles (Johnson et al., 2017; Swen et al., 2011).

3.1.3 *CYP2C19*

Currently, genetic testing for *CYP2C19* is usually performed to predict response to clopidogrel therapy and multiple studies are ongoing to investigate whether genotyping of *CYP2C19* can lead to an improvement in antiplatelet therapy with clopidogrel (Cavallari et al., 2017). The most frequently tested variants in the *CYP2C19* gene are **2*, **3* (which were also found on the Amplichip platform), and **17*. Commercially available assays for *CYP2C19* such as the INFINITI platform by AutoGenomics (AutoGenomics, Inc., Vista, CA), the xTag 2C19 Mutation Detection Kit by Luminex (Luminex Molecular Diagnostics, Austin, TX), and the GenMark (GenMark Diagnostics, Carlsbad, CA) have a broad coverage of genetic variants, whereas in-house assays developed by clinical laboratories usually include **2*, **3*, and **17*.

3.1.4 CYP3A5

The most frequent variants found among the (Caucasian) population are the **3* and **6* alleles, encoding for a nonfunctional protein, whereas the functional variant *1 is relatively uncommon in this population with an MAF of 0.078. In African Americans the *1 is more common than the **3* and **6* alleles (Birdwell et al., 2015; Swen et al., 2011). A systematic review of the literature has shown that patients that are hetero- or homozygous carriers of the *1 variant of the *CYP3A5* gene require a significantly higher dose (175%–250%) than patients carrying two nonfunctional copies (Birdwell et al., 2015; Swen et al., 2011). However, clinical studies investigating the use of the *CYP3A5* genotype to personalize tacrolimus dosing have shown mixed results whether genotyping can improve pharmacotherapy with tacrolimus compared to standard care (often comprising of therapeutic drug monitoring) (Shuker et al., 2016; Thervet et al., 2010). Currently, AutoGenomics (AutoGenomics, Inc., Vista, CA) and GenMark provide commercial platforms for *CYP3A5* in combination with the *CYP3A4* gene with both platforms providing a coverage of eight alleles for CYP3A5, whereas the assays developed in laboratories usually include the **3* and **6* alleles.

3.1.5 DPYD

Although genetic testing for *DPYD* is widespread in routine care in some countries for multiple years (e.g., the Netherlands), it has only recently been incorporated into the Clinical Practice Guidelines of the European Society for Medical Oncology or the American Society for Clinical Oncology. Screening for relevant genetic variants in *DPYD* before starting capecitabine or 5-fluorouracil is increasingly becoming part of the standard of care when treating patients with fluoropyrimidine derivatives (Lunenburg, van Staveren, Gelderblom, Guchelaar, & Swen, 2016; Toffoli et al., 2015). In recent years, literature has been accumulated on genetic variants in *DPYD* and their effects on the functionality of the DPD enzyme. For instance, the evidence for a 50% dose reduction among heterozygous carriers of the IVS14+1G>A (*2A) has been established in many studies (Bank, Guchelaar, & Swen, 2014). Efforts by Meulendijks et al. and Offer et al. and initiatives as the DPWG and CPIC have resulted in a consensus on the variants on the *2A, 1679T>G (*13) and the 2846A>T variants having no (*2A and *13) or reduced activity (2846A>T), respectively (Caudle et al., 2013; Meulendijks et al., 2015; Offer et al., 2014; Swen et al., 2011). Until recently there was a discordance between the CPIC and the DPWG concerning the classification of the 1236G>A/HapB3 variant. In the guidelines of the DPWG is mentioned that this variant leads to decreased fluoropyrimidine clearance and to increased toxicity, while in their 2013 guideline the CPIC had not yet assigned a status to this variant (Bank, Caudle, et al., 2018; Caudle et al., 2013; Swen et al., 2011). However, this difference has currently been resolved by an update of the *DPYD* guideline published in February 2018 in which the gene–activity score for *DPYD* has also been adopted (Amstutz et al., 2018). In the Netherlands assays developed by clinical laboratories usually included the four SNPs described by Meulendijks et al. (Lunenburg et al., 2016; Meulendijks et al., 2015).

3.1.6 TPMT

The first guidelines published by the CPIC covered the interpretation of genetic variations found in the *TPMT* gene to genetic predicted phenotypes and therapeutic recommendations for dosing of azathioprine, 6-mercaptopurine, and thioguanine in case of actionable *TPMT* genotypes (Relling et al., 2011). In an update of the guideline published in 2013 a total of 33 variants in the *TPMT* gene are described; however, the alleles **2*, **3A*, **3B*, and **3C* appear to be the most relevant as this set of alleles explains 95% of the variance found in TPMT in terms of frequency (Relling et al., 2013). Most clinical laboratories that have developed their own assay will commonly use the three SNPs found in **2*, **3B*, and **3C*. As the *TPMT*3A* haplotype is comprised of both rs1800460 (**3B*) and rs1142345 (**3C*) this combination of SNPs can thus also be used to detect the **3A* haplotype (Relling et al., 2013).

3.1.7 Panel-Based Approach

With the advancement of the field of biotechnology with a concurrent decrease of costs of techniques the screening of multiple (pharmaco)genes simultaneously (panel-based) approach has become available for use in a clinical setting. As multiple large implementation studies in secondary care have shown that patients are often (>90%–95%) carriers of at least one actionable phenotype, a panel-based screening of multiple pharmacogenes appears to be the next step in PGx testing. The genes *CYP2C19*, *CYP2C6*, *SLCO1B1*, and *TPMT* were included in panels by all large studies, whereas *CYP2C9/VKORC1* and *CYP3A5* are included two of the three implementation projects (Dunnenberger et al., 2015; Hoffman et al., 2014; O'Donnell et al., 2014; Van Driest et al., 2014). Van Driest et al. have shown in the Vanderbilt Pharmacogenomic Resource for Enhanced Decisions in

Care and Treatment (PREDICT) program that using a panel reduced the number of tests by 60% compared to a reactive single-gene assay (Van Driest et al., 2014). Currently, multiple platforms can be used for a preemptive panel approach. One of the first high-throughput genotyping methods available for analysis of multiple pharmacogenes was the Drug Metabolizing Enzymes and Transporters (DMET) Plus array by Affymetrix using Genechip platform (Affymetrix, Santa Clara, CA). Fernandez et al. showed a high concordance with other genotyping methods (Fernandez et al., 2012). The disadvantages of the DMET plus array include the length of a single run (~48 h spread out over 3 days), the inability to detect certain copy number variants (e.g., heterozygous carriers of *the CYP2D6**5* and duplications of the *CYP2D6*), and recently discovered but clinically relevant alleles such as the 2846A > T and 1236G > A/HapB3 in the *DPYD* gene are missing. In case the DMET plus platform is used to guide pharmacotherapy in a clinical setting; this platform has to be supplemented with additional test depending on the genes incorporated in the desired panel (Bank, Swen, Schaap, et al., 2017; Hoffman et al., 2014).

In the PREDICT program the VeraCode ADME core panel (Illumina, San Diego, CA) was used (Van Driest et al., 2014). This platform detects 184 genetic markers in 34 ADME (Lin, Yeakley, McDaniel, & Shen, 2009). Similar to the DMET platform the VeraCode platform is not able to detect duplications of this gene (although it can detect the *5 allele). Furthermore, important SNPs in the *DPYD* gene (2846A > T and 1236G > A/HapB3 and *13) are absent in the panel of 184 genetic variants and would have to be supplemented if the panel would be used for the characterization of *CYP2D6* and *DPYD* (Bank, Swen, Schaap, et al., 2017).

In addition to fixed selections of genetic variants found on the DMET plus and the VeraCode ADME core panel laboratories may choose to select the pharmacogenes and an associated panel of genetic variants based on their own criteria. Although Thermo Fisher (Thermo Fisher, Waltham, MA) did offer a prefabricated array that tests for 158 variants in 29 Phase I/II and transporter genes, a custom platform based on Taqman assays can also designed. A downside to the array similar to the DMET platform is that the Taqman cannot detect copy number variants and an additional qPCR has to be performed if genes with known duplication and/or deletions as *CYP2D6* and *UGT2B7* are included in the desired panel.

3.1.8 Genome-Wide Approaches

In the last decade whole exome screening (WES) and whole genome screening (WGS) have become available for use in the clinical setting as a result of the advances in the field of biotechnology. Although WES and WGS are still relatively costly and therefore mainly used by clinical geneticists as an end-of-line method to diagnose hereditary diseases, information on genetic variants found in pharmacogenes can be considered a useful by-product of the use of these methods. Along with Genome-Wide Association (GWA) methods, WES and WGS are currently mostly used in a research setting to detect novel genetic variants in pharmacogenes.

3.2 Providing Data on Diagnostic Criteria of PGx Testing

Currently, outcomes of (GWA) studies related to PGx are often reported as odds/hazard ratios or associations, where an individual carrying a certain genetic variant in a gene has a higher risk on a negative outcome of therapy or a lack of response. However, odds/hazards ratios and associations do not provide information about the analytical validity, clinical validity, and clinical utility of genetic tests or panels which are important objective factors in determining whether the test can lead to a clinically relevant improvement in healthcare (Tonk, Gurwitz, Maitland-van der Zee, & Janssens, 2017). The analytical validity is the ability to identify the genetic variants of interest and is expressed as the analytical sensitivity and specificity of the test. The analytical sensitivity and specificity are generally required to be higher than 98% and 99.5%, respectively (Palomaki, FitzSimmons, & Haddow, 2004; Palomaki et al., 2003). The clinical validity concerns the correlation of the genetic marker with a clinical phenotype or outcome. Parameters for clinical validity are clinical sensitivity, clinical specificity, and the amount of change in a person's risk for a certain event between the wild-type genotype and a variant genotype. The final parameter for the reliability of a genetic marker is the clinical utility. Clinical utility relates to whether the genetic information would lead to change in treatment that improves drug efficacy or safety (i.e., the impact on healthcare) (Burke, 2014). Currently, relevant data concerning clinical validity and clinically utility are scarcely reported despite the need for this information to answer the question whether implementation of a specific genetic test or a panel in clinical practice can lead to a significant benefit of healthcare (Tonk et al., 2017). A manner to obtain information regarding the clinical validity (such as negative and positive predicting values) is to reassess existing literature and extract these relevant data. With this information clinicians and other decision makers in healthcare can more objectively guide the decision-making process regarding the question whether genetic tests are useful in clinical practice (Janssens & Deverka, 2014; Tonk et al., 2017).

Jansen et al. have shown for example that for the gene–drug pair *SLCO1B1* and statins, a systematic review of the literature could provide the desired information on diagnostic criteria.

3.3 Guidelines Directing the Clinical Use of PGx Test Results

In 2010 the most important barrier for the implementation of PGx into clinical practice identified by clinicians was the translation of PGx test results into clinical action (Relling, Altman, Goetz, & Evans, 2010; Relling & Klein, 2011; Swen et al., 2007). Two consortia, the CPIC® and the DPWG, both anticipated a near future where patients would confront their treating physician and pharmacists with their own genotype and started with the translation of information found in the scientific literature into tools usable by clinicians. The guidelines of both groups provide recommendations for treatment of patients where an actionable genetic predicted phenotype is known at start of pharmacotherapy, rather than indicating which gene should be tested (see Table 1) (Relling & Klein, 2011; Swen et al., 2008). Up to date, CPIC has published guidelines which cover 40 gene–drug pairs and the DPWG has reviewed 86 candidate gene–drug pairs in their guidelines and provide therapeutic recommendations for 47 gene–drug pairs (Bank, Caudle, et al., 2018).

When guidelines of the CPIC and the DPWG on the same gene–drug pairs are compared there is substantial agreement between the guidelines in terms of therapeutic recommendations for certain phenotypes. The most common explanation for observed discordances in therapeutic recommendations between the CPIC and the DPWG is the use of different methodologies to support dosing advices. Whereas the CPIC used a consensus-based approach from a panel of experts on the subject, the DPWG calculates dosing advices with aid of pharmacokinetic data. Other explanations for differences can be found based on the date of literature review (Bank, Caudle, et al., 2018).

Another important difference is the discordance in the translation of genotypes to genetic predicted phenotypes. Similar to the therapeutic recommendations these discordances in translation can be explained by a difference of interpretation of *CYP2D6* genetic predicted phenotypes in the literature combined with the use of different model substrates by the CPIC and the DPWG. This in turn led to a difference in the interpretation of the *CYP2D6* intermediate metabolizer phenotype. Currently an international working group of experts on the subject including members from the CPIC and the DPWG has recently begun to standardize the translation from genotype to phenotype (Bank, Caudle, et al., 2018).

To aid in the personalization of pharmacotherapy the guidelines should not only be available in the form of published articles or chapters in books but also should be an integral part of the workflow of healthcare professionals. In the Netherlands the first therapeutic dose recommendations of the DWPG were integrated in the national drug database (G-standard) in 2006, making medication surveillance based on actionable genetic predicted phenotypes available on a national level for healthcare professionals in both primary and secondary care through CDS in drug prescribing and dispensing systems (Swen et al., 2008). In other nations where there is no national drug database available, multiple reports describe the integration of PGx into CDS at an institutional level in both primary and secondary care (Dawes et al., 2016; Elliott et al., 2017; Hicks, Dunnenberger, Gumpper, Haidar, & Hoffman, 2016; Hicks, Stowe, et al., 2016; Hinderer et al., 2017; Rohrer Vitek et al., 2017). Alternatively, in situations where electronic medication surveillance is not (yet) possible a mobile-enabled CDS could aid healthcare professionals in adjusting pharmacotherapy based on a patient's PGx profile (Blagec, Romagnoli, Boyce, & Samwald, 2016; Samwald, Minarro-Gimenez, Blagec, & Adlassnig, 2014). Evidence suggest that medication surveillance based on a patient's PGx profile indeed leads to a change in behavior among physicians reducing the number of high PGx risk (O'Donnell et al., 2017).

3.4 Providing Scientific Evidence for Improvement in Patient Care by PGx Testing

The body of evidence that is required to justify the implementation of routine PGx testing in clinical practice has been subject of debate (Altman, 2011; Khoury, Gwinn, Dotson, & Bowen, 2011; Pirmohamed & Hughes, 2013). The evidence-based medicine paradigm would require evidence to prove that a new technique or treatment would indeed lead to increased safety or efficacy or a same performance for lower costs before it can be implemented into clinical practice with a randomized controlled trial (RCT) considered the gold standard. The evidence-based model would require RCTs for genotype-guided therapy for each individual gene–drug pair or a panel approach. However, there are multiple arguments against the demand for RCTs to deliver evidence for genotype-guided therapy for each gene–drug pair.

From one point of view there is no pharmacological argument to see adjustments for a gene–drug pair any different than adjustments for many other relevant clinical factors such as impaired renal function. Dosing adjustments for clinical factors are usually based on data from observational studies and case-reports/series; however, regulatory authorities do not enforce a requirement of RCTs to deliver evidence that adjustments based on clinical parameters lead to an improvement of clinical outcomes (Pirmohamed & Hughes, 2013). Additionally, if there is sufficient observational evidence available that pharmacogenomic screening can reduce significant morbidity or prevent mortality RCTs can be considered unethical as patients with nonwild-type genotypes in the standard arm are knowingly exposed to suboptimal treatment which can lead to adverse events (Frueh, 2009). Another argument against a RCT for each gene–drug pair is the cost aspect. As RCTs are highly expensive this would require an enormous investment to finance the required trials for all relevant gene–drug pairs. As stated earlier, in case of novel drugs RCTs are financed as part of the research and development by the innovative pharmaceutical companies that hold the patent for the marketed drug. However, many of the drugs with a known interaction with a polymorphic pharmacogene are drugs with a well-known pharmacology which are already produced by generic pharmaceutical companies which do not have any gain by financing additional research concerning their pharmaceutical in their portfolio.

However, despite this rationale clinicians seemed hesitant to implement this new concept of pharmacology in clinical practice as evidence for an improvement of pharmacotherapy by PGx in the previous decade was lacking (Stanek et al., 2012). Fortunately, in the last years several clinical studies for single gene–drug pairs have already been performed providing evidence for implementation of genotype-guided therapy in case of these gene–drug pairs. A landmark RCT performed by Mallal et al. in 2008 showed that genotyping for the **5701* allele in the *HLA-B* gene could lower the incidence of abacavir-induced hypersensitivity reactions from 7.8% in the control group to 3.4% in the control group ($P < 0.001$) (Mallal et al., 2008). Additionally, Coenen et al. studied in a multicenter study whether genotyping for the *TPMT* would lead to a reduction of hematologic adverse drug reactions (ADRs) in treatment of inflammatory bowel disease using thiopurines. Although the study could not detect a reduction in the proportion in hematologic ADRs between the screening arm and the control arm (7.4% vs 7.9%, 95% confidence interval: 0.57–1.52) a 10-fold reduction in the hematological ADRs among carriers of TPMT variants was observed in the intervention group compared to the same population in the control group (2.6% vs 22.9%, 95% confidence interval 0.01–0.85) (Coenen et al., 2015). A third example of a multicenter study to investigate the clinical utility of a PGx test was performed by Deenen et al. Unlike the two previous studies this group did not use a RCT design, but compared a prospectively genotype-guided cohort to a historical cohort to show that screening for the **2A* variant in the *DPYD* gene can reduce the risk of toxicity of grade 3 or higher from 73% to 28% ($P<0.001$). Furthermore, the proportion of patients that died because of the fluoropyrimidine was reduced from 10% to 0% (Deenen et al., 2016). In case of the gene–drug pairs *HLA-B*57:01* and abacavir, *DPYD* and fluoropyrimidines, and *TPMT* and thiopurines the results of the performed studies helped to provide evidence to justify implementation of routine screening in clinical practice.

In addition to studies investigating whether routine genetic screening of a single pharmacogene can lead to an improvement of healthcare, a number of studies tests for a panel of multiple pharmacogenes simultaneously (a panel approach). Using a case-control study consisting of 205 genotyped patients receiving genotype-guided dosing through CDS and 820 matched controls Brixner et al. showed that a preemptive screening using a panel approach resulted in a significant reduction in hospitalizations (9.8% vs 16.1%, $P=0.027$) and patient visits to the emergency department (4.4% vs 15.4%, $P=0.0002$) (Brixner et al., 2016). Similar to the results of Brixner et al. a prospective pilot RCT performed by Elliot et al. found a reduction of in the number of rehospitalizations at 60 days in the intervention group compared to the group receiving regular care. In the intervention arm of the study patients were preemptively genotyped for *CYP2C9*, *CYP2C19*, *CYP2D6*, *CYP3A4*, and *CYP3A5* followed by optimization of pharmacotherapy using CDS whereas the control population received regular care (Elliott et al., 2017). In addition, the Ubiquitous PGx Consortium is currently enrolling patients in the PREemptive PGx testing for prevention of Adverse drug Reactions (PREPARE) study in sites across seven European countries as part of a Horizon2020-funded program with the aim to provide evidence to support routine implementation of preemptive panel-based PGx screening (van der Wouden et al., 2017). Overall, the body of evidence supporting the implementation of PGx in clinical practice is growing, mostly by the efforts of academic hospitals or specialized research institutions.

3.5 Providing Information on Cost-Effectiveness and Cost-Consequences of PGx Testing

In addition to information about the analytical validity, clinical validity, and clinical utility an important aspect for the implementation in clinical care is data about cost-effectiveness and cost-consequences of PGx tests. The information on the cost-effectiveness is especially relevant in the case of implementation of PGx testing in primary as health insurers will require this information in their decision to reimburse specific (pharmaco)genomic testing. In secondary and tertiary care cost-effectiveness is slightly less relevant as in a hospital setting a laboratory test is usually part of integral treatment plans and are not reimbursed directly by health insurers.

Ironically, most of the cost-effectiveness analysis (CEA) relating to PGx tests has been performed for gene–drug interactions concerning drugs that are mostly initiated in a hospital setting. For fluoropyrimidines the studies performed by Deenen et al. and Cortejoso et al. show that genotyping for variants in *DPYD* can reduce the number of patients admitted to the intensive care unit with severe fluoropyrimidine-induced toxicity (Cortejoso et al., 2016; Deenen et al., 2016). Other gene–drug pairs where the body of evidence concerning the cost-effectiveness is growing are *HLA-B*5701* and abacavir and *CYP2C19* and clopidogrel by reducing the number of patients suffering from hypersensitivity reaction or stent thrombosis, respectively (Borse et al., 2017; Deiman et al., 2016; Patel et al., 2014; Schackman et al., 2008).

Up to date the evidence supporting cost-effectiveness of routine screening for genetic variants in pharmacogenes associated with prescription drugs which are frequently prescribed in primary care such as antidepressants (CYP2D6 and CYP2C19), statins (SLCO1B1), and coumarins (CYP2C9 and VKORC1) has only been shown in a number of studies despite the amount of literature published on these gene–drug pairs (Patrick, Avorn, & Choudhry, 2009; Verhoef et al., 2016). As a result, health insurance companies are not likely to reimburse routine PGx testing for these single gene–drug pairs in primary care. However, evidence for cost-effectiveness for each individual gene–drug may not be necessary when using a panel approach. Brixner et al. have shown in their study that simultaneous screening for *CYP2C19*, *CYP2C9*, *CYP2D6*, *CYP3A4*, and *CYP3A5* can lead to savings in healthcare as a result of a reduction in hospitalizations and patient visits to the emergency department (Brixner et al., 2016). Similarly, the U-PGx project will also perform an analysis to determine whether preemptive screening of 50 variants in 13 pharmacogenes will lead to a decrease in costs in the healthcare system (van der Wouden et al., 2017). Finally, with the rapid developments in biotechnology and the concurrent rapid decrease in costs of genotyping techniques such as genome-wide screening as WES or WGS might become cost-efficient in the next decade.

3.6 Improving Acceptance of PGx Testing

In addition to the scientific evidence, the integration of any laboratory test or clinical procedure is dependent on the adoption by healthcare professionals and patients. With the rapid progression of the field of PGx in the last decades healthcare professionals are advent of an era where there is a significant chance they will be confronted with (pharmaco)genomic information from patients and are expected to optimize the patients' treatment based on this information. A survey performed among US physicians has shown that although doctors believe in the concept of heritable drug response only 10.3% feels adequately informed about the availability of PGx testing and the place of PGx testing within pharmacotherapy (Stanek et al., 2012). Similarly, a questionnaire among Canadian pharmacists revealed a high expectation of PGx to improve safety and effectiveness of drug therapy; only 7.7% of the responders felt comfortable, interpreting, and advising upon PGx test results. Furthermore, virtually all (96.6%) of the surveyed pharmacist would like additional education on the subject (de Denus et al., 2013). Both studies indicate a knowledge gap relating to PGx is present among healthcare professionals.

With the integration of therapeutic recommendations for patients with known actionable genotypes into CDS in electronic drug prescribing and dispensing systems it was anticipated that a knowledge gap relating to PGx among healthcare professionals would be circumvented. In contrast, a questionnaire performed among Dutch pharmacists showed that this was not the case. Knowledge of the guidelines of the DPWG and their integration in the CDS was not associated with feeling informed about PGx testing or PGx test adoption (Bank, Swen, & Guchelaar, 2017b). Additionally, the percentages of responders that felt informed about PGx testing (14.7%), that would like to follow additional training on the subject (88.8%) and that had adopted a PGx test (14.1%) were similar to previous studies (Bank, Swen, & Guchelaar, 2017b; de Denus et al., 2013; Stanek et al., 2012). Further research performed among pharmacy students revealed a similar percentage of 12.8% of participants that felt adequately informed despite almost all of the students (96.6%) having followed some form of education on the subject (Bank, Swen, & Guchelaar, 2018). The results from the latter study indicate that the current traditional form education on PGx as part of the curriculum is not sufficient and may result in a future knowledge gap.

The results from these studies indicate that a lack of knowledge on PGx testing is one of the remaining barriers hindering implementation. To remove this barrier more education on the subject for (future) healthcare professionals is required and should be presented in an alternate manner. In one initiative reported by Weitzel et al. students obtain their own pharmacogenomic profile and use this information in an education setting. This form of education using hands-on experience-based learning appears to increase understanding of PGx markers and allows students to get used to the idea to act on (pharmaco)genomic markers (Weitzel, Aquilante, Johnson, Kisor, & Empey, 2016). Training on the subject for practicing healthcare professionals could be provided in the form of postacademic education where in addition to basic information about (pharmaco)genomics, the existence of guidelines containing therapeutic recommendations and evidence for implementation of genetic testing is discussed. One survey found a link between this form of education and the future use of PGx testing (Bank, Swen, & Guchelaar, 2017b).

A current challenge is that certain practicing healthcare professionals do not often receive the opportunity to gain experience in adjusting medication based on PGx markers. As the body of evidence for genetic screening for gene–drug pairs occurring in primary care is not as large compared to fields in secondary care (e.g., oncology) general practitioners and community pharmacists do not routinely use PGx markers to adjust therapy. As a result, they probably do not feel qualified to adjust pharmacotherapy based on PGx markers (Bank, Swen, & Guchelaar, 2017b). In the Implementation of Pharmacogenomics in to Primary care Project (IP3) community pharmacists were offered free ordering of a PGx panel consisting of 8 genes (*CYP2C9*, *CYP2C19*, *CYP2D6*, *CYP3A5*, *DPYD*, *SLCO1B1*, *TPMT*, and *VKORC1*) and gain experience with genotype-guided dosing of 10 drugs frequently prescribed in primary care (Bank, Swen, Schaap, et al., 2017). In line with previous implementation projects the IP3 showed that the majority of patients (90%) carried at least one actionable genotype in the panel and combinations of actionable genotypes with relevant drugs were common (31.0%). And although not significant ($P=0.112$) there was an increase in the percentage of surveyed community pharmacists and general practitioners that felt qualified to interpret and act on PGx data (15.2% before vs 28.3% after) (Bank, Swen, Schaap, et al., 2017).

The combination of the frequencies of actionable genotypes from this panel of eight genes along with prescription data from 95% of the community pharmacies in the Netherlands projects that 23.6% of all patients receiving incident prescriptions from a selection of 45 drugs associated with the genes in the panel experience a gene–drug. In a possible future scenario where patients are routinely genotyped for this panel of clinically relevant pharmacogenes community pharmacists are likely required to perform an intervention in 5.4% of therapy and strictly monitor an additional 18.2%. To execute this role as key user of PGx data pharmacists will need to be comfortable with adjusting therapy based on genetic markers (Bank, Swen, & Guchelaar, 2017a).

4. CONCLUSION

In the last decades the field of PGx has provided a wealth of information from research on SNPs in candidate genes up to studies using hypothesis-free testing in the form of GWA studies and next-generation sequencing powered by the advances in molecular technology. In the last years assays have been developed that are usable in the clinical settings and by efforts of the CPIC and the DPWG the vast amount of scientific literature concerning many gene–drug pairs has been reviewed and condensed into actionable therapeutic recommendations usable in the clinic. Multiple studies have shown that implementation of PGx testing (using a panel approach) in clinical practice is feasible and several RCTs have delivered evidence for the routine implementation of PGx testing for a number of gene–drug pairs such as *DPYD* and *TPMT*. Currently, studies providing the clinical utility and cost-effectiveness of panel-based screening are ongoing which might deliver the final evidence required for widespread implementation of PGx in clinical care. One barrier which still appears to be remaining are healthcare provides themselves which indicate that they hindered by a knowledge gap on the subject. A change in the current curriculum might prevent lack of knowledge among future healthcare professionals whereas postacademic education will resolve the knowledge gap among current practicing colleagues.

ACKNOWLEDGMENTS

This work was supported by unrestricted grants from The Royal Dutch Pharmacist's Association, The Hague (KNMP), the Netherlands.

CONFLICT OF INTEREST

The authors declare no conflict of interest.

REFERENCES

Altman, R. B. (2011). Pharmacogenomics: "Noninferiority" is sufficient for initial implementation. *Clinical Pharmacology and Therapeutics*, *89*(3), 348–350. https://doi.org/10.1038/clpt.2010.310.

Amstutz, U., Henricks, L. M., Offer, S. M., Barbarino, J., Schellens, J. H. M., Swen, J. J., et al. (2018). Clinical Pharmacogenetics Implementation Consortium (CPIC) guideline for dihydropyrimidine dehydrogenase genotype and fluoropyrimidine dosing: 2017 update. *Clinical Pharmacology and Therapeutics*, *103*(2), 210–216. https://doi.org/10.1002/cpt.911.

Bank, P. C., Caudle, K. E., Swen, J. J., Gammal, R. S., Whirl-Carrillo, M., Klein, T. E., et al. (2018). Comparison of the guidelines of the Clinical Pharmacogenetics Implementation Consortium and the Dutch Pharmacogenetics Working Group. *Clinical Pharmacology and Therapeutics*, *103*(4), 599–618. https://doi.org/10.1002/cpt.762.

Bank, P. C., Guchelaar, H. J., & Swen, J. J. (2014). Fluoropyrimidine toxicity in patients with dihydropyrimidine dehydrogenase (DPD) splice site variant: The need for further revision of dose and schedule. *Internal and Emergency Medicine*, *9*(4), 481–482. https://doi.org/10.1007/s11739-013-1027-6.

Bank, P. C., Swen, J. J., & Guchelaar, H. J. (2017a). Nation-wide impact of implementing a preemptive pharmacogenetic panel approach to guide drug prescribing in primary care in the Netherlands. *Clinical Pharmacology and Therapeutics*. submitted.

Bank, P. C., Swen, J. J., & Guchelaar, H. J. (2017b). A nationwide survey of pharmacists' perception of pharmacogenetics in the context of a clinical decision support system containing pharmacogenetics dosing recommendations. *Pharmacogenomics*, *18*(3), 215–225. https://doi.org/10.2217/pgs-2016-0138.

Bank, P. C., Swen, J. J., & Guchelaar, H. J. (2018). A nationwide cross-sectional survey of pharmacy students on knowledge of, experience with, and attitudes towards pharmacogenetics. *Pharmacogenomics*, *19*(4), 311–319. https://doi.org/10.2217/pgs-2017-0175.

Bank, P. C., Swen, J. J., Guchelaar, H. J., & van der Straaten, T. (2015). GenoChip CYP2D6 macroarray as a method to genotype for CYP2D6 variants: Results of a validation study in a Caucasian population. *Pharmacogenomics*, *16*(7), 681–687. https://doi.org/10.2217/pgs.15.30.

Bank, P. C., Swen, J. J., Schaap, R. D., Klootwijk, D. B., Baak-Pablo, R. F., & Guchelaar, H. J. (2017). Results of the implementation of pharmacogenomics into primary care project. *Clinical Pharmacology and Therapeutics*, *101*(Suppl. 1), 6.

Birdwell, K. A., Decker, B., Barbarino, J. M., Peterson, J. F., Stein, C. M., Sadee, W., et al. (2015). Clinical Pharmacogenetics Implementation Consortium (CPIC) guidelines for CYP3A5 genotype and tacrolimus dosing. *Clinical Pharmacology and Therapeutics*, *98*(1), 19–24. https://doi.org/10.1002/cpt.113.

Blagec, K., Romagnoli, K. M., Boyce, R. D., & Samwald, M. (2016). Examining perceptions of the usefulness and usability of a mobile-based system for pharmacogenomics clinical decision support: A mixed methods study. *PeerJ*, *4*, e1671. https://doi.org/10.7717/peerj.1671.

Borse, M. S., Dong, O. M., Polasek, M. J., Farley, J. F., Stouffer, G. A., & Lee, C. R. (2017). CYP2C19-guided antiplatelet therapy: A cost-effectiveness analysis of 30-day and 1-year outcomes following percutaneous coronary intervention. *Pharmacogenomics*, *18*(12), 1155–1166. https://doi.org/10.2217/pgs-2017-0075.

Brixner, D., Biltaji, E., Bress, A., Unni, S., Ye, X., Mamiya, T., et al. (2016). The effect of pharmacogenetic profiling with a clinical decision support tool on healthcare resource utilization and estimated costs in the elderly exposed to polypharmacy. *Journal of Medical Economics*, *19*(3), 213–228. https://doi.org/10.3111/13696998.2015.1110160.

Buermans, H. P., Vossen, R. H., Anvar, S. Y., Allard, W. G., Guchelaar, H. J., White, S. J., et al. (2017). Flexible and scalable full-length CYP2D6 long amplicon PacBio sequencing. *Human Mutation*, *38*(3), 310–316. https://doi.org/10.1002/humu.23166.

Burke, W. (2014). Genetic tests: Clinical validity and clinical utility. *Current Protocols in Human Genetics*, *81*, 9.15.11–18. https://doi.org/10.1002/0471142905.hg0915s81.

Caudle, K. E., Thorn, C. F., Klein, T. E., Swen, J. J., McLeod, H. L., Diasio, R. B., et al. (2013). Clinical Pharmacogenetics Implementation Consortium guidelines for dihydropyrimidine dehydrogenase genotype and fluoropyrimidine dosing. *Clinical Pharmacology and Therapeutics*, *94*(6), 640–645. https://doi.org/10.1038/clpt.2013.172.

Cavallari, L. H., Weitzel, K. W., Elsey, A. R., Liu, X., Mosley, S. A., Smith, D. M., et al. (2017). Institutional profile: University of Florida Health Personalized Medicine Program. *Pharmacogenomics*, *18*(5), 421–426. https://doi.org/10.2217/pgs-2017-0028.

Coenen, M. J., de Jong, D. J., van Marrewijk, C. J., Derijks, L. J., Vermeulen, S. H., Wong, D. R., et al. (2015). Identification of patients with variants in TPMT and dose reduction reduces hematologic events during thiopurine treatment of inflammatory bowel disease. *Gastroenterology*, *149*(4), 907–917. https://doi.org/10.1053/j.gastro.2015.06.002.

Cortejoso, L., Garcia-Gonzalez, X., Garcia, M. I., Garcia-Alfonso, P., Sanjurjo, M., & Lopez-Fernandez, L. A. (2016). Cost-effectiveness of screening for DPYD polymorphisms to prevent neutropenia in cancer patients treated with fluoropyrimidines. *Pharmacogenomics*, *17*(9), 979–984. https://doi.org/10.2217/pgs-2016-0006.

Dawes, M., Aloise, M. N., Ang, J. S., Cullis, P., Dawes, D., Fraser, R., et al. (2016). Introducing pharmacogenetic testing with clinical decision support into primary care: A feasibility study. *CMAJ Open*, *4*(3), E528–e534. https://doi.org/10.9778/cmajo.20150070.

de Denus, S., Letarte, N., Hurlimann, T., Lambert, J. P., Lavoie, A., Robb, L., et al. (2013). An evaluation of pharmacists' expectations towards pharmacogenomics. *Pharmacogenomics*, *14*(2), 165–175. https://doi.org/10.2217/pgs.12.197.

Deenen, M. J., Meulendijks, D., Cats, A., Sechterberger, M. K., Severens, J. L., Boot, H., et al. (2016). Upfront genotyping of DPYD*2A to individualize fluoropyrimidine therapy: A safety and cost analysis. *Journal of Clinical Oncology*, *34*(3), 227–234. https://doi.org/10.1200/JCO.2015.63.1325.

Deiman, B. A., Tonino, P. A., Kouhestani, K., Schrover, C. E., Scharnhorst, V., Dekker, L. R., et al. (2016). Reduced number of cardiovascular events and increased cost-effectiveness by genotype-guided antiplatelet therapy in patients undergoing percutaneous coronary interventions in the Netherlands. *Netherlands Heart Journal*, *24*(10), 589–599. https://doi.org/10.1007/s12471-016-0873-z.

Dodgen, T. M., Hochfeld, W. E., Fickl, H., Asfaha, S. M., Durandt, C., Rheeder, P., et al. (2013). Introduction of the AmpliChip CYP450 Test to a South African cohort: A platform comparative prospective cohort study. *BMC Medical Genetics*, *14*, 20. https://doi.org/10.1186/1471-2350-14-20.

Dunnenberger, H. M., Crews, K. R., Hoffman, J. M., Caudle, K. E., Broeckel, U., Howard, S. C., et al. (2015). Preemptive clinical pharmacogenetics implementation: Current programs in five US medical centers. *Annual Review of Pharmacology and Toxicology*, *55*, 89–106. https://doi.org/10.1146/annurev-pharmtox-010814-124835.

Ehmann, F., Caneva, L., Prasad, K., Paulmichl, M., Maliepaard, M., Llerena, A., et al. (2015). Pharmacogenomic information in drug labels: European Medicines Agency perspective. *The Pharmacogenomics Journal*, *15*(3), 201–210. https://doi.org/10.1038/tpj.2014.86.

Eichelbaum, M., Spannbrucker, N., Steincke, B., & Dengler, H. J. (1979). Defective N-oxidation of sparteine in man: A new pharmacogenetic defect. *European Journal of Clinical Pharmacology*, *16*(3), 183–187.

Elliott, L. S., Henderson, J. C., Neradilek, M. B., Moyer, N. A., Ashcraft, K. C., & Thirumaran, R. K. (2017). Clinical impact of pharmacogenetic profiling with a clinical decision support tool in polypharmacy home health patients: A prospective pilot randomized controlled trial. *PLoS One*, *12*(2), e0170905. https://doi.org/10.1371/journal.pone.0170905.

FDA Approvals of Brand-Name Prescription Drugs in 2014. (2015). *American Health & Drug Benefits*, *8*(Spec Feature), 22–35.

Fernandez, C. A., Smith, C., Yang, W., Lorier, R., Crews, K. R., Kornegay, N., et al. (2012). Concordance of DMET plus genotyping results with those of orthogonal genotyping methods. *Clinical Pharmacology and Therapeutics*, *92*(3), 360–365. https://doi.org/10.1038/clpt.2012.95.

Frueh, F. W. (2009). Back to the future: Why randomized controlled trials cannot be the answer to pharmacogenomics and personalized medicine. *Pharmacogenomics*, *10*(7), 1077–1081. https://doi.org/10.2217/pgs.09.62.

Fukuyoshi, S., Kometani, M., Watanabe, Y., Hiratsuka, M., Yamaotsu, N., Hirono, S., et al. (2016). Molecular dynamics simulations to investigate the influences of amino acid mutations on protein three-dimensional structures of cytochrome P450 2D6.1, 2, 10, 14A, 51, and 62. *PLoS One*, *11*(4), e0152946. https://doi.org/10.1371/journal.pone.0152946.

Gaedigk, A., Garcia-Ribera, C., Jeong, H. E., Shin, J. G., & Hernandez-Sanchez, J. (2014). Resolution of a clinical AmpliChip CYP450 Test no call: Discovery and characterization of novel CYP2D6*1 haplotypes. *Pharmacogenomics*, *15*(9), 1175–1184. https://doi.org/10.2217/pgs.14.94.

Gaedigk, A., Hernandez, J., Garcia-Solaesa, V., Sanchez, S., & Isidoro-Garcia, M. (2011). Detection and characterization of the CYP2D6*9x2 gene duplication in two Spanish populations: Resolution of AmpliChip CYP450 test no-calls. *Pharmacogenomics*, *12*(11), 1617–1622. https://doi.org/10.2217/pgs.11.107.

Gaedigk, A., Ndjountche, L., Divakaran, K., Dianne Bradford, L., Zineh, I., Oberlander, T. F., et al. (2007). Cytochrome P4502D6 (CYP2D6) gene locus heterogeneity: Characterization of gene duplication events. *Clinical Pharmacology and Therapeutics*, *81*(2), 242–251. https://doi.org/10.1038/sj.clpt.6100033.

Gaedigk, A., Riffel, A. K., Berrocal, B. G., Solaesa, V. G., Davila, I., & Isidoro-Garcia, M. (2014). Characterization of a complex CYP2D6 genotype that caused an AmpliChip CYP450 Test no-call in the clinical setting. *Clinical Chemistry and Laboratory Medicine*, *52*(6), 799–807. https://doi.org/10.1515/cclm-2013-0943.

Hicks, J. K., Dunnenberger, H. M., Gumpper, K. F., Haidar, C. E., & Hoffman, J. M. (2016). Integrating pharmacogenomics into electronic health records with clinical decision support. *American Journal of Health-System Pharmacy*, *73*(23), 1967–1976. https://doi.org/10.2146/ajhp160030.

Hicks, J. K., Stowe, D., Willner, M. A., Wai, M., Daly, T., Gordon, S. M., et al. (2016). Implementation of clinical pharmacogenomics within a large health system: From electronic health record decision support to consultation services. *Pharmacotherapy*, *36*(8), 940–948. https://doi.org/10.1002/phar.1786.

Hinderer, M., Boeker, M., Wagner, S. A., Binder, H., Uckert, F., Newe, S., et al. (2017). The experience of physicians in pharmacogenomic clinical decision support within eight German university hospitals. *Pharmacogenomics*, *18*(8), 773–785. https://doi.org/10.2217/pgs-2017-0027.

Hoffman, J. M., Haidar, C. E., Wilkinson, M. R., Crews, K. R., Baker, D. K., Kornegay, N. M., et al. (2014). PG4KDS: A model for the clinical implementation of pre-emptive pharmacogenetics. *American Journal of Medical Genetics. Part C, Seminars in Medical Genetics*, *166C*(1), 45–55. https://doi.org/10.1002/ajmg.c.31391.

Janssens, A. C., & Deverka, P. A. (2014). Useless until proven effective: The clinical utility of preemptive pharmacogenetic testing. *Clinical Pharmacology and Therapeutics*, *96*(6), 652–654. https://doi.org/10.1038/clpt.2014.186.

Johnson, J. A., Caudle, K. E., Gong, L., Whirl-Carrillo, M., Stein, C. M., Scott, S. A., et al. (2017). Clinical Pharmacogenetics Implementation Consortium (CPIC) guideline for pharmacogenetics-guided warfarin dosing: 2017 update. *Clinical Pharmacology and Therapeutics*, *102*(3), 397–404. https://doi.org/10.1002/cpt. 668.

Khoury, M. J., Gwinn, M., Dotson, W. D., & Bowen, M. S. (2011). Is there a need for PGxceptionalism? *Genetics in Medicine*, *13*(10), 866–867. https://doi.org/10.1097/GIM.0b013e3182265bed.

Lin, C. H., Yeakley, J. M., McDaniel, T. K., & Shen, R. (2009). Medium- to high-throughput SNP genotyping using VeraCode microbeads. *Methods in Molecular Biology*, *496*, 129–142. https://doi.org/10.1007/978-1-59745-553-4_10.

Lunenburg, C. A., van Staveren, M. C., Gelderblom, H., Guchelaar, H. J., & Swen, J. J. (2016). Evaluation of clinical implementation of prospective DPYD genotyping in 5-fluorouracil- or capecitabine-treated patients. *Pharmacogenomics*, *17*(7), 721–729. https://doi.org/10.2217/pgs-2016-0013.

Mahgoub, A., Idle, J. R., Dring, L. G., Lancaster, R., & Smith, R. L. (1977). Polymorphic hydroxylation of debrisoquine in man. *Lancet*, *2*(8038), 584–586.

Mallal, S., Phillips, E., Carosi, G., Molina, J. M., Workman, C., Tomazic, J., et al. (2008). HLA-B*5701 screening for hypersensitivity to abacavir. *The New England Journal of Medicine*, *358*(6), 568–579. https://doi.org/10.1056/NEJMoa0706135.

McCarthy, D. J., Humburg, P., Kanapin, A., Rivas, M. A., Gaulton, K., Cazier, J. B., et al. (2014). Choice of transcripts and software has a large effect on variant annotation. *Genome Medicine*, *6*(3), 26. https://doi.org/10.1186/gm543.

Meulendijks, D., Henricks, L. M., Sonke, G. S., Deenen, M. J., Froehlich, T. K., Amstutz, U., et al. (2015). Clinical relevance of DPYD variants c.1679T>G, c.1236G>A/HapB3, and c.1601G>A as predictors of severe fluoropyrimidine-associated toxicity: A systematic review and meta-analysis of individual patient data. *The Lancet Oncology*, *16*(16), 1639–1650. https://doi.org/10.1016/s1470-2045(15)00286-7.

O'Daniel, J., Lucas, J., Deverka, P., Ermentrout, D., Silvey, G., Lobach, D. F., et al. (2010). Factors influencing uptake of pharmacogenetic testing in a diverse patient population. *Public Health Genomics*, *13*(1), 48–54. https://doi.org/10.1159/000217795.

O'Donnell, P. H., Bush, A., Spitz, J., Danahey, K., Saner, D., Das, S., et al. (2012). The 1200 patients project: Creating a new medical model system for clinical implementation of pharmacogenomics. *Clinical Pharmacology and Therapeutics*, *92*(4), 446–449. https://doi.org/10.1038/clpt.2012.117.

O'Donnell, P. H., Danahey, K., Jacobs, M., Wadhwa, N. R., Yuen, S., Bush, A., et al. (2014). Adoption of a clinical pharmacogenomics implementation program during outpatient care—Initial results of the University of Chicago "1,200 Patients Project" *American Journal of Medical Genetics. Part C, Seminars in Medical Genetics*, *166C*(1), 68–75. https://doi.org/10.1002/ajmg.c.31385.

O'Donnell, P. H., Wadhwa, N., Danahey, K., Borden, B. A., Lee, S. M., Hall, J. P., et al. (2017). Pharmacogenomics-based point-of-care clinical decision support significantly alters drug prescribing. *Clinical Pharmacology and Therapeutics*, *102*(5), 859–869. https://doi.org/10.1002/cpt.709.

Offer, S. M., Fossum, C. C., Wegner, N. J., Stuflesser, A. J., Butterfield, G. L., & Diasio, R. B. (2014). Comparative functional analysis of DPYD variants of potential clinical relevance to dihydropyrimidine dehydrogenase activity. *Cancer Research*, *74*(9), 2545–2554. https://doi.org/10.1158/0008-5472.can-13-2482.

Owen, R. P., Sangkuhl, K., Klein, T. E., & Altman, R. B. (2009). Cytochrome P450 2D6. *Pharmacogenetics and Genomics*, *19*(7), 559–562. https://doi.org/10.1097/FPC.0b013e32832e0e97.

Palomaki, G. E., FitzSimmons, S. C., & Haddow, J. E. (2004). Clinical sensitivity of prenatal screening for cystic fibrosis via CFTR carrier testing in a United States panethnic population. *Genetics in Medicine*, *6*(5), 405–414. https://doi.org/10.109701.GIM.0000139505.06194.39.

Palomaki, G. E., Haddow, J. E., Bradley, L. A., Richards, C. S., Stenzel, T. T., & Grody, W. W. (2003). Estimated analytic validity of HFE C282Y mutation testing in population screening: The potential value of confirmatory testing. *Genetics in Medicine*, *5*(6), 440–443. https://doi.org/10.1097/01.GIM.0000096500.66084.85.

Patel, V., Lin, F. J., Ojo, O., Rao, S., Yu, S., Zhan, L., et al. (2014). Cost-utility analysis of genotype-guided antiplatelet therapy in patients with moderate-to-high risk acute coronary syndrome and planned percutaneous coronary intervention. *Pharmacy Practice (Granada)*, *12*(3), 438.

Patrick, A. R., Avorn, J., & Choudhry, N. K. (2009). Cost-effectiveness of genotype-guided warfarin dosing for patients with atrial fibrillation. *Circulation. Cardiovascular Quality and Outcomes*, *2*(5), 429–436. https://doi.org/10.1161/circoutcomes.108.808592.

Pirmohamed, M., & Hughes, D. A. (2013). Pharmacogenetic tests: The need for a level playing field. *Nature Reviews. Drug Discovery*, *12*(1), 3–4. https://doi.org/10.1038/nrd3921.

Pratt, V. M., Zehnbauer, B., Wilson, J. A., Baak, R., Babic, N., Bettinotti, M., et al. (2010). Characterization of 107 genomic DNA reference materials for CYP2D6, CYP2C19, CYP2C9, VKORC1, and UGT1A1: A GeT-RM and Association for Molecular Pathology collaborative project. *The Journal of Molecular Diagnostics*, *12*(6), 835–846. https://doi.org/10.2353/jmoldx.2010.100090.

Raimundo, S., Toscano, C., Klein, K., Fischer, J., Griese, E. U., Eichelbaum, M., et al. (2004). A novel intronic mutation, 2988G > A, with high predictivity for impaired function of cytochrome P450 2D6 in white subjects. *Clinical Pharmacology and Therapeutics*, *76*(2), 128–138. https://doi.org/10.1016/j.clpt.2004.04.009.

Relling, M. V., Altman, R. B., Goetz, M. P., & Evans, W. E. (2010). Clinical implementation of pharmacogenomics: Overcoming genetic exceptionalism. *The Lancet Oncology*, *11*(6), 507–509. https://doi.org/10.1016/S1470-2045(10)70097-8.

Relling, M. V., Gardner, E. E., Sandborn, W. J., Schmiegelow, K., Pui, C. H., Yee, S. W., et al. (2011). Clinical Pharmacogenetics Implementation Consortium guidelines for thiopurine methyltransferase genotype and thiopurine dosing. *Clinical Pharmacology and Therapeutics*, *89*(3), 387–391. https://doi.org/10.1038/clpt.2010.320.

Relling, M. V., Gardner, E. E., Sandborn, W. J., Schmiegelow, K., Pui, C. H., Yee, S. W., et al. (2013). Clinical Pharmacogenetics Implementation Consortium guidelines for thiopurine methyltransferase genotype and thiopurine dosing: 2013 update. *Clinical Pharmacology and Therapeutics*, *93*(4), 324–325. https://doi.org/10.1038/clpt.2013.4.

Relling, M. V., & Klein, T. E. (2011). CPIC: Clinical Pharmacogenetics Implementation Consortium of the Pharmacogenomics Research Network. *Clinical Pharmacology and Therapeutics*, *89*(3), 464–467. https://doi.org/10.1038/clpt.2010.279.

Roche Diagnostics, Inc. (2005). *AmpliChip™ CYP450 package insert.*

Rohrer Vitek, C. R., Abul-Husn, N. S., Connolly, J. J., Hartzler, A. L., Kitchner, T., Peterson, J. F., et al. (2017). Healthcare provider education to support integration of pharmacogenomics in practice: The eMERGE Network experience. *Pharmacogenomics*, *18*(10), 1013–1025. https://doi.org/10.2217/pgs-2017-0038.

Rosell, R., Moran, T., Queralt, C., Porta, R., Cardenal, F., Camps, C., et al. (2009). Screening for epidermal growth factor receptor mutations in lung cancer. *The New England Journal of Medicine*, *361*(10), 958–967. https://doi.org/10.1056/NEJMoa0904554.

Samwald, M., Minarro-Gimenez, J. A., Blagec, K., & Adlassnig, K. P. (2014). Towards a global IT system for personalized medicine: The Medicine Safety Code initiative. *Studies in Health Technology and Informatics, 205*, 261–265.

Schackman, B. R., Scott, C. A., Walensky, R. P., Losina, E., Freedberg, K. A., & Sax, P. E. (2008). The cost-effectiveness of HLA-B*5701 genetic screening to guide initial antiretroviral therapy for HIV. *AIDS, 22*(15), 2025–2033. https://doi.org/10.1097/QAD.0b013e3283103ce6.

Shuker, N., Bouamar, R., van Schaik, R. H., Clahsen-van Groningen, M. C., Damman, J., Baan, C. C., et al. (2016). A randomized controlled trial comparing the efficacy of Cyp3a5 genotype-based with body-weight-based tacrolimus dosing after living donor kidney transplantation. *American Journal of Transplantation, 16*(7), 2085–2096. https://doi.org/10.1111/ajt.13691.

Sim, S. C., & Ingelman-Sundberg, M. (2006). The human cytochrome P450 Allele Nomenclature Committee Web site: Submission criteria, procedures, and objectives. *Methods in Molecular Biology, 320*, 183–191. https://doi.org/10.1385/1-59259-998-2:183.

Stanek, E. J., Sanders, C. L., Taber, K. A., Khalid, M., Patel, A., Verbrugge, R. R., et al. (2012). Adoption of pharmacogenomic testing by US physicians: Results of a nationwide survey. *Clinical Pharmacology and Therapeutics, 91*(3), 450–458. https://doi.org/10.1038/clpt.2011.306.

Swen, J. J., Huizinga, T. W., Gelderblom, H., de Vries, E. G., Assendelft, W. J., Kirchheiner, J., et al. (2007). Translating pharmacogenomics: Challenges on the road to the clinic. *PLoS Medicine, 4*(8), e209. https://doi.org/10.1371/journal.pmed.0040209.

Swen, J. J., Nijenhuis, M., de Boer, A., Grandia, L., Maitland-van der Zee, A. H., Mulder, H., et al. (2011). Pharmacogenetics: From bench to byte—An update of guidelines. *Clinical Pharmacology and Therapeutics, 89*(5), 662–673. https://doi.org/10.1038/clpt.2011.34.

Swen, J. J., Wilting, I., de Goede, A. L., Grandia, L., Mulder, H., Touw, D. J., et al. (2008). Pharmacogenetics: From bench to byte. *Clinical Pharmacology and Therapeutics, 83*(5), 781–787. https://doi.org/10.1038/sj.clpt.6100507.

Thervet, E., Loriot, M. A., Barbier, S., Buchler, M., Ficheux, M., Choukroun, G., et al. (2010). Optimization of initial tacrolimus dose using pharmacogenetic testing. *Clinical Pharmacology and Therapeutics, 87*(6), 721–726. https://doi.org/10.1038/clpt.2010.17.

Toffoli, G., Giodini, L., Buonadonna, A., Berretta, M., De Paoli, A., Scalone, S., et al. (2015). Clinical validity of a DPYD-based pharmacogenetic test to predict severe toxicity to fluoropyrimidines. *International Journal of Cancer, 137*(12), 2971–2980. https://doi.org/10.1002/ijc.29654.

Tonk, E. C. M., Gurwitz, D., Maitland-van der Zee, A. H., & Janssens, A. (2017). Assessment of pharmacogenetic tests: Presenting measures of clinical validity and potential population impact in association studies. *The Pharmacogenomics Journal, 17*(4), 386–392. https://doi.org/10.1038/tpj.2016.34.

Toscano, C., Klein, K., Blievernicht, J., Schaeffeler, E., Saussele, T., Raimundo, S., et al. (2006). Impaired expression of CYP2D6 in intermediate metabolizers carrying the *41 allele caused by the intronic SNP 2988G > A: Evidence for modulation of splicing events. *Pharmacogenetics and Genomics, 16*(10), 755–766. https://doi.org/10.1097/01.fpc.0000230112.96086.e0.

van der Straaten, T., Swen, J., Baak-Pablo, R., & Guchelaar, H. J. (2008). Use of plasmid-derived external quality control samples in pharmacogenetic testing. *Pharmacogenomics, 9*(9), 1261–1266. https://doi.org/10.2217/14622416.9.9.1261.

van der Wouden, C. H., Cambon-Thomsen, A., Cecchin, E., Cheung, K. C., Lucia Davila-Fajardo, C., Deneer, V. H., et al. (2017). Implementing Pharmacogenomics in Europe: Design and Implementation Strategy of the Ubiquitous Pharmacogenomics Consortium. *Clinical Pharmacology and Therapeutics, 101*(3), 341–358. https://doi.org/10.1002/cpt.602.

Van Driest, S. L., Shi, Y., Bowton, E. A., Schildcrout, J. S., Peterson, J. F., Pulley, J., et al. (2014). Clinically actionable genotypes among 10,000 patients with preemptive pharmacogenomic testing. *Clinical Pharmacology and Therapeutics*, *95*(4), 423–431. https://doi.org/10.1038/clpt.2013.229.

Verhoef, T. I., Redekop, W. K., Langenskiold, S., Kamali, F., Wadelius, M., Burnside, G., et al. (2016). Cost-effectiveness of pharmacogenetic-guided dosing of warfarin in the United Kingdom and Sweden. *The Pharmacogenomics Journal*, *16*(5), 478–484. https://doi.org/10.1038/tpj.2016.41.

Weitzel, K. W., Aquilante, C. L., Johnson, S., Kisor, D. F., & Empey, P. E. (2016). Educational strategies to enable expansion of pharmacogenomics-based care. *American Journal of Health-System Pharmacy*, *73*(23), 1986–1998. https://doi.org/10.2146/ajhp160104.

Whirl-Carrillo, M., McDonagh, E. M., Hebert, J. M., Gong, L., Sangkuhl, K., Thorn, C. F., et al. (2012). Pharmacogenomics knowledge for personalized medicine. *Clinical Pharmacology and Therapeutics*, *92*(4), 414–417. https://doi.org/10.1038/clpt.2012.96.

CHAPTER TEN

Pharmacogenetics in Pain Treatment

Ana M. Peiró[1]
Clinical Pharmacology Unit, Department of Health of Alicante-General Hospital, Alicante, Spain
Neuropharmacology on Pain (NED), Alicante Institute for Health and Biomedical Research (ISABIAL-FISABIO Foundation), Alicante, Spain
[1]Corresponding author: e-mail address: peiro_ana@gva.es

Contents

1. Introduction 248
   1.1 Why Is Pharmacogenetics Necessary? 249
   1.2 Individual Genetic Variability 251
   1.3 Genetic and Epigenetic Research 252
2. Pharmacogenetics Applied to the Treatment of Pain 253
   2.1 WHO Analgesic Ladder First Step: Nonopioid Analgesics 254
   2.2 WHO Analgesic Ladder Second Step: Tramadol and Codeine 259
   2.3 WHO Analgesic Ladder Third Step: Opioid Analgesics 260
   2.4 Research, Ethics, and Legislation in Pharmacogenetics 266
3. Conclusion 267
Acknowledgments 268
References 268
Further Reading 272

Abstract

Pain is an unpleasant feeling usually resulting from tissue damage that can persist along weeks, months, or even years after the injury, turning into pathological chronic pain, the leading cause of disability. Currently, pharmacology interventions are usually the first-line therapy but there is a highly variable analgesic drug response. Pharmacogenetics (PGx) offers a means to identify genetic biomarkers that can predict individual analgesic response opening doors to precision medicine. PGx analyze the way in which the presence of variations in the DNA sequence (single-nucleotide polymorphisms, SNPs) could be responsible for portions of the population reaching different levels of pain relief (phenotype) due to gene interference in the drug mechanism of action (pharmacodynamics) and/or its concentration at the place of action (pharmacokinetics). SNPs in the cytochrome P450 enzymes genes (*CYP2D6*) influence metabolism of codeine, tramadol, hydrocodone, oxycodone, and tricyclic antidepressants. Blood concentrations of some NSAIDs depend on CYP2C9 and/or CYP2C8 activity. Additional candidate genes encode for opioid receptors, transporters, and other molecules important for pharmacotherapy in pain management. However, PGx studies are often contradictory, slowing the uptake

Advances in Pharmacology, Volume 83
ISSN 1054-3589
https://doi.org/10.1016/bs.apha.2018.04.004

of this information. This is likely due, in large part, to a lack of robust evidence demonstrating clinical utility and to its polygenic response modulated by other exogenous or epigenetics factors. Novel therapies, including targeting of epigenetic changes and gene therapy-based approaches, broaden future options to improve understanding of pain and the treatment of people who suffer it.

ABBREVIATIONS

CB1 cannabinoid receptor
COMT catechol-*O*-methyltransferase
COX cyclooxygenase
EPOS European Pharmacogenetic Opioid Study
FDA Food and Drug Agency
FEDRA Spanish pharmacovigilance system
GCH1 guanosine triphosphate cyclohydrolase 1
GPCRs G protein-coupled receptors
GWAS genome-wide association studies
ICH International Conference on Harmonization
KCNJ6 potassium ion channels named Kir3.2
MRP multidrug resistance protein
NSAID nonsteroidal antiinflammatory drugs
OPRM1 *mu* opioid receptor
PharmGKB pharmacogenetics and pharmacogenomics knowledge base
PGx pharmacogenetics
SNP single-nucleotide polymorphism
UGT2B7 UDP-glucuronyl transferase gene
UM ultrarapid metabolizers

1. INTRODUCTION

Pain is the most common presenting physical symptom in medicine and accounts for a substantial burden for the individual patient, health care, and society in general. Its persistence and response to analgesic drugs show toward pain varies according to several and complex factors with unresolved questions. Chronic pain is an unpleasant sensory and emotional experience, without apparent biological value, that persists beyond normal tissue healing. It is a global health problem underestimated for decades that affects 20% of the adult population chronically and despite the fact that about half of them receive some analgesic treatment, 64% fail to control it (Hardt, Jacobsen, Goldberg, Nickel, & Buchwald, 2008). Thus, the scenario for chronic pain management is unsatisfactory, with many patients suffering from pain up to their maximum tolerance level, huge impact on their own quality of life and a large variability of pharmacological combinations used to treat them (Pérez et al., 2013).

How can an individual have a very different sensory experience and drug response to another person receiving a similar sensory input and treatment? It could be said that one of the reasons for which people are receiving an ineffective drug to treat their pain are the interindividual genetic differences that generate a polygenic responses modulated by exogenous factors (epigenetics, "epi" means "above" in Greek). The field that addresses pharmacogenetics (PGx) is developing an understanding of such differences and the mechanisms that support them are the base to optimize treatment on an individual-by-individual focus. PGx analyze the way in which the presence of variations in the DNA sequence could be responsible for a proportion of the population reaching a different pain relief by interfering with its mechanism of action and/or its concentration in the place of action (Cazacu, Mogosan, & Loghin, 2015).

The concept that "one size fits all" has been replaced by the idea of precision medicine, which foresees the use of molecular data to treat patients with more specificity and efficacy but fewer adverse events. So hopefully, patients with an unsatisfactory response to analgesic treatment will have a ray of hope thanks to PGx (Webster & Belfer, 2016). However, the translation of its results to the "real world" remains scarce (Langley, 2011).

1.1 Why Is Pharmacogenetics Necessary?

The disciplines that study the relationships between genes and the response to drugs are PGx and pharmacogenomics. Both versions were used as synonyms until 2007, when at the proposal of the International Council for Harmonization of Technical Requirements for Pharmaceuticals for Human Use (ICH, http://www.ich.org), PGx was defined as the study of the influence of changes in the DNA sequence on the response to drugs; and pharmacogenomics as the investigation of DNA and RNA variations in relation to drug response. Discovery efforts have been assisted by robust accessible reference databases that classify and annotate genetic variations, as for example, the single-nucleotide polymorphism (SNP) database/genomic structural variation database, ClinVar, and Online Mendelian Inheritance in Man (OMIM) database (Hoffman et al., 2016).

From an evolutionary point of view, these differences would behave as a biological security because they function as a survival reserve, to the extent that they facilitate the adaptation of the species as a whole to a changing environment. Thus, a specific genetic endowment of the individual (inherited SNP in block or haplotype), modulated by physiological, pathological, or environmental factors (epigenetics), could explain, in part or totally, the variations in the drug action or the concentration reached on its place of action (Vuilleumier, Stamer, & Landau, 2012).

Genes can affect pharmacodynamics based on variations in drug target receptors and downstream signal, transduction pathways (i.e., the *mu* opioid receptor (OPRM1), catechol-*O*-methyltransferase (*COMT*)). On the other hand, other genes affect pharmacokinetics altering drug metabolism and/or elimination (i.e., CYP450 family of enzymes, enzymes responsible for glucuronidation, drug transporter proteins, and COX enzyme), modifying the relationship between drug dose and concentration at target organ. In addition, the interaction of the drug with each category of proteins can be affected by other medications or factors related with the patient as physiological (sex, age, or pregnancy) or environmental (diet, exercise, tobacco, or alcohol) (Kadiev et al., 2008; Kirchheiner et al., 2007).

PGx research could be used to: (a) explain the variability of the response observed among participants in clinical studies, as well as unexpected adverse events; (b) determine eligibility to participate in clinical trials (preselection) in order to optimize the study design; (c) develop diagnostic tests linked to the drug to identify patients with higher or lower probability of benefiting from a treatment, or who may be at risk of suffering adverse events; (d) have better understanding of the mechanism of action or the metabolism of new and existing drugs, as well as of the mechanisms of disease and individual doses (Hajj, Khabbaz, Laplanche, & Peoc'h, 2013). However, nowadays, the interpretation and translation of these genetic results to the clinic is still under discussion.

The following considerations should be taken in account: whether PGx test results are actionable, the level of evidence needed for implementation of PGx, the sources of information regarding the interpretation of PGx data, and the need to move from local national clinical guidelines to international ones. Clinical guidelines as structured and coded knowledge sources will facilitate their adoption and implementation by reducing the amount of expertise and effort required for transforming the knowledge into technical specifications. Concerted efforts like an open active cooperation with industry are required in order to facilitate translation and commercialization of genetic testings (Peiró et al., 2016). In addition, payers need to be convinced about the positive cost–benefit of PGx-guided healthcare, and professionals need to be trained and reassured on the availability and utility of genetic testing, even more when 30% of the medicinal products centrally approved in the Europe Union, since 1995, contain a genetic biomarker in their product label (Ehmann et al., 2015; Friedman, Wong, & Blumenthal, 2010).

1.2 Individual Genetic Variability

The genetic information is encoded in the molecular structure of the nucleic acids, which in turn, is formed by a sugar molecule, a phosphate group that allows binding to other nucleotides, and a nitrogenous base. Therefore, a nucleotide is the phosphate ester of a nucleoside. Depending on the nature of the pentose, two types of nucleic acids are distinguished: ribonucleic acid (RNA) that carries D-ribose and deoxyribonucleic acid (DNA) containing 2-deoxy-D-ribose. The bases that are involved in the formation of DNA are called adenine (A), cytosine (C), guanine (G), and thymine (T). RNA contains the three first and uracil (U) instead of thymine. The genetic information is contained in these nucleotide sequences along a chain, as ATGCTAGTCTGTAAA.

Genetic polymorphism is the term for genes structural variations and can be classified into five major classes: RFLP (restriction fragment length polymorphism), VNTR (variable number of tandem repeat), STR (short tandem repeat or microsatellite), SNP, and CNV (copy-number variation) (Nakamura, 2009). A SNP is the most common altered gene form.

In humans, it is estimated that there are more than 10 million SNPs (i.e., 1 in 300 base pairs on average) with an observed minor allele frequency of $\geq$1% in the population. In a SNP, the change of a single nucleotide in the genomic sequence gives rise to different alleles. They can be changed (substitution), removed (deletions), or added (insertion) to a polynucleotide sequence (Baroy, Misceo, & Frengen, 2008). Remarkably, insertions and deletions are also abundant in the human genome with sizes ranging from single to several million base pairs (Mullaney, Mills, Pittard, & Devine, 2010). Usually, these variants are silent (synonymous, no change in amino acid sequence or change in amino acid that does not affect the phenotype), while others are missense (different amino acid) or nonsense (premature stop codon) variants (nonsynonymous, they change an amino acid in the protein encoded by the gene) being the main source of interindividual genetic variability (Ng & Henikoff, 2006).

However, the great advantage of SNPs over other types of markers is the possibility of analyzing them using large-scale automated methods. In 1986, the Department of Energy of the United States led the Human Genome Initiative and launched the Human Genome Project (http://www.genome.gov) with the objective of developing tools capable of achieving the complete sequence of the human genome. Since multiple large-scale SNP genotyping platforms were developed around 2003, construction of an international consortium for making a SNP database for three major populations had been discussed and the International HapMap project was organized in 2003.The International HapMap Project proposed to identify the most frequent SNPs in the human genome in individuals from different ethnic groups. Genetic linkage analysis, construction of the international SNP database, and development of high-throughput SNP genotyping platforms, are used to perform genome-wide association studies (GWAS), which have identified genes susceptible to common diseases or associated with drug responses (Dalca & Brudno, 2010).

1.3 Genetic and Epigenetic Research

1.3.1 Genome-Wide Association Studies

GWAS have identified hundreds of genetic variants associated with complex human diseases and traits scanning markers across the DNA. However, they rarely reported or even measured the experienced pain. This might be due to the lack of reliable and cheap pain level measurement tools, and, also, because of the fluctuations in the personal pain experience that makes very hard to detect true average pain intensity in cross-sectional studies (Peters et al., 2013). Most variants identified so far conferred relatively small increments in risk and explained only a small proportion of familial clustering, leading to question how the remaining "missing" heritability could be explained. However, most of the studies compared the cooccurrence of the painful disease itself, and not the experienced pain states. Induced pain under laboratory circumstances can provide slightly better measurements of the heritability rate of pain vulnerability, which is estimated among 22%–60% (Manolio et al., 2009). The rare exception of the multilevel GWAS of chronic widespread pain resulted in the association of rheumatic pain with 5p12.2 chromosomal region (Peters et al., 2013). These results might facilitate other research to consider experienced pain as a target for GWAS. In addition, novel therapies, including targeting of epigenetic changes and gene therapy-based approaches, are further broadening future options for pain (Pirmohamed, 2014).

1.3.2 Epigenetic Modifications

Epigenetic modifications, such as DNA methylation and histone modifications (e.g., acetylation and phosphorylation), are known to cause stable gene expression changes via chromatin remodeling. These mechanisms have a role not only in the determination of developmental cell fates but also in the physiological and pathological processes in the nervous system. There is evidence that injury-induced changes in chromatin structure drive stable changes in gene expression and neural function, which may cause symptoms, including allodynia, hyperalgesia, anxiety, and depression (Descalzi et al., 2015).

Recent findings on epigenetic changes in the spinal cord and brain during chronic pain may guide fundamental advances in new treatments. DNA methylation is an epigenetic mechanism for long-term regulation of gene expression. Alterations in DNA methylation, an enzymatic covalent modification of cytosine bases in the DNA, could serve as a "genomic" memory of pain in the adult cortex mediating the long-term consequences of painful experiences and embed them into the genome. Neuronal plasticity at the neuroanatomical, functional, morphological, physiological, and molecular levels has been demonstrated throughout the neuroaxis in response to persistent pain, including in the adult prefrontal cortex (Kim & Kaang, 2017), thereby contributing to the alterations in both, pain sensitivity and pharmacological efficacy in neuropathic pain (Ueda & Uchida, 2015).

At this point, it is important to understand that structural and functional aspects are integrated into a "dynamic" model and it must be taken into account that it is also possible to regulate the expression of genes without changing their DNA sequence, because it may vary due to the function of the RNA molecules themselves (noncoding RNA transcripts, microRNAs), due to their interactions with DNA and/or proteins, or by alterations in the chromatin.

2. PHARMACOGENETICS APPLIED TO THE TREATMENT OF PAIN

A multitude of candidate genes related to different pain neurotransmission pathways have been described. Most relevant are those that encode for the *OPRM1* gene which variants can give rise to a receptor three times more active and to a request of higher doses of morphine; *COMT* gene, which can decrease its enzymatic activity three to four times; cytochrome

P450 complex especially in *CYP2D6* and UDP-glucuronyl transferase (enconded by the *UGT2B7* gene) where SNPs are the general rule that can lead to a loss of metabolic function and toxicity. The functional variants of the cited genes are described associated with the WHO analgesic ladder three-step approach (Světlík, Hronová, Bakhouche, Matoušková, & Slanař, 2013) (Tables 1 and 2).

2.1 WHO Analgesic Ladder First Step: Nonopioid Analgesics

Nonopioid analgesics such as analgesics and nonsteroidal antiinflammatory drugs (NSAIDs) are very accessible drugs (5.5% of total prescriptions). All of them exert their effect through the inhibition of the COX enzyme blocking the activation of peripheral nerve fibers and decreasing the number of impulses that reach the central nervous system. Its metabolism occurs mainly in the liver especially by conjugation with glucuronic acid and oxidation through CYP450. Only *CYP2C9* gene has more than 33 variants capable of modifying NSAIDs pharmacology such as diclofenac, ibuprofen, naproxen, tenoxicam, piroxicam, or celecoxib (Stamer, Zhang, & Stuber, 2010).

2.1.1 NSAIDs as COX Inhibitors: Balancing Benefit/Risk

The COX inhibitors are used very commonly in noncancer pain. However, they are often proved to be ineffective in severe pain, as well as, they present dangerous cardiorenal and gastrointestinal long-term side effects even more in elderly, at higher doses, and with long-term use. Following recommendations of the United States Food and Drug Administration (FDA), "NSAIDs should be administered at the lowest effective dose for the shortest duration consistent with individual treatment goals" (Enthoven, Roelofs, Deyo, Tulder, & Koes, 2016; Fine, 2013).

COX is a product of the enzyme responsible for the synthesis of prostaglandins (*prostaglandin-endoperoxide synthase* gene, *PTGS*). SNPs on this enzyme have been associated with lower response to the antiplatelet effect of acetylsalicylic acid (−842G, *PTGS1* gene) and at a lower risk of suffering severe oncological pain (837C, rs5275, *PTGS2* gene). However, its expression is very variable (−36% to +300%) after surgery (Wyatt, Pettit, & Harirforoosh, 2012). In relation to its metabolism, UDP-Glucuronosyltransferase enzyme as UGT1A6*2/2 associated a faster conjugation of acetylsalicylic acid modifying its antiaggregant effect (Chen et al., 2007). Other NSAIDs, such as ibuprofen, naproxen, tenoxicam, and celecoxib, suffered a reduction of up to 70% in their clearance in carriers CYP2C9*3 (rs1057910), in some cases together with

Table 1 Pharmacogenetics Applied to the Drugs Most Used in Pain Treatment

Drug	Gene and Genetic Variability	Patients/Design	Clinical Effect
AAS	*PTGS1, −842G*	n=101 (♀25 ♂76) patients scheduled for percutaneous coronary intervention. Observational study. Prospective	Less response to antiaggregant effect (100 mg/d)
	PTGS2, 837T	n=667 non-Hispanic whites with lung cancer. Cases and controls study n=1149 targets with lung cancer. Observational study. Retrospective	Lower risk of severe pain
	*UGT1A6*2/2*	n=28 healthy volunteers. Observational study. Prospective	Modification of the antiaggregant effect (650 mg/d)
NSAID	*CYP2C9*2* *CYP2C9*3* (rs1057910) *CYP2C8*3* (rs10509681, rs11572080)	n=335 (♀182 ♂153) healthy Spanish volunteers n=134 patients with hemorrhages and 177 without adverse effects. Transversal study	Decreased clearance (ibuprofen, tenoxicam, celecoxib) and increased risk of bleeding, peptic ulcer, and kidney disorders
	*CYP2C9*1,*2,*3* *CYP2C8*1,*3*	n=35 (♀11 ♂24) healthy Brazilian volunteers	Decreased clearance of piroxicam and increased COX1 inhibition
	*CYP2C8*3,*4*	n=142 healthy white Spanish volunteers	Changes in renal elimination
	*HLA-DQA1*0102*	n=41 patients with liver injury and 176 without injury. Cases and controls study	Increased risk of severe hepatotoxicity
Tramadol Codeíne	*CYP2D6*	n=300 patients after abdominal surgery n=250 Korean patients with gonarthrosis. Prospective observational studies n=13 cases after adenotonsillectomy	Less analgesia in slow metabolizers and greater toxicity in ultrarapid metabolizers

Continued

Table 1 Pharmacogenetics Applied to the Drugs Most Used in Pain Treatment—cont'd

Drug	Gene and Genetic Variability	Patients/Design	Clinical Effect
Opioids	*OPRM1, A118G* (rs1799971)	$n=80$ ♀ programmed for hysterectomy. Observational study $n=167$ healthy volunteers, experimental pain	Lower dose of morphine and fewer analgesic rescues
	OPRM1, −172G (rs6912029), *−1510G* (rs12205732)	$n=183$ ♂ with dependence on opioids of Arab origin. Observational study	Worst response to detoxification treatment
	OPRD1, 80T (rs1042114)	$n=735$ (♀443 ♂292) healthy American volunteers of European origin (50%), African (23%), Hispanic (11%), or Asian (14%)	Less sensitivity to pain
	OPRD1 (rs678849)	$n=643$ patients with dependence on North American opioids of European origin (88%), African (12%). Observational study	Better response to treatment with methadone, worse with buprenorphine
	OPRK1, 36G (rs1051660)	$n=176$ subjects (106 whites from Eastern countries with heroin dependence and 70 healthy volunteers) Estudio de casos y controles	Greater vulnerability dependency behaviors
	*CYP3A4*1G* *CYP3A5*1/*3* *CYP3A5*3/*3*	$n=203$ ♀ programmed for total hysterectomy. Abdominal or myomectomy. Observational study. Prospective $n=25$ cases analyzed (22 whites, 1 African-American, and 2 Americans)	Lower dose requirement and possible predictive factor for fentanyl toxicity

	UGT2B7, 802C > T (rs7439366) *−840G*	$n=20$ patients with sickle cell disease. Transversal study	Increased conjugation for buprenorphine and minor with morphine
	ABCB1, 3435C (rs1045642)	$n=33$ healthy volunteers, experimental pain $n=228$ oncological patients. Observational study	Lower dose required
	ABCB1, 2677A (rs2032582), *3435T* (rs1045642)		Variable risk of nausea and vomiting, increased with morphine and minor with oxycodone
	ABCB1, 1236T (rs1128503), *2677T* (rs2032582), *3435T* (rs1045642)		Increased risk of miosis with loperamide and respiratory depression with fentanyl
	COMT (rs6269A > G, rs4633T > C, rs4818C > G, rs4680G > A)	$n=202$ ♀ healthy volunteers, experimental pain (85% of European or American origin, 15% African, Asian, or Hispanic)	Phenotypes of sensitivity to pain
	COMT (rs4633T, rs4680G, rs165722C)	$n=2294$ oncological patients. Observational study. Retrospective	Protective factor nausea and vomiting
	GCH1, haplotipo	$n=251$ (♀109 ♂142) oncological patients. Observational study. Retrospective	Less sensitivity to pain and later onset of cancer pain treatment
	DRD2, 1174 C 1192C	$n=194$ whites (85 patients with opioid dependence and 99 healthy volunteers). Cases and controls study	Greater doses of methadone and fewer responders to. Detoxification treatment with methadone

Table 2 Pharmacogenetics Applied to the Metabolism of Drugs: Substrate, Inducers, and Inhibitors Drugs Metabolized by Cytochrome P450

CYP	1A2	2B6	2C9	2C19	2D6	3A4
Substrates	Acetaminophen	Bupropion	Celecoxib	Diazepam	Codeine	Alprazolam
	Melatonin	Methadone	Piroxicam	Carisoprodol	Tramadol	Midazolam
	Caffeine	Phenobarbital	Ibuprofen	Rifampin	Oxycodone	Methadone
	Tobacco		Warfarin		Hydrocodone	Fentanyl
			St. John's Wort			Buprenorphine
					Rifampin	Phenobarbital
Inducers	Cannabinoid		Rifampin	Gingko	Dexamethasone	Rifampin
	Oxcarbazepine		Ritonavir	Prednisone		Butalbital
	Carbamazepine					
	Phenobarbital					
Inhibitors	Ciprofloxacin	Paroxetine	Fluoxetine	Fluoxetine	Duloxetine	Clarithromycin
	Caffeine	Venlafaxine	Fluconazole		Paroxetine	Erythromycin
	Grapefruit				Fluoxetine	Grapefruit
					Goldenseal	Indinavir
					Bupropion	Ritonavir

CYP22C8*3 (rs10509681 and rs11572080), and in a way independent to CYP2C9*2 (rs1799853) whose isolated presence is able to reduce it up to 96% (Tracy et al., 2002). This led to a greater risk of gastric and renal toxicity. Similarly, piroxicam has been associated with worse clearance and greater COX1 inhibition in CYP2C9*1/*2 or CYP2C9*1/*3, and diclofenac in native subjects CYP2C8*1 (Martínez et al., 2005). However, these effects are not similar for other NSAIDs.

2.2 WHO Analgesic Ladder Second Step: Tramadol and Codeine

In this step, we incorporate weak opioid analgesics such as tramadol, the most prescribed for moderate pain intensity, and codeine, one of the most used in pediatrics in countries like Canada. Both are OPRM1 agonists, being tramadol, in addition, capable of inhibiting the reuptake of noradrenaline and serotonin. Its bioactivation is carried out, above all, through CYP2D6. Thus, decreases in CYP2D6 activity may lead to reduced conversion of prodrugs into their more active metabolites, causing inadequate analgesia and the need for increased opioid medication. Conversely, increased CYP2D6 activity can lead to elevated levels of active metabolites in the blood, increasing the risk of adverse outcomes (such as an overdose) (Kirchheiner et al., 2007; Paar, Poche, Gerloff, & Dengler, 1997). This cytochrome has about 80 described variants that are grouped into four phenotypes according to their metabolizing activity (De Gregori et al., 2001): (i) slow (individuals poor metabolizers, PM, very diminished enzymatic activity) that require 30% more tramadol, (ii) intermediate (intermediate metabolizers), (iii) rapid (extensive metabolizers), or (iv) ultrarapid (ultrarapid metabolizers, UM), when presenting multiple copies of the functional gene, that may increase the risk of toxicity due to drowsiness, confusion, or respiratory depression (Crews et al., 2012).

Tramadol is metabolized through CYP2D6 and its analgesic effect may change according to polymorphisms (Chidambaran, Sadhasivam, & Mahmoud, 2017; Matic, de Wildt, Tibboel, & van Schaik, 2017) with a lower degree of analgesia in PM with acute postoperative pain and an increase in nausea and vomiting in osteoarthritis (Kim, Choi, Kang, & Bae, 2010). Also, SNPs in *CYP2D6* lead to the inability to convert codeine to morphine, thus making codeine ineffective as an analgesic but in UM cases, high concentrations of morphine can be observed inducing major adverse events. In fact, the FDA warned of cases of severe respiratory depression and death in children with UM phenotype after adenoidectomy or tonsillectomy (Racoosin, Roberson, Pacanowski, & Nielsen, 2013).

2.3 WHO Analgesic Ladder Third Step: Opioid Analgesics

Opioids with their central mechanisms of action are controversial drugs in noncancer pain treatment. Apart from the most-discussed abuse potential and the tolerance developed after chronic administration are also limiting the usage of opioids against pain (Furlan et al., 2010).

Opioids modulate nociception by stimulating OPRM1, the major molecular gate for opioid analgesia (Kieffer & Gaveriaux-Ruff, 2002). Several other strategies have been developed to try to reduce opioids adverse effects, such as using agonists of other opioid receptors (Vanderah, 2010) or peripheral *mu* antagonists (Webster & Belfer, 2016). However, the former ones produce a limited analgesia (Riviere, 2004) and the latter ones need to be coprescribed with opioids and prevent constipation. Recently, using a different strategy, it has been demonstrated that the K+ channel TREK-1 is a crucial contributor of morphine-induced analgesia in mice, while it is not involved in morphine-induced constipation, respiratory depression, and/or dependence. These observations suggest that TREK-1 channel, acting downstream from the *mu* receptor, might have strong analgesic effects without opioids-like adverse effects (Rodrigues et al., 2014).

2.3.1 Pharmacodynamics

Some candidate genes are implied either directly (opioid receptors) or indirectly into the opioid transduction pathways when signal is transmitted to a variety of effectors (e.g., adenylate cyclase or calcium and potassium ion channels named Kir3.2, *KCNJ6*).

2.3.1.1 Opioid Receptors

Opioid receptors belong to the family of G protein-coupled receptors (GPCRs). There are three types of classical receptors: *mu, kappa*, and *delta*. They share a high degree of homology containing an extracellular N-terminus domain, seven-transmembrane domains, and an intracellular C-terminus domain. Most variations are found in the N-terminal domain and the extracellular loops. Splice variations of opioid receptor mRNA have been shown to produce receptor subtypes that may be of functional importance (Dietis, Rowbotham, & Lambert, 2011).

OPRM1 gene represents the first line candidate for evaluating the role of polymorphisms in the clinical effects of morphine. Studies in mice established that this receptor is essential for morphine analgesia, physical dependence, and reward (Lancaster, Linden, & Heerey, 2012). More than 100 SNPs are localized in the C-terminal (Shabalina et al., 2009). The most common polymorphism A118AG (rs1799971, A118G), leading to an asparagine to aspartate substitution at amino acid 40 (Asn40Asp), with an allelic frequency varying from 2% to 50% according to ethnic groups, has been extensively studied (Brunton, Chabner, & Knollman, 2011). This polymorphism is responsible for the loss of a putative N-linked glycosylation site in the N-terminal domain and is associated with modified response to opiates. Indeed, the variant protein exhibits three-times greater binding affinity for the endopeptide β-endorphin, whereas binding to substances such as morphine, methadone, and naloxone is unaffected in vitro (Chou, Wang, et al., 2006, Chou, Yang, et al., 2006; Kreek, Bart, Lilly, LaForge, & Nielsen, 2005). Furthermore, this variant presents reduced analgesic response to alfentanil and morphine-6-glucuronide (Romberg et al., 2005; Skarke, Darimont, Schmidt, Geisslinger, & Lotsch, 2003), requiring higher doses of morphine for pain relief or associating a decreased *OPRM1* expression in both mRNA expression and translation into a functional protein (Bond et al., 1998). Also, lower mRNA expression in human brain tissue and in transfected cells was found in 118AG-allele carriers (Zhang, Wang, Johnson, Papp, & Sadee, 2005).

The largest genetic association study in pain was the European Pharmacogenetic Opioid Study (EPOS, $n=2.294$), which included 112 SNPs of 25 genes, the most analyzed being A118G (rs1799971, *OPRM1* gene). This variant increases its affinity for endogenous opioids, with a decrease in pain perception and lower cortical response to the painful stimulus. The homozygous 118-G allele subjects required lower doses of morphine and a lower number of analgesic rescues (Klepstad et al., 2011). However, a significant association between genetic profile, opioid dose, and analgesia could not be shown.

In addition, there is a large number of studies according to the gender or origin of the population in relation to the sensitivity to experimental painful stimuli (Hastie et al., 2012), opioid-dependence behaviors (Mistry, Bawor, Desai, Marsh, & Samaan, 2014), or to response to opioids deprescription (AL-Eitan, Jaradat, Su, Tay, & Hulse, 2012). However, further pharmacogenetic studies in larger cohorts of patients are needed to confirm these findings.

2.3.1.2 Opioid Transduction Pathways

β-Arrestin 2 is an intracellular protein that is integral to *mu* receptor inactivation and internalization (Zhang, Xiong, Lin, Ma, & Yu, 2009). On binding, opioid receptor agonists differentially trigger receptor phosphorylation and recruitment of β-arrestin. Knockout studies have shown that mice lacking *β-arrestin 2* (*ARRB2*) gene exhibit prolonged analgesia with morphine lower doses and variants have been associated with overall response to opioid switching (Branford, Droney, & Ross, 2012).

2.3.2 Pharmacokinetics

Some genes are implicated in cellular transport and metabolism of the molecules, which aims to convert lipophilic compounds into more readily excreted hydrophilic products (mainly cytochrome CYP2D6, CYP3A4, and CYP2B6; and UGT2B7) (Table 2 and Fig. 1).

2.3.2.1 Opioid Metabolism

(a) Phase 1 opioid metabolism

Cytochrome P450 2D6 (*CYP2D6*) *gene*: *CYP2D6* is highly polymorphic and expression of different variants results in several phenotypes. The prevalence of variant alleles exhibits considerable interethnic differences in CYP distribution: as PM present in 2% in Asians, 6%–10% Caucasians, and >10% African or UM most frequent in the Middle East and North Africa (Rajman, Knapp, Morgan, & Masimirembwa, 2017).

Concomitant use of CYP inhibitors (e.g., paroxetine, fluoxetine, and bupropion) or inducers (e.g., carbamazepine, phenobarbital, and phenytoin) could counteract the clinical effect or trigger side effects of analgesics in the same manner as genetically determined differences in CYP2D6-mediated metabolism of many opioids (Table 2). Moreover, combination treatment with drugs that inhibit or induce P-glycoprotein (ABCB1), a blood–brain barrier efflux transporter, may alter the amount (dose) of opioids distributed to the brain. At the pharmacodynamic level, it is crucial to be aware of the potential risk of interaction causing serotonergic syndrome when combining opioids and antidepressants inhibiting serotonin reuptake (Solhaug & Molden, 2017).

Drug–Gene CYP Interactions: Many of the common medicines used in pain and adjuvant medications, such as antidepressants are metabolized through the CYP450 system and can significantly inhibit the activity and, therefore, influence the effect of opioids. Verbeurgt, Mamiya, and Oesterheld (2015) looked at a sample of 1143 patients, where the total number of medications prescribed ranged from 1 to 44, with a mean of 8.4 and a median of 7 medications with a drug

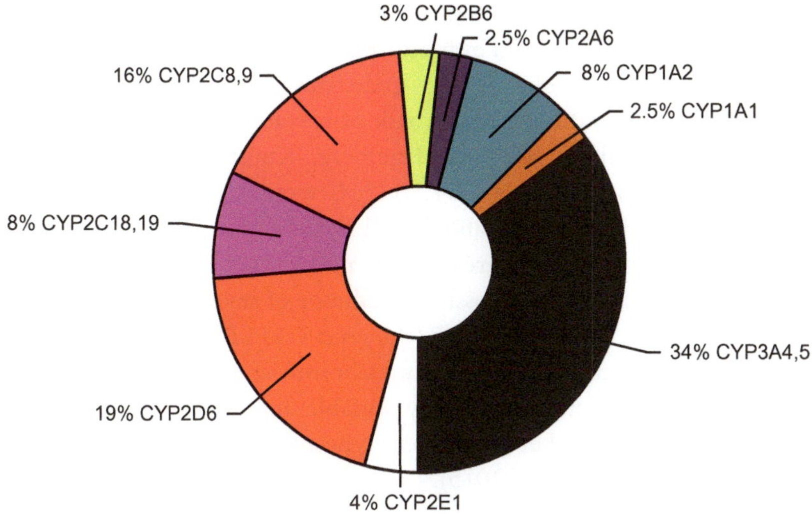

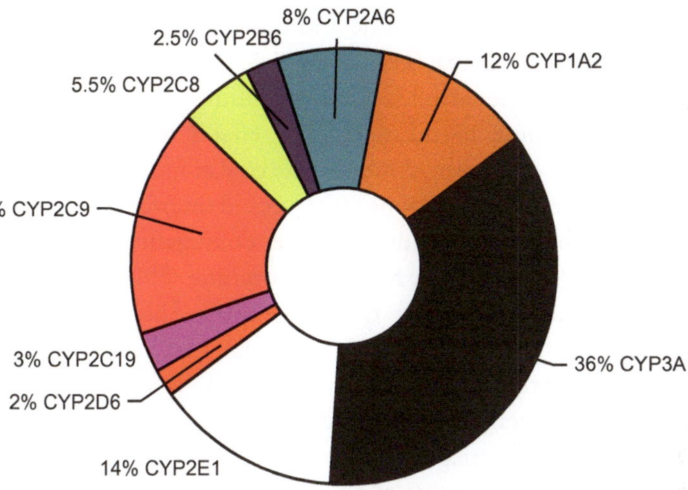

Fig. 1 Pharmacogenetics applied to the metabolism of drugs: proportion of drugs metabolized by cytochrome P450 and abundance in the liver. *Adapted from Rendic, S., & Di Carlo, F. J. (1997). Human cytochrome P450 enzymes: A status report summarizing their reactions, substrates, inducers, and inhibitors.* Drug Metabolism Reviews, *29(1–2), 413–580.*

interaction (–drug, –gene, or drug–gene) between 12% and 31% of the patients (Agarwal, Udoji, & Trescot, 2017).

Cytochrome P450 3A (CYP3A4) gene: The CYP3A4 enzyme is localized in the liver and small intestine and, thus, contributes to first-pass and systemic metabolism of opiates regulating the excretion of fentanyl, methadone, and buprenorphine. PM patients who are taking oral *CYP3A4* inhibitors (e.g., grapefruit juice, verapamil, diltiazem, clarithromycin) have higher risk of elevated blood levels and subsequent toxicity (Liukas, Hagelberg, Kuusniemi, Neuvonen, & Olkkola, 2011). Asian CYP3A4*1G women required lower doses of fentanyl after total abdominal hysterectomy or myomectomy. This effect could be greater if CYP3A5*1/*3 or CYP3A5*3/*3 is also presented as a possible predictor of severe fentanyl toxicity. *Cytochrome P450 2B6* (*CYP2B6*) *gene*: *CYP2B6* gene is a major isoform implied in methadone metabolism and clearance. However, although its activity is highly variable among individuals, and no clear correlation between a genotype and a phenotype has yet been established (Li et al., 2015).

(b) Phase 2 metabolism

UGT2B7 gene: UGT2B7 insures the glucuronidation of morphine to morphine-6-glucuronide and morphine-3-glucuronide metabolites (Campa, Gioia, Tomei, Poli, & Barale, 2008). Even though, morphine-3-glucuronide has little affinity for opioid receptors, it may contribute to the excitatory effects of morphine (Trescot, Datta, Lee, & Hansen, 2008). In the case of morphine, some variants of UGT2B7 (homozygous 802T) could interfere in the production of their metabolites, induce a lower conjugation (−840G) but that can be 10 times higher for buprenorphine (802T, rs7439366) (Jin, Gock, Jannetto, Jentzen, & Wong, 2005; Zhang et al., 2011).

Multidrug resistance gene: P-glycoprotein 1 also known as multidrug resistance protein 1 (MRP1 or ABCB1) is an important protein of the cell membrane involved in multidrug resistance. It is responsible for decreased drug accumulation in multidrug-resistant cells and also functions as a transporter in the blood–brain barrier (Hodges et al., 2011). It is associated with higher brain concentration of opioids (methadone, morphine), lower dose requirement (allele 3435C, rs1045642), variable risk of nausea/vomiting (alleles 2677A, rs2032582, 3435T), increased risk of miosis, respiratory depression with fentanyl (homozygotes 1236T, rs1128503, 2677T, rs2032582, and 3435T), and in children with toxicity after tonsillectomy (allele G, rs9282564) (Sadhasivam et al., 2015). Also, there has been noted to be an association between *ABCB1* and *OPRM1* gene polymorphisms related to morphine pain relief (Sia, Sng, Lim, Law, & Tan, 2010).

2.3.2.2 Modifying Systems Genes

(a) *Catechol-O-methyltransferase* (*COMT*): The involvement of catecholamines in pain modulation is known from both clinical and experimental studies. COMT is a key modulator of dopaminergic and adrenergic neurotransmission, and, as a consequence, in the reward signaling response to opioids. The C472G > A SNP (rs4680, Val158Met) causes a valine to methionine substitution at codon 158 of the enzyme. The Met allele leads to an enzyme that is up to four times less active than the Val allele (Niemi & Breivik, 2002). Research also indicates that *COMT* and *OPRM1* variants synergistically interact, affecting analgesia. Both genes have additional functional variants that may further shape analgesic effects. Thus, combined *COMT* Met/Met in Val158Met and *OPRM1* A/A in A118G polymorphisms required less morphine; however, differences were not significant (De Gregori et al., 2013; Matic et al., 2014). Moreover, *COMT* haplotypes are associated with great differences in enzymatic activity that may predict analgesia induced by beta blockers in patients with chronic musculoskeletal pain. Thus, variants may influence analgesia independently or in combination (Webster & Belfer, 2016).

(b) *Potassium channel*: This channel allows a greater flow of potassium into the cell than out of it. These proteins modulate physiological processes, including neuronal activity, through GPCR stimulation and it has been shown to participate in the modulation of analgesic on postsynaptic transmission and miosis under opioids (Rhodin et al., 2013). Several SNPs have been related to opioid response (postoperative analgesia, required dose) but negative findings have been published as well (Matic et al., 2017).

(c) *Serotonin transporter*: Preliminary work in pain research is now emerging, with published studies that examine genotypic influence *serotonin transporter* (*5HTT*) gene polymorphisms on opioid analgesia in healthy volunteers, in response to antidepressants (Jimenez & Galinkin, 2015) and also in the severity of depressive symptoms in adults with chronic pain (Hooten, Townsend, & Sletten, 2017). Future research is warranted in order to characterize these moderating effects.

2.3.3 Genetic Modulation of Nociception

It is well known that nociceptive mechanisms are complex. Tissue injury, for example, induces the release of large numbers of proinflammatory mediators, such as substance P, that activate receptors in the cell membrane of the primary afferent and permeabilize it for calcium and sodium. Other mediators, such as serotonin, the peptide related to the calcitonin (*CGRP*) gene, or histamine, are able to increase the activity of adenylate cyclase and thus increase intracellular cAMP which further depolarizes the neuronal membrane and activates a large population of voltage-dependent ionotropic channels that increase their excitability and painful sensation. In addition, pain intensity can vary depending on the nociceptive pathway, leading to its inhibition (OPRM1, transient receptor potential caption channel subfamily V member 1, guanosine triphosphate cyclohydrolase 1 (GCH1)) or its activation (fatty acid amide hydrolase, COMT; ADRB adrenergic receptor B2, B3).

In a subanalysis of the EPOS study conducted with 1579 patients who presented nausea and vomiting, the presence of three SNPs (rs4633T, rs4680G, rs165722C) was found to be a protective factor. A haplotype with 15 SNPs of the *GTP-cyclohydrolase* (*GCH1*) gene has also been configured where there is a phenotype of lower sensitivity to pain and some variants are associated with a later onset of the opioids treatment in oncological pain ($n=251$). In relation to dopamine receptors, variants in the *DRD2* gene have been associated with a need for higher opioids doses (1174-C allele) and a higher rate of nonresponders to methadone detoxification in Caucasians (1192-C allele) (Doehring et al., 2009).

2.4 Research, Ethics, and Legislation in Pharmacogenetics

The PGx would make possible to improve the classic therapeutic scheme based on the "trial–error" method by incorporating the genetic profile of the individual for choosing and optimizing the treatment. This point is relevant since obtaining samples for DNA has become a key component of clinical development. Its clinical implementation is an aspect of high social, ethical, and legal impact, forcing health authorities to take regulatory actions and being a field of research for programs of pharmacovigilance, pharmaceutical companies, research groups, and networks (http://who.int/genomics/elsi/en).

Regulatory authorities may require that PGx information accompany applications for new drug approvals and its incorporation into drug labeling (http://www.fda.gov/cder/genomics). In fact, the pharmacogenetics and pharmacogenomics knowledge base, (PharmGKB project, http://www.pharmgkb.org) describes a series of "very important pharmacogenes" that correspond to genes with a relevance associated with safety or therapeutic efficacy (Table 2).

Due to the bioethical and sensitive nature of the genetic information, PGx studies require an informed and express consent of the patient or legal representative, separate, and express declaration of anonymization of biological samples, right to the information derived from them, to which respect you will not to be informed, the custody of the genetic data and genetic counseling, among others. A significant number of guidelines and regulatory documents have been published, which are available at: http://www.i-pwg.org. The Universal Declaration on the Human Genome establishes its special protection has been published in line with current legislation (Organic Law 15/1999, Biomedical. Research Law, 2007; Declaration of Helsinki, 2013). All provides guidance as to how these tasks can be achieved.

3. CONCLUSION

Each person carries his or her own genetic imprint for the risk of more severe or more chronic pain, pain perception, and response to analgesics. Ideally, PGx studies aim to aid in the selection and dosing of an optimal drug therapy for a specific patient. However, patients are very commonly prescribed several medications for multiple comorbidities and genetics can only partially explain the variability in patient responses to analgesic drugs. Nowadays, the studies reviewed show that there is little evidence to determine the contribution of genetic factors to the variability in the patient's response to analgesic treatment. Probably because the response to drugs is a complex process involving a large number of proteins encoded by several genes, whose expression may also be the result of mechanisms independent of DNA (DNA methylation, histone modification in chromatin, or microRNAs).

For this, it is necessary to promote research, to train experts in the clinical application of these techniques, and to prescribing physicians, in the meaning and limitations of the PGx application. Also, it will be necessary to demonstrate that the findings in a specific population group can be extrapolated to others, defining the percentage of people who would benefit from the genetic test. All this without forgetting that PGx information should be just another element of judgment to try to predict the response to a drug in a patient with pain. Concerted efforts, open and active cooperation with industry, are required in order to facilitate translation and commercialization, avoiding to stuck PGx biomarkers in the discovery phase. Additionally, the knowledge and acceptance of new approaches to determine drug targets by clinicians, regulators, patients, and the public will be important in determining future success.

The future of PGx in pain management depends on a united group of professionals from governments, academia, private industry, and caregivers turning PGx information in standard of care for pain physicians (Table 2).

ACKNOWLEDGMENTS

We acknowledge the help received from Dr. María-del-Mar Inda (Alicante General Hospital Pain Research Coordinator), Dr. César Margarit (Alicante General Hospital Pain Unit chief), and Dr. Adrián LLerena (Director of the Clinical Research Center in the University Hospital Infanta Cristina en Badajoz Spain) for their help and support.

CONFLICT OF INTEREST

The authors have no conflicts of interest to declare.

REFERENCES

Agarwal, D., Udoji, M. A., & Trescot, A. (2017). Genetic testing for opioid pain management: A primer. *Pain and Therapy*, *6*, 93–105.

AL-Eitan, L. N., Jaradat, S. A., Su, S. Y., Tay, G. K., & Hulse, G. K. (2012). Mu opioid receptor (OPRM1) as a predictor of treatment outcome in opiate-dependent individuals of Arab descent. *Pharmacogenomics and Personalized Medicine*, *5*, 99.

Baroy, T., Misceo, D., & Frengen, E. (2008). Structural variation in the human genome contributes to variation of traits. *Tidsskrift for den Norske Lægeforening*, *128*(17), 1951–1955.

Bond, C., LaForge, K. S., Tian, M., Melia, D., Zhang, S., Borg, L., et al. (1998). Single-nucleotide polymorphism in the human mu opioid receptor gene alters beta-endorphin binding and activity: Possible implications for opiate addiction. *Proceedings of the National Academy of Sciences of the United States of America*, *95*, 9608–9613.

Branford, R., Droney, J., & Ross, J. R. (2012). Opioid genetics: The key to personalized pain control? *Clinical Genetics*, *82*, 301–310.

Brunton, L., Chabner, B., & Knollman, B. (2011). *Goodman and Gilman's the pharmacological basis of therapeutics* (12th ed.). New York: McGraw-Hill Education.

Campa, D., Gioia, A., Tomei, A., Poli, P., & Barale, R. (2008). Association of ABCB1/MDR1 and OPRM1 gene polymorphisms with morphine pain relief. *Clinical Pharmacology and Therapeutics*, *83*, 559–566.

Cazacu, I., Mogosan, C., & Loghin, F. (2015). Safety issues of current analgesics: An update. *Clujul Medical*, *88*, 128–136.

Chen, Y., Kuehl, G. E., Bigler, J., Rimorin, C. F., Schwarz, Y., Shen, D. D., et al. (2007). UGT1A6 polymorphismands alicylicacid glucuronidation following aspirin. *Pharmacogenetics and Genomics*, *17*, 571–579.

Chidambaran, V., Sadhasivam, S., & Mahmoud, M. (2017). Codeine and opioid metabolism: implications and alternatives for pediatric pain management. *Current Opinion in Anaesthesiology*, *30*, 349–356.

Chou, W. Y., Wang, C. H., Liu, P. H., Liu, C. C., Tseng, C. C., & Jawan, B. (2006). Human opioid receptor A118G polymorphism affects intravenous patient-controlled analgesia morphine consumption after total abdominal hysterectomy. *Anesthesiology*, *105*, 334–337.

Chou, W. Y., Yang, L. C., Lu, H. F., Ko, J. Y., Wang, C. H., Lin, S. H., et al. (2006). Association of mu-opioid receptor gene polymorphism (A118G) with variations in morphine consumption for analgesia after total. Knee arthroplasty. *Acta Anaesthesiologica Scandinavica, 50*, 787–792.

Crews, K. R., Gaedigk, A., Dunnenberger, H. M., Klein, T. E., Shen, D. D., Callaghan, J. T., et al. (2012). Clinical Pharmacogenetics Implementation Consortium (CPIC) guidelines for codeine therapy in the context of cytochrome P450 2D6 (CYP2D6) genotype. *Clinical Pharmacology and Therapeutics, 91*, 321–326.

Dalca, A. V., & Brudno, M. (2010). Genome variation discovery with high-throughput sequencing data. *Briefings in Bioinformatics, 11*(1), 3–14.

De Gregori, M., Allegri, M., De Gregori, S., Garbin, G., Tinelli, C., Regazzi, M., et al. (2001). How and why to screen for CYP2D6 interindividual variability in patients under pharmacological treatments. *Current Drug Metabolism, 11*, 276–282.

De Gregori, M., Garbin, G., De Gregori, S., Minella, C. E., Bugada, D., Lisa, A., et al. (2013). Genetic variability at COMT but not at OPRM1 and UGT2B7 loci modulates morphine analgesic response in acute postoperative pain. *European Journal of Clinical Pharmacology, 69*, 1651–1658.

Descalzi, G., Ikegami, D., Ushijima, T., Nestler, E. J., Zachariou, V., & Narita, M. (2015). Epigenetic mechanisms of chronic pain. *Trends in Neurosciences, 38*, 237–246.

Dietis, N., Rowbotham, D. J., & Lambert, D. G. (2011). Opioid receptor subtypes: Fact or artifact? *British Journal of Anaesthesia, 107*, 8–18.

Doehring, A., Hentig, N., Graff, J., Salamat, S., Schmidt, M., Geisslinger, G., et al. (2009). Genetic variants altering dopamine D2 receptor expression or function modulate the risk of opiate addiction and the dose requirements of methadone substitution. *Pharmacogenetics and Genomics, 19*, 407–414.

Ehmann, F., Caneva, L., Prasad, K., Ehmann, F., Caneva, L., Prasad, K., et al. (2015). Pharmacogenomic information in drug labels: European medicines agency perspective. *The Pharmacogenomics Journal, 15*, 201–210.

Enthoven, W. T., Roelofs, P. D., Deyo, R. A., van Tulder, M. W., & Koes, B. W. (2016). Non-steroidal anti-inflammatory drugs for chronic low back pain. *The Cochrane Database of Systematic Review, 2*, CD012087.

Fine, M. (2013). Quantifying the impact of NSAID-associated adverse events. *The American Journal of Managed Care, 19*, s267–s272.

Friedman, C., Wong, A., & Blumenthal, K. (2010). Achieving a nationwide learning health system. *Science Translational Medicine, 2*, 57.

Furlan, A. D., Reardon, R., Weppler, C., & National Opioid Use Guideline G (2010). Opioids for chronic noncancer pain: A new Canadian practice guideline. *Canadian Medical Association Journal, 182*, 923–930.

Hajj, A., Khabbaz, L., Laplanche, J. L., & Peoc'h, K. (2013). Pharmacogenetics of opiates in clinical practice: The visible tip of the iceberg. *Pharmacogenomics, 14*, 575–585.

Hardt, J., Jacobsen, C., Goldberg, J., Nickel, R., & Buchwald, D. (2008). Prevalence of chronic pain in a representative sample in the United States. *Pain Medicine, 9*, 803–812.

Hastie, B. A., Riley, J. L., 3rd, Kaplan, L., Herrera, D. G., Campbell, C. M., Virtusio, K., et al. (2012). Ethnicity interacts with the OPRM1 gene in experimental pain sensitivity. *Pain, 153*(8), 1610–1619.

Hodges, L. M., Markova, S. M., Chinn, L. W., Gow, J. M., Kroetz, D. L., Klein, T. E., et al. (2011). Very important pharmacogene summary: ABCB1 (MDR1, P-glycoprotein). *Pharmacogenetics and Genomics, 21*(3), 152.

Hoffman, J. M., Dunnenberger, H. M., Hicks, J., Caudle, K. E., Carrillo, M., Freimuth, R. R., et al. (2016). Developing knowledge resources to support precision medicine: Principles from the Clinical Pharmacogenetics Implementation Consortium (CPIC). *Journal of the American Medical Informatics Association, 23*, 796–801.

Hooten, W. M., Townsend, C. O., & Sletten, C. D. (2017). The triallelic serotonin transporter gene polymorphism is associated with depressive symptoms in adults with chronic pain. *Journal of Pain Research*, *10*, 1071.

Jimenez, N., & Galinkin, J. L. (2015). Personalizing pediatric pain medicine: Using population-specific pharmacogenetics, genomics, and other -omics approaches to predict response. *Anesthesia and Analgesia*, *121*, 183–187.

Jin, M., Gock, S. B., Jannetto, P. J., Jentzen, J. M., & Wong, S. H. (2005). Pharmacogenomics as molecular autopsy for forensic toxicology: Genotyping cytochrome P450 3A4*1B and 3A5*3 for 25 fentanyl cases. *Journal of Analytical Toxicology*, *29*, 590–598.

Kadiev, E., Patel, V., Rad, P., Thankachan, L., Tram, A., Weinlein, M., et al. (2008). Role of pharmacogenetics in variable response to drugs: Focus on opioids. *Expert Opinion on Drug Metabolism & Toxicology*, *4*, 77–91.

Kieffer, B. L., & Gaveriaux-Ruff, C. (2002). Exploring the opioid system by gene knockout. *Progress in Neurobiology*, *66*, 285–306.

Kim, E., Choi, C. B., Kang, C., & Bae, S. C. (2010). Adverse events in analgesic treatment with tramadol associated with CYP2D6 extensive-metaboliser and OPRM1 high-expression variants. *Annals of the Rheumatic Diseases*, *69*, 1889–1890.

Kim, S., & Kaang, B. K. (2017). Epigenetic regulation and chromatin remodeling in learning and memory. *Experimental & Molecular Medicine*, *49*, e281.

Kirchheiner, J., Schmidt, H., Tzvetkov, M., Keulen, J. T., Lotsch, J., Roots, I., et al. (2007). Pharmacokinetics of codeine and its metabolite morphine in ultra-rapid metabolizers due to CYP2D6 duplication. *The Pharmacogenomics Journal*, 7(4), 257–265.

Klepstad, P., Fladvad, T., Skorpen, F., Bjordal, K., Caraceni, A., Dale, O., et al. (2011). Influence from genetic variability on opioid use for cancer pain: A European genetic association study of 2294 cancer pain patients. *Pain*, *152*, 1139–1145.

Kreek, M. J., Bart, G., Lilly, C., LaForge, K. S., & Nielsen, D. A. (2005). Pharmacogenetics and human molecular genetics of opiate and cocaine addictions and their treatments. *Pharmacological Reviews*, *57*, 1–26.

Lancaster, T. M., Linden, D. E., & Heerey, E. A. (2012). COMT val158met predicts reward responsiveness in humans. *Genes, Brain, and Behavior*, *11*, 986–992.

Langley, P. (2011). The prevalence, correlates and treatment of pain in the European Union. *Current Medical Research and Opinion*, *27*, 463–480.

Li, Y., Jackson, K. A., Slon, B., Hardy, J. R., Franco, M., William, L., et al. (2015). CYP2B6*6 allele and age substantially reduce steady-state ketamine clearance in chronic pain patients: Impact on adverse effects. *British Journal of Clinical Pharmacology*, *80*(2), 276–284.

Liukas, A., Hagelberg, N. M., Kuusniemi, K., Neuvonen, P. J., & Olkkola, K. T. (2011). Inhibition of cytochrome P450 3A by clarithromycin uniformly affects the pharmacokinetics and pharmacodynamics of oxycodone in young and elderly volunteers. *Journal of Clinical Psychopharmacology*, *31*, 302–308.

Manolio, T. A., Collins, F. S., Cox, N. J., Goldstein, D. B., Hindorff, L. A., Hunter, D. J., et al. (2009). Finding the missing heritability of complex diseases. *Nature*, *461*, 747–753.

Martínez, C., García-Martín, E., Blanco, G., Gamito, F., Ladero, J. M., & Agúndez, A. G. (2005). The effect of the cytochrome P450 CYP2C8 polymorphism on the disposition of (R)-ibuprofen enantiomer in healthy subjects. *British Journal of Clinical Pharmacology*, *59*, 62–68.

Matic, M., de Wildt, S. N., Tibboel, D., & van Schaik, R. H. N. (2017). Analgesia and opioids: A pharmacogenetics shortlist for implementation in clinical practice. *Clinical Chemistry*, *63*, 1204–1213.

Matic, M., Simons, S. H., van Lingen, R. A., van Rosmalen, J., Elens, L., de Wildt, S. N., et al. (2014). Rescue morphine in mechanically ventilated newborns associated with combined OPRM1 and COMT genotype. *Pharmacogenomics*, *15*, 1287–1295.

Mistry, C. J., Bawor, M., Desai, D., Marsh, D. C., & Samaan, Z. (2014). Genetics of opioid dependence: A review of the genetic contribution to opioid dependence. *Current Psychiatry Reviews*, *10*(2), 156–167.

Mullaney, J. M., Mills, R. E., Pittard, W. S., & Devine, S. E. (2010). Small insertions and deletions (INDELs) in human genomes. *Human Molecular Genetics*, *19*(R2), R131–136.

Nakamura, Y. (2009). DNA variations in human and medical genetics: 25 years of my experience. *Journal of Human Genetics*, *54*(1), 1–8.

Ng, P. C., & Henikoff, S. (2006). Predicting the effects of amino acid substitutions on protein function. *Annual Review of Genomics and Human Genetics*, 7, 61–80.

Niemi, G., & Breivik, H. (2002). Epinephrine markedly improves thoracic epidural analgesia produced by a small-dose infusion of ropivacaine, fentanyl, and epinephrine after major thoracic or abdominal surgery: A randomized, double-blinded crossover study with and without epinephrine. *Anesthesia and Analgesia*, *94*, 1598–1605.

Paar, W. D., Poche, S., Gerloff, J., & Dengler, H. J. (1997). Polymorphic CYP2D6 mediates O-demethylation of the opioid analgesic tramadol. *European Journal of Clinical Pharmacology*, *53*(3–4), 235–239.

Peiró, A. M., Planelles, B., Juhasz, G., Bagdy, G., Libert, F., Eschalier, A., et al. (2016). Pharmacogenomics in pain treatment. *Drug Metabolism and Personalized Therapy*, *31*, 131–142.

Pérez, C., Margarit, C., Serrano, M., & Spanish group of Change Pain patient survey. (2013). Survey of European patients assessing their own noncancer chronic pain: Results from Spain. *Current Medical Research and Opinion*, *29*, 643–651.

Peters, M. J., Broer, L., Willemen, H. L., Eiriksdottir, G., Hocking, L. J., Holliday, K. L., et al. (2013). Genome-wide association study meta-analysis of chronic widespread pain: Evidence for involvement of the 5p15.2 region. *Annals of the Rheumatic Diseases*, *72*, 427–436.

Pirmohamed, M. (2014). Personalized pharmacogenomics: Predicting efficacy and adverse drug reactions. *Annual Review of Genomics and Human Genetics*, *15*, 349–370.

Racoosin, J. A., Roberson, D. W., Pacanowski, M. A., & Nielsen, D. R. (2013). New evidence about an old drug—Risk with codeine after adenotonsillectomy. *The New England Journal of Medicine*, *368*, 2155–2157.

Rajman, I., Knapp, L., Morgan, T., & Masimirembwa, C. (2017). African genetic diversity: Implications for cytochrome P450-mediated drug metabolism and drug development. *eBioMedicine*, *17*, 67–74.

Rhodin, A., Gronbladh, A., Ginya, H., Nilsson, K. W., Rosenblad, A., Zhou, Q., et al. (2013). Combined analysis of circulating beta-endorphin with gene polymorphisms in OPRM1, CACNAD2 and ABCB1 reveals correlation with pain, opioid sensitivity and opioid-related side effects. *Molecular Brain*, *12*, 8.

Riviere, P. J. (2004). Peripheral kappa-opioid agonists for visceral pain. *British Journal of Pharmacology*, *141*, 1331–1334.

Rodrigues, N., Bennis, K., Vivier, D., Pereira, V., Chatelain, F. C., Chapuy, E., et al. (2014). Synthesis and structure–activity relationship study of substituted caffeate esters as antinociceptive agentsmodulating the TREK-1 channel. *European Journal of Medicinal Chemistry*, *75*, 391–402.

Romberg, R. R., Olofsen, E., Bijl, H., Taschner, P. E., Teppema, L. J., Sarton, E. Y., et al. (2005). Polymorphism of mu-opioid receptor gene (OPRM1:c.118A > G) does not protect against opioid-induced respiratory depression despite reduced analgesic response. *Anesthesiology*, *102*, 522–530.

Sadhasivam, S., Chidambaran, V., Zhang, X., Meller, J., Esslinger, H., Zhang, K., et al. (2015). Opioid-induced respiratory depression: ABCB1 transporter pharmacogenetics. *The Pharmacogenomics Journal*, *15*, 119–126.

Shabalina, S. A., Zaykin, D. V., Gris, P., Ogurtsov, A. Y., Gauthier, J., Shibata, K., et al. (2009). Expansion of the human mu-opioid receptor gene architecture: Novel functional variants. *Human Molecular Genetics*, *18*, 1037–1051.

Sia, A. T., Sng, B. L., Lim, E. C., Law, H., & Tan, E. C. (2010). The influence of ATP-binding cassette sub-family B member-1 (ABCB1) genetic polymorphisms on acute and chronic pain after intrathecal morphine for caesarean section: A prospective cohort study. *International Journal of Obstetric Anesthesia*, *19*, 254–260.

Skarke, C., Darimont, J., Schmidt, H., Geisslinger, G., & Lotsch, J. (2003). Analgesic effects of morphine and morphine-6-glucuronide in a transcutaneous electrical pain model in healthy volunteers. *Clinical Pharmacology and Therapeutics*, *73*, 107–121.

Solhaug, V., & Molden, E. (2017). Individual variability in clinical effect and tolerability of opioid analgesics—Importance of drug interactions and pharmacogenetics. *Scandinavian Journal of Pain*, *17*, 193–200.

Stamer, U. M., Zhang, L., & Stuber, F. (2010). Personalized therapy in pain management: Where do we stand? *Pharmacogenomics*, *11*, 843–864.

Světlík, S., Hronová, K., Bakhouche, H., Matoušková, O., & Slanař, O. (2013). Pharmacogenetics of chronic pain and its treatment. *Mediators of Inflammation*, *2013*, 864319.

Tracy, T. S., Hutzler, J. M., Haining, R. L., Rettie, A. E., Hummel, M. A., & Dickmann, L. J. (2002). Polymorphic variants (CYP2C9*3 and CYP2C9*5) and the F114L active site mutation of CYP2C9: Effect on atypical kinetic metabolism profiles. *Drug Metabolism and Disposition*, *30*, 385–390.

Trescot, A. M., Datta, S., Lee, M., & Hansen, H. (2008). Opioid pharmacology. *Pain Physician*, *11*, S133–53.

Ueda, H., & Uchida, H. (2015). Epigenetic modification in neuropathic pain. *Current Pharmaceutical Design*, *21*, 849–867.

Vanderah, T. W. (2010). Delta and kappa opioid receptors as suitable drug targets for pain. *The Clinical Journal of Pain*, *26*, S10–15.

Verbeurgt, P., Mamiya, T., & Oesterheld, J. (2015). How common are drug and gene interactions? Prevalence in a sample of 1143 patients with CYP2C9, CYP2C19 and CYP2D6 genotyping. *Pharmacogenomics*, *15*, 655–665.

Vuilleumier, P. H., Stamer, U. M., & Landau, R. (2012). Pharmacogenomic considerations in opioid analgesia. *Pharmgenomics and Perssonalized Medicine*, *5*, 73–87.

Webster, L. R., & Belfer, I. (2016). Pharmacogenetics and personalized medicine in pain management. *Clinics in Laboratory Medicine*, *36*, 493–506.

Wyatt, J. E., Pettit, W. L., & Harirforoosh, S. (2012). Pharmacogenetics of nonsteroidal anti-inflammatory drugs. *The Pharmacogenomics Journal*, *12*, 462–467.

Zhang, Y., Wang, D., Johnson, A. D., Papp, A. C., & Sadee, W. (2005). Allelic expression imbalance of human mu opioid receptor (OPRM1) caused by variant A118G. *The Journal of Biological Chemistry*, *280*, 32618–32624.

Zhang, Y., Xiong, W., Lin, X., Ma, X., & Yu, L. C. (2009). Receptor trafficking induced by mu-opioid-receptor phosphorylation. *Neuroscience and Biobehavioral Reviews*, *33*, 1192–1197.

Zhang, W., Yuan, J. J., Kan, Q. C., Zhang, L. R., Chang, Y. Z., Wang, Z. Y., et al. (2011). Influence of CYP3A5*3 polymorphism and interaction between CYP3A5*3 and CYP3A4*1G polymorphisms on post-operative fentanyl analgesia in Chinese patients undergoing gynaecological surgery. *European Journal of Anaesthesiology*, *28*, 245–250.

FURTHER READING

Barriere, D. A., Mallet, C., Blomgren, A., Simonsen, C., Daulhac, L., Libert, F., et al. (2013). Fatty acid amide hydrolase-dependent generation of antinociceptive drug metabolites acting on TRPV1 in the brain. *PLoS One*, *8*, e70690.

Dalmann, R., Daulhac, L., Antri, M., Eschalier, A., & Mallet, C. (2015). Supraspinal. FAAH is required for the analgesic action of paracetamol in an inflammatory context. *Neuropharmacology*, *91*, 63–70.

Desmond-Hellmann, S. (2012). Toward precision medicine: A new social. Contract? *Science Translational Medicine*, *4*, 129ed3.

Fillingim, R. B., Kaplan, L., Staud, R., Ness, T. J., Glover, T. L., Campbell, C. M., et al. (2005). The A118G single nucleotide polymorphism of the muopioid receptor gene (OPRM1) is associated with pressure pain sensitivity in humans. *The Journal of Pain*, *6*, 159–167.

Kerckhove, N., Mallet, C., Francois, A., Boudes, M., Chemin, J., Voets, T., et al. (2014). Ca(v)3.2 calcium channels: The key protagonist in the supraspinal effect of paracetamol. *Pain*, *155*, 764–772.

Lotsch, J., Pruss, H., Veh, R. W., & Doehring, A. (2010). A KCNJ6 (Kir3.2, GIRK2) gene polymorphism modulates opioid effects on analgesia and addiction but not on pupil size. *Pharmacogenetics and Genomics*, *20*, 291–297.

Mallet, C., Daulhac, L., Bonnefont, J., Ledent, C., Etienne, M., Chapuy, E., et al. (2008). Endocannabinoid and serotonergic systems are needed for acetaminophen-induced analgesia. *Pain*, *139*, 190–200.

Peiró, A. M., Margarit, C., Gimenez, P., & Horga, J. F. (2010). Pharmacogenetic testing is of limited utility for predicting analgesic response to morphine. *Journal of Pain and Symptom Management*, *39*, e8–e11.

Peters, M. J., Broer, L., Willemen, H. L., Eiriksdottir, G., Hocking, L. J., Manolio, T. A., et al. (2009). Finding the missing heritability of complex diseases. *Nature*, *461*, 747–753.

Pickering, G., Esteve, V., Loriot, M. A., Eschalier, A., & Dubray, C. (2008). Acetaminophen reinforces descending inhibitory pain pathways. *Clinical Pharmacology and Therapeutics*, *84*, 47–51.

Yoon, J. H., Abdelmohsen, K., & Gorospe, M. (2014). Functional interactions among microRNAs and long noncoding RNAs. *Seminars in Cell & Developmental Biology*, *34*, 9–14.

CHAPTER ELEVEN

The Pharmacogenetics of Immune-Modulating Therapy

Ingolf Cascorbi[1]

Institute of Experimental and Clinical Pharmacology, University Hospital Schleswig-Holstein, Kiel, Germany

[1]Corresponding author: e-mail address: cascorbi@pharmakologie.uni-kiel.de

Contents

1. Introduction 276
2. Azathioprine/Mercaptopurine 277
3. Methotrexate 280
4. Mycophenolate 281
5. Calcineurin Inhibitors 283
   5.1 Cyclosporine A 283
   5.2 Tacrolimus 286
   5.3 Pharmacogenetics Affecting the Pharmacodynamics of Calcineurin Inhibitors 287
6. Sirolimus 288
7. Conclusion 288
References 291

Abstract

Immunosuppressive drugs are a prerequisite in organ transplantation to prevent rejection and are also widely used in inflammatory diseases such as inflammatory bowel disease (IBD) or also in some hematologic malignancies—depending on the mode of action. For thiopurine analogs the polymorphic thiopurine *S*-methyltransferase (TPMT) was early detected to be associated with thiopurine-induced leukopenia; recent studies identified also NUDT15 to be related to this severe side effect. For drugs like methotrexate and mycophenolate mofetil a number of ADME genes like UDP-glucuronosyltransferases (UGTs) and ABC efflux transporters were investigated, however, with partly contradicting results. For calcineurin inhibitors like cyclosporine and in particular tacrolimus however, cytochrome P450 3A4 and 3A5 variants were found to significantly affect the pharmacokinetics. Genetic variants in genes encoding relevant pharmacodynamic proteins, however, lacked compelling evidence to affect the clinical outcome.

This chapter reviews the current evidence on the association of pharmacogenetic traits to dose finding and clinical outcome of small-molecule immunosuppressants.

Advances in Pharmacology, Volume 83
ISSN 1054-3589
https://doi.org/10.1016/bs.apha.2018.02.004

Moreover this chapter critically summarizes suitability to apply pharmacogenetics in clinical practice in order to optimize immunosuppressant therapy.

ABBREVIATIONS

ABCB1 ATP-binding cassette transporter B1, P-glycoprotein, P-gp
ABCC2 ATP-binding cassette transporter C2, multidrug resistance-related protein 2, MRP2
ABCG2 ATP-binding cassette transporter G2, breast cancer-related protein, BCRP
ADME absorption, distribution, metabolism, excretion
CYP3A4 cytochrome P450 3A4
CYP3A5 cytochrome P450 3A5
IBD inflammatory bowel disease
IMPDH inosine-5′-monophosphate dehydrogenase
MMF mycophenolate mofetil
MPA mycophenolic acid
mTOR mammalian target of rapamycin
MTX methotrexate
NUDT15 nucleoside diphosphate-linked moiety X-type motif 15
PK pharmacokinetic
POR cytochrome P450 oxidoreductase
PPARA peroxisome proliferator-activated receptor alpha
PXR pregnane X receptor
SLCO1B1 solute carrier organic anion transporter family member 1B1, organic anion transporter, OATP1B1
SNP single-nucleotide polymorphism
TPMT thiopurine *S*-methyltransferase
UGT1A9 UGT-glucuronosyltransferase 1A9

1. INTRODUCTION

The introduction of immune-modulating drugs led to a tremendous success in the prevention of transplant rejection but also in the treatment of inflammatory and autoimmune diseases. The invention of orally available small molecules like thiopurine analogs was the first successful approach to treat inflammatory bowel disease (IBD) but also acute lymphatic leukemia (Elion, 1989). Later on, the calcineurin inhibitors cyclosporine and tacrolimus or mTOR inhibitors such as sirolimus allowed stable suppression of the immune systems without completely compromising antibacterial or antiviral defense. Such drugs are most often used in combination with antiproliferative drugs such as mycophenolate and glucocorticoids. However, the need of sufficient plasma concentrations to avoid transplant rejection on the one side and prevention from toxic concentration leading, e.g., to kidney toxicity or infection risk on the other side is an ongoing problem (van Gelder, van Schaik, & Hesselink, 2014).

Many immunosuppressants provide varying intra- and inter-bioavailability, impeding proper dose finding and making frequent plasma concentration determinations mandatory. Since most of the nonbiological immunosuppressants are substrates of membrane transporters and drug-metabolizing enzymes, many studies aimed to investigate whether hereditary variants in ADME genes may contribute to the observation of varying pharmacokinetics, whether such traits are suitable to predict proper dosing, to avoid adverse drug events, and finally whether pharmacogenetics should be applied to improve the clinical outcome, e.g., with respect to prevention of transplant rejection.

This review gives an overview on the impact of genetic variants on pharmacokinetics of small-molecule immunosuppressants and whether pharmacogenetics is a suitable tool to predict toxic effects and transplant rejection.

2. AZATHIOPRINE/MERCAPTOPURINE

Azathioprine is a purine analog approved as immunosuppressant in the treatment of IBDs or transplant medicine. Its direct metabolite mercaptopurine is also used to treat acute lymphatic leukemia. The compounds are metabolized through hypoxanthine phosphoribosyltransferase to 6-thioguanosines (6-TGNs), acting as antimetabolites, but the majority is detoxified to inactive metabolites by thiopurine *S*-methyltransferase (TPMT) and to a minor extent by xanthine oxidase (XO) (Fig. 1A). There is a close relationship between TPMT activity and occurrence of rare but serious side effects (Weinshilboum, 1992). Among enzyme-deficient patients, the alternative pathway via hypoxanthine phosphoribosyltransferase is accelerated, leading to high amounts of 6-TGN which in turn may cause myelosuppression or even pancytopenia. In Caucasian IBD patients the frequency of patients suffering from a thiopurine-associated leukopenia is estimated to be 5% (Fraser, Orchard, & Jewell, 2002). The severity of hematologic side effects correlates directly with 6-TGN plasma concentrations, whereas intestinal adverse events occurred independently (Schwab et al., 2002).

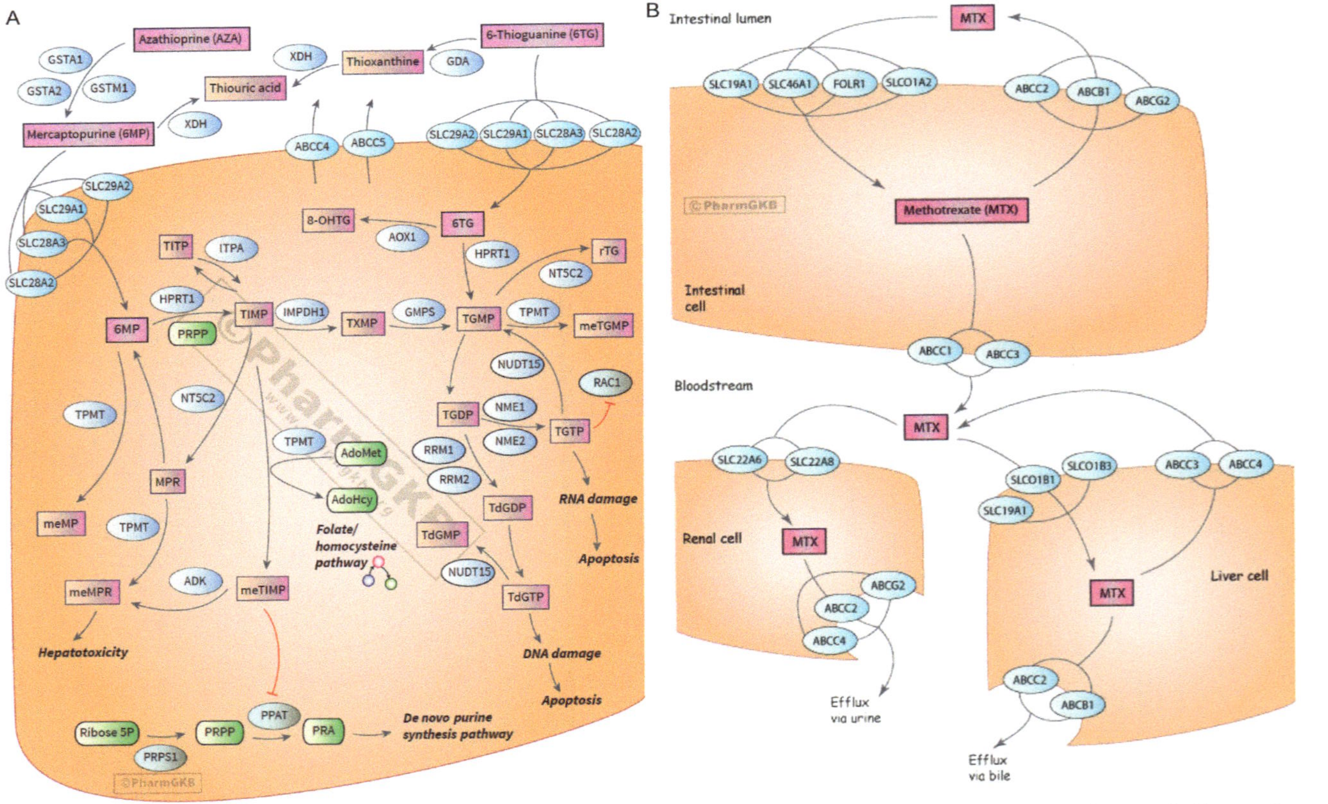

Fig. 1 (A) Diagrammatic representation of a nontissue-specific cancer cell displaying candidate genes involved in the metabolism and action of thiopurines. TPMT and NUDT15 are highly significant susceptibility factors of thiopurine-induced leukopenia (Zaza et al., 2010). (B) Methotrexate cellular disposition and effects (Mikkelsen et al., 2011). *Panel (A): From https://www.pharmgkb.org/pathway/PA2040. Panel (B): From https://www.pharmgkb.org/pathway/PA165816349. Permission has been given by PharmGKB and Stanford University.*

The activity of TPMT has a trimodal distribution with 89.5% normal to high methylators, 9.9% intermediates, and 0.6% deficient methylators (Schaeffeler et al., 2004). The TPMT activity can be easily determined by ex vivo phenotyping procedures, but just three genetic variants in the TMPT gene (rs12201199, rs1142345, and rs1800460) account for more than 90% of inactivating alleles (Relling et al., 2011). Moreover consideration of rare genetic variations applying modern technologies allows a reliable prediction of TMPT status by means of genotyping, as the genetically driven TPMT activity is exclusively dependent on variants in the TPMT gene (Liu et al., 2017). Aside from genetic causes however, TPMT activity can also be diminished by the concomitant use of allopurinol which inhibits thiopurine excretion. Hence, allopurinol should be avoided in azathioprine/mercaptopurine-treated patients, or the dose of the immunosuppressant should be reduced to avoid subsequent elevated thiopurine levels (Teml, Schaeffeler, Herrlinger, Klotz, & Schwab, 2007).

Despite safety concerns, also some cost–benefit analyses recommended assessment of TPMT activity prior to thiopurine therapy in IBD patients; however, more recent economic evaluations gave only inconclusive evidence (Plumpton, Roberts, Pirmohamed, & Hughes, 2016). One of the reasons may be the fact that only about a quarter of IBD patients who develop thiopurine-associated leukopenia are carriers of TPMT genetic variants. Moreover, the above mentioned TPMT frequencies and dosing recommendations are based on investigation mainly in Caucasian populations. In Asians, TPMT variants are even rarer than in Caucasians (3% vs 10%), but leukopenia occurs more often (Kim et al., 2010). An immunochip-based study in Korean IBD patients identified a nonsynonymous variant p.Arg139Cys in the NUDT15 (nucleoside diphosphate-linked moiety X-type motif 15) gene to be significantly associated to the risk of thiopurine-related leukopenia (odds ratio $=35.6$; $P=4.88\times 10^{-94}$) (Yang et al., 2014). It catalyzes the hydrolysis of nucleoside diphosphates and can induce base mispairing during DNA replication, causing transversions. The association with NUDT15 could be confirmed in subsequent studies in Japanese (Kakuta et al., 2016) and Chinese (Chao et al., 2017) IBD patients. The role of NUDT15 in thiopurine-induced leukopenia was in particular confirmed also in children with ALL (Moriyama et al., 2017; Yang et al., 2015). Hence aside TPMT, at least NUDT15 must be considered as an additional susceptibility factor for leukopenia risk (Moriyama et al., 2016).

So far, there are guidelines to consider TMPT variants in routine therapy. A dose reduction to 10% of standard dose is recommended for homozygote TPMT-poor metabolizers, and the frequency of application should be reduced to thrice a week instead of daily. Also in heterozygous carriers a dose reduction to 30%–70% of the starting dose is recommended; for details, see Relling et al. (2011, 2013).

Finally, also drug–drug interactions bear the risk of elevated thiopurine toxicity. Allopurinol, used in the treatment of throat, inhibits XO, one of the pathways of detoxification of mercaptopurine (Fig. 1). Hence, in case of allopurinol prescription, it is recommended to reduce the thiopurine dose by 75% in order to avoid elevated toxicity.

3. METHOTREXATE

Methotrexate (MTX) is a folic acid analog that inhibits the dihydrofolate reductase. At lower concentrations this leads to inhibition of thymidylate synthase and at higher concentration to inhibition of purine synthesis. In addition, MTX causes an increase of intracellular of deoxyadenosine triphosphate thereby inhibiting polynucleotide ligase, an enzyme involved in DNA synthesis and repair. As a consequence proliferation in particular of lymphocytes and subsequent release of cytokines are reduced. MTX is a basic immunosuppressive medication in the treatment of rheumatoid arthritis but also used within complex treatments of acute lymphatic leukemia, non-Hodgkin lymphoma, malignant trophoblast tumors, and other malignancies.

MTX causes a number of partly severe side effects. Starting with nausea and vomiting, dermatitis, stomatitis, liver injuries, and increased infection risk may occur. Most endangering is the risk of myelosuppression which may have a fatal course. Hence, depending on the dose regimen daily or weekly blood cell count is obligatory. Since MTX is mainly renally excreted, kidney function has to be considered. A creatinine clearance of less than 60 mL/min is a contraindication of MTX administration.

The renal excretion is mediated glomerularly and via secretion. One of the main contributing efflux transporters is ABCC2 (MRP2). MTX is both a substrate and an inhibitor of ABCC2; this explains to some extent the observed time-dependent pharmacokinetic through functional modification of MRP2 over time, thereby modifying its own elimination rate (Woillard et al., 2017) (Fig. 1B). Moreover, ABCC2 is a gene consisting of clinically relevant polymorphisms that have been shown to be associated with reduced protein function and expression (Cascorbi & Haenisch, 2010). Most extensively studied SNPs are the 5′-UTR c.−24C>T (rs717620), the exon 11 variant c.1249G > A (p.V417I) (rs2273697), and a nonsynonymous exon 28 variant c.3972C > T (rs3740066). ABCC2 −24C > T is associated with decreased mRNA expression in vitro (Laechelt et al., 2011) and in vivo (Haenisch et al., 2007).

In 2006 Rau et al. reported a significant impact of ABCC2 −24C > T on MTX plasma concentrations at high-dose therapies in German children suffering from ALL (Rau et al., 2006), and a study from Lebanon in children with ALL confirmed an impact on dose requirement (Zgheib et al., 2014). Another recently performed study in Hungarian children with osteosarcoma found −24C > T to be associated with MTX-related hepato- and myelotoxicity (Hegyi et al., 2017). Interestingly, the same study did not observe any impact of this ABCC2 variant on the PK, but variants in other transporters such as ABCB1 and ABCC3 as well as in the pregnane X receptor gene NR1I2 and the gamma-glutamyl-hydrolase GGH. PXR is a nuclear receptor known to be involved in the induction of ABC transporters, and GGH hydrolyzes polyglutamated MTX derivatives to facilitate elimination (Galivan et al., 2000). Toxicity was also mediated by ABCC1. Many other SNPs in candidate genes were investigated in further studies; however, the study size was often too small to make any further conclusions. Concluding there are some associations, but pharmacogenetics does not seem to be suitable to predict MTX-related side effects with enough confidence. In any case regular blood cell count as major monitoring parameter remains obligatory.

4. MYCOPHENOLATE

Mycophenolic acid (MPA), administered as ester such as mycophenolate mofetil (MMF) or as sodium salt, is a selective, noncompetitive, and reversible inhibitor of inosine monophosphate dehydrogenase. As a consequence the drug exerts immunosuppressive properties, since de novo synthesis of guanosine nucleotides which is essential in particular in T and B lymphocytes is inhibited. Due to its much better safety profile, MPA derivatives have almost replaced azathioprine in solid organ transplantation.

MMF is rapidly absorbed in the intestine and undergoes a complete presystemic metabolization to the active metabolite MPA. The immunosuppressive efficacy correlates with the MPA plasma concentration. Only neglectable amounts of MPA (less than 1%) can be found in the urine. The vast majority is excreted renally as MPA glucuronide via organic anion transporters OATP and ATP efflux transporters such as ABCC2 (MRP2) and ABCG2 (BCRP). MPA glucuronide is not pharmacologically active. ABCB1 (P-glycoprotein, MDR1) is involved in the intestinal transport of MPA, but only to a minor extent. Since there is a broad interindividual but also some intraindividual variability in the bioavailability of MPA, there was a major interest in the role of genetic variants on the genes of the above mentioned conjugating enzymes and transporters.

First of all, the conjugation of MPA with glucuronic acid via UGT1A9 is crucial to enable excretion via the above mentioned transporters. The −2152C>T (rs17868320) and −275T>A (rs6714486) variants in the UGT1A9 promoter region are associated with significantly reduced MPA plasma levels at early kidney transplant stages (Kuypers, Naesens, Vermeire, & Vanrenterghem, 2005; van Schaik et al., 2009) due to elevated expression of this phase II enzyme (Girard et al., 2004). Other variants in UGT1A9 and in UGT2B7 were shown to have an impact in Chinese healthy volunteers (Guo et al., 2013), but further research did not reveal a major impact on MPA or MPA glucuronide (MPA-G) plasma concentrations as compared to UGT1A9 −2152C>T and −275T>A.

The transport of the conjugated product MPA-G into kidney epithelial cells is facilitated by organic uptake transporters such as SLCO1B1 (OATP1B1) or 1B3. In vitro research in transfected human embryonic kidney cells could demonstrate that the OATP1B3 polymorphism 334T>G (rs4149117) leads to a reduced uptake (Picard et al., 2010), studies in Chinese healthy volunteers and patients revealed some influence on MPA plasma concentrations (Geng et al., 2012), and others did not confirm this observation in clinical studies (Miura et al., 2011).

MPA-G is further a substrate of the ABC efflux transporter ABCC2. Possibly the lowered efflux explained the 25% increase in acyl MPA glucuronide plasma levels observed in Caucasian healthy volunteers carrying the −24T allele compared to −24C carriers, who received a single dose of 1.5 g MMF (Levesque, Benoit-Biancamano, Delage, Couture, & Guillemette, 2008). However, studies in Caucasian or Asian renal transplant recipients did not confirm this observation (Baldelli et al., 2007; Miura et al., 2007; Zhang et al., 2008) or showed even the opposite effect under steady-state conditions (Naesens, Kuypers, Verbeke, & Vanrenterghem, 2006).

In addition it was supposed that ABCG2 (breast cancer-related protein, BCRP) contributes to the excretion of MPA-G. The transporter belongs to the major mediators of drug resistances in humans with a profound impact on the pharmacokinetics of drugs and other xenobiotics. Various genetic variants located in the coding region have been associated with function, expression, or mRNA stability (Bruhn & Cascorbi, 2014). However, there is only weak evidence if any on a significant impact of ABCG2 variants on MPA kinetics or clinical outcome (Geng et al., 2012; Miura et al., 2011).

Overall, the influence of genetic variants on the pharmacokinetics of MFF and its derivatives seems to be modest and does not have a significant impact on the clinical outcome of solid organ transplantation. Consideration of pharmacodynamics features such as the target of MPA, namely, Type I and II inosine monophosphate dehydrogenases (IMPDHs), however, disclosed biopsy-proven acute rejection and a higher risk of leucopenia over the first year posttransplantation associated with the IMPDH I rs2278294 SNP (Gensburger et al., 2010). Another study revealed additional variants, possibly associated with MPA efficacy and toxicity (Wu et al., 2010); however, further data are sparse.

5. CALCINEURIN INHIBITORS

Calcineurin inhibitors such as cyclosporine and tacrolimus are widely used in solid organ transplantation of the kidney, liver, and heart. Cyclosporine is also approved in bone marrow transplantation and for the treatment of inflammatory diseases such as rheumatoid arthritis, psoriasis, and Crohn's disease. Application of tacrolimus in kidney organ transplantation led to a 5-year graft survival of 80% and low rates of acute organ rejection. These tremendous successes in organ transplantation are compromised by a narrow therapeutic window making continuous therapeutic drug monitoring necessary to avoid too low trough concentrations bearing the risk of long-term allograft failure on the one side and too high peak concentrations causing adverse effects such as calcineurin inhibitor-related nephrotoxicity requiring regular therapeutic drug monitoring to optimize the clinical outcome (Hariharan et al., 2000; Staatz & Tett, 2004).

Since some genetic traits were shown to significantly affect the pharmacokinetics, the question arose whether application could contribute to improvement of rapid dose adaptation with the goal of a decrease of toxicity and organ rejection (Elens et al., 2014).

5.1 Cyclosporine A

Cyclosporine A is a large cyclic organic molecule that was first isolated in 1971 from the fungus *Tolypocladium inflatum*. Through binding to cyclophilin it inhibits the phosphatase activity of calcineurin. As a consequence, NFATc (nuclear factor of activated T cell) is not activated and interleukin-2 expression is suppressed. Cyclosporine is approved for prophylactic prevention of allogenic organ transplant rejection, treatment of cellular transplant rejection after failure of other immunosuppressants, as well as for the prevention of bone marrow transplant rejection and prevention and treatment of graft vs host diseases. Cyclosporine is extensively metabolized preferentially via CYP3A4 and to a minor extent through CYP3A5 (Kronbach, Fischer, & Meyer, 1988) (Fig. 2A). CYP3A4 consists of a large number of coding and noncoding variations, but only few are clinically relevant (Werk & Cascorbi, 2014). So far, there is only one frequent (5%–7% in Caucasians) variant in the *CYP3A4* locus, namely, **22* (rs35599367) that was found to be associated with about 20% reduced CYP3A4 activity (Wang, Guo, Wrighton, Cooke, & Sadee, 2011) in kidney transplant patients. Studies on other CYP3A4 alleles such as *1B or rs4646437 revealed inconsistent results (Hesselink et al., 2004; Sun et al., 2017). However, there are some hints that the missense variant L293P present in *CYP3A4*18* occurring only in Asian populations affects cyclosporine dosages (Tao et al., 2015). Interestingly, *CYP3A4*22* did not significantly affect kidney graft survival, but was associated with a reduced risk of cancer in those patients (Traynor et al., 2015).

Despite drug metabolism, cyclosporine is an established substrate and inhibitor of P-glycoprotein (ABCB1), an efflux transporter that is expressed at many interfaces such as the intestine, liver, and kidneys. The impact of genetic variants of ABCB1 on the pharmacokinetics of drugs is modest or even neglectable (Cascorbi, 2011); however, there are a large number of studies investigating the association of ABCB1 SNPs to cyclosporine dose requirements or the risk of transplant rejection. Many results are conflicting and some positive results could not be reproduced (Elens et al., 2014). Since ABCB1 expression of the transplanted organ is, however, of major importance for local immunosuppression and toxicity, the genotype of the donor was also taken into account. Well-conducted studies considering both donors and recipients are rare. Interestingly, one study investigating DNA from 227 kidney transplant donors disclosed a higher risk of graft loss for ABCB1 triple variant carriers 1236T/2677T/3435T (rs1128503, rs2032582, rs1045642) (Woillard et al., 2010), a haplotype that was assumed to have low P-gp expression. This result could not be explained from a mechanistic point of view, since high efflux would be expected to lead to inefficient immunosuppression. Other studies pointed into the opposite direction (Bandur et al., 2008). A study in liver transplant patients did not reveal any significant association to any investigated ADME gene

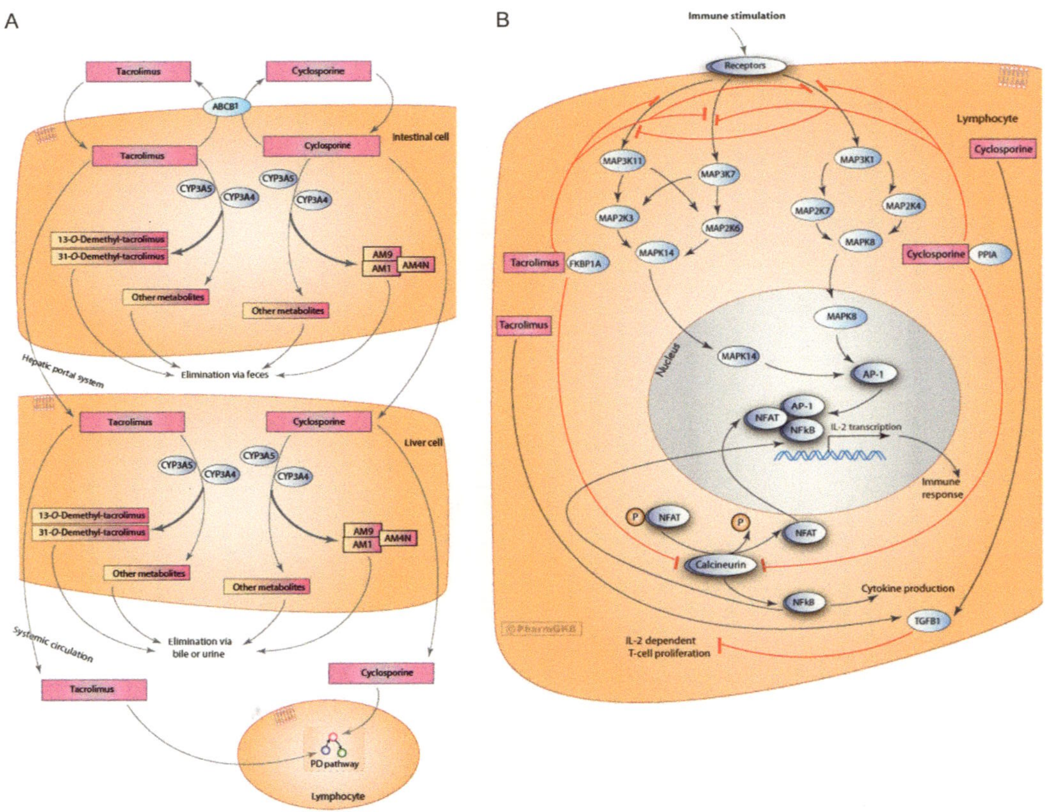

Fig. 2 (A) Schematic representation of tacrolimus and cyclosporine metabolism (Barbarino, Staatz, Venkataramanan, Klein, & Altman, 2013). (B) Stylized cell depicting the mechanism of action of tacrolimus and cyclosporine, as well as the candidate genes believed to interact with the two drugs (Barbarino et al., 2013). *Panel (A): From https://www.pharmgkb.org/pathway/PA165986114. Panel (B): From https://www.pharmgkb.org/pathway/PA165985892. Permission has been given by PharmGKB and Stanford University.*

(Debette-Gratien et al., 2016). Overall it can be concluded that neither the recipient ABCB1 genotype nor the donor genotype plays a significant role if any for dose requirements, risk of transplant rejection, or cyclosporine-associated toxicity.

5.2 Tacrolimus

Tacrolimus (also termed FK506) is a macrolide lactone isolated from *Streptomyces tsukubaensis* approved for the prevention of solid organ rejection of the kidney, liver, and heart. Likewise cyclosporine it inhibits cyclophilin, however, through binding to FK512. A major determinant of interindividual variation in the pharmacokinetics of tacrolimus is CYP3A5 (Renders et al., 2007) and to a smaller extent CYP3A4 (Fig. 2B). The contribution of further genetic variants in genes controlling the activity of the CYP3A4 locus such as cytochrome P450 oxidoreductase (POR) (Barraclough et al., 2012; Zhang, Zhang, Ding, Ma, & Miao, 2013), the pregnane X receptor (PXR/NR1/2) (Barraclough et al., 2012), or PPAR alpha (*PPARA*) (Klein et al., 2012) has been considered more recently in various clinical studies. As cyclosporine, tacrolimus is also a substrate of P-glycoprotein (ABCB1) (Staatz, Goodman, & Tett, 2010) and many studies put genotypes of ABCB1 into consideration. To make a long story short, most studies failed to prove a significant association (Elens et al., 2014), and as for cyclosporine, ABCB1 genotypes should not be recommended for pharmacogenetic diagnostics of tacrolimus dosing.

Numerous genetic association studies on tacrolimus PK revealed that CYP3A5 expressers (carriers of at least one *CYP3A5*1* allele) require up to twofold higher tacrolimus doses to reach similar blood trough concentrations than subject having no CYP3A5 activity (Anglicheau et al., 2004; Renders et al., 2007). These nonexpressers are mostly carriers of *CYP3A5*3* (rs776746) and *CYP3A5*6* (rs10264272) (Kuehl et al., 2001). From an evolutionary point of view it is an interesting fact that about 80% of Caucasians are nonexpressers due to homozygous presence of **3*, whereas *CYP3A5*3* has a frequency of 12%–33% in African populations. *CYP3A5*6*, however, is absent in Caucasians, but occurs up to 23% in Africans (Bains et al., 2013; Hustert et al., 2001). The impact of these main genotypes on tacrolimus trough/dose ratio could be shown in various ethnicities in kidney, liver, and heart transplant patients (van Gelder et al., 2014).

Further progress to better predict interindividual variability was made after consideration of *CYP3A4*22* (rs35599367). Studies in kidney transplant patients demonstrated that this trait contributed significantly to tacrolimus dose requirements independent of the *CYP3A5* genotype (Elens et al., 2011, 2013). In our own study, *CYP3A4*22* was only a significant factor when considering presence or absence of CYP3A5 activity. Strongest differences appear when comparing patients being CYP3A5 expressers and having high-active CYP3A4 and those carrying *CYP3A5*3/*3* and *CYP3A4*22*. The first group required 165% higher doses to reach similar plasma concentrations than low-active metabolizers (Bruckmueller et al., 2015). In the same study, we could rule out that *NR1I2*, *POR*, or *PPAR alpha* played any major role. The impact of combined consideration of *CYP3A4*22* and *CYP3A5*3* was confirmed by further studies (Lloberas et al., 2017), who also denied the influence of genetic variants in other candidate genes. However, total absence of CYP3A activity may also occur in rare cases. We were asked to investigate reasons for extremely low tacrolimus dose requirement in a kidney transplant patient. This subject was identified to be homozygous for *CYP3A5*3* and homozygous for a premature stop-codon in the *CYP3A4* locus, later termed *CYP3A4*26*, contributing to the clinical explanation of minimal tacrolimus requirement to keep optimal trough levels (Werk et al., 2014).

Based on the above discussed experience, Elens and Haufroid (2017) recommended to distinguish three genetically distinct groups, namely, carriers of (a) *CYP3A5*3/*3* + *CYP3A4*22* requiring 0.14 mg/kg/day, (b) *CYP3A5*3/*3* + *CYP3A4*1/*1* requiring 0.2–0.25 mg/kg/day, and (c) *CYP3A5*1* + *CYP3A4**1/*1* requiring 0.3–0.4 mg/kg/day tacrolimus (Elens & Haufroid, 2017) and to replace current CPIC guidelines on tacrolimus that only consider *CYP3A5* genotypes (Birdwell et al., 2015).

As mentioned above for cyclosporine, not only the recipient genotype but also the donor genotype could have an influence on the clinical outcome. A study among liver transplant patients, however, interestingly showed no effect of the donor *CYP3A4/5* genotypes on survival probability without graft loss, but a significant association to the genotype of the recipient. It was hypothesized that in particular CYP3A5*1 expression in the recipient's intestine led to hepatic tacrolimus levels in the first time after liver transplantation and consequently underexposure of the new organ with the calcineurin inhibitor (Debette-Gratien et al., 2016).

5.3 Pharmacogenetics Affecting the Pharmacodynamics of Calcineurin Inhibitors

The above outlined approaches take only parameters into account, affecting the pharmacokinetics of cyclosporine or tacrolimus. However, due to therapeutic drug monitoring, variation of trough levels can be corrected by dose adaptation. So, most studies did not show any significant association of ADME gene variants on c_0 levels. The question whether genetic variants in the calcineurin pathway have any impact on the clinical outcome was investigated in a large study in 381 renal transplant patients. The investigators genotyped 13 genes encoding proteins expressed in T cells, namely, cyclophilin A (*PPIA*), FKBP12 (*FKBP1A*), calmodulin 1–3 isoforms (*CALM1–3*), calcineurin A (α- and β-subunits, *PPP3CA*, *PPP3CB*) and B (α-subunit, *PP3R1*), nuclear factor of activated T cells (*NFATC1, 2, 3*), interleukin-2 (*IL-2*), and the IL-2 α-chain receptor (*IL-2RA*). As a result, multivariate survival analyses did not reveal any significant association of any genetic variant to any outcome parameter (Pouche et al., 2016).

6. SIROLIMUS

The mTOR inhibitor sirolimus is structurally closely related to tacrolimus and produced by the bacteria strain *Streptomyces hygroscopicus*. In combination with cyclosporine and glucocorticoids it is approved for the prevention of organ rejection after kidney transplantation. Sirolimus is also used as antiproliferative agent in coated cardiac stents. Due to its similarity to tacrolimus, the pharmacokinetics are also driven by metabolism via CYP3A4 (and to a minor extent by CYP3A5) and efflux transport via ABCB1. A PK/PD model considering also genetic variants disclosed a significant, but small impact of *CYP3A5*3* on sirolimus PK (Emoto, Fukuda, Venkatasubramanian, & Vinks, 2015). Similar results were obtained in a recent small Chinese study (Zhang et al., 2013). In a study by our own group in 20 kidney transplant patient treated with sirolimus, there was however lack of any association of sirolimus dose/trough concentrations to variants in CYP3A5, ABCB1, and ABCC2 (Renders et al., 2007). CYP3A4 was not included into the study.

So far, the impact of pharmacogenetics on sirolimus kinetics seems to be modest and data on the clinical outcome are not yet available.

7. CONCLUSION

So far, the best established pharmacogenetics marker in immunosuppression is TPMT in azathioprine and mercaptopurine treatment. The product information contains recommendations to consider either genotype or phenotype patients for TPMT. Due to the fact that TPMT-poor metabolizers have a 100% risk to suffer from leukopenia if the standard dose is applied, this recommendation has to be taken seriously. However, the regulatory authorities make it very clear that TPMT testing cannot substitute for complete blood count monitoring in patients receiving thiopurine analogs, since leukopenia may occur also in TPMT wild types. Accordingly NUDT15 should be a further genetic parameter that should be taken into consideration.

As far as all other immunosuppressants are concerned, only those which are metabolized to a major extent by CYP3A5 showed a clear and significant association of pharmacogenetic traits to pharmacokinetic properties. The evidence on the influence of *CYP3A5*3* and to a minor extent of *CYP3A4*22* could be made preferentially on tacrolimus dosing in kidney, liver, and heart transplant patients. Data on significant impact on the clinical outcome such as nephrotoxicity and transplant function or rejection are sparse. So far there is no convincing evidence that early consideration of pharmacogenetics could improve the outcome. This may be due to the fact pharmacogenetics explains only part of the overall variability. In a recent study on tacrolimus in kidney transplant patients from Denmark and Germany, the final multiple linear regression model for trough concentration/dose ratio including CYP3A5, CYP3A4, and age explained only 18.3% of the interindividual variability of tacrolimus trough concentration/dose ratios ($P = 8.8 \times 10^{-10}$) (Bruckmueller et al., 2015). Hence although dose recommendations are available, these have not yet been considered in the product information of the various tacrolimus formulations, but regular therapeutic drug monitoring is strongly required. Moreover, acute cellular rejection also occurs when tacrolimus trough concentration is within the therapeutic window. It is hypothesized that determination of intracellular and/or unbound tacrolimus or monitoring of pharmacodynamic features could be better tools for adequate tacrolimus exposure (Picard et al., 2016).

For MTX and MMF the evidence of pharmacogenetics in dose optimization is weak. Although a number of genetic associations on ADME genes were reported, results remain partly uncertain and in particular, no proof is available that application of genetic markers could improve the clinical outcome so far. Therefore for these immunosuppressive drugs, no recommendations to consider any pharmacogenetic trait can currently be made (Table 1).

Table 1 Association of Variant ADME Genes or Others (and Most Important Variants) to Drug-Related Toxicity or Pharmacokinetics of Selected Small-Molecule Immunosuppressants: +++ Very Strong Evidence, ++ Strong Evidence, + Some Evidence, (+) Conflicting Data, – Lack of Association

	Phase I Enzymes		**Phase II Enzymes**		**Uptake Transporters**	**ABC Transporters**		**Others**	
	CYP3A4	CYP3A5	TPMT	UGT1A9	OATP1B1/3	ABCB1	ABCC2	NUDT15	IMPDH I/II
	rs35599367	rs776746, rs10264272	rs12201199, rs1142345, rs1800460	rs17868320, rs6714486	rs4149056/ rs4149117	rs1128503, rs2032582, rs1045642	rs717620	rs116855232	rs2278293, rs2278294/ rs11706052
Drug									
Azathioprine	–	–	+++	–		–	–	+++	–
Methotrexate	–	–	–	–		(+)	+	–	
Mycophenolic acid	–	–	–	+	(+)	–	(+)	–	+
Cyclosporine	(+)	–	–	–	–	(+)	–	–	–
Tacrolimus	+	++	–	–	–	(+)	–	–	–
Sirolimus	(+)	–	–	–	–	–	–	–	–

Possibly the discovery of rare but functional genetic variants may further contribute to the interpretation of interindividual variation in drug response (Kozyra, Ingelman-Sundberg, & Lauschke, 2017; Lauschke & Ingelman-Sundberg, 2016). Today a number of other biomarkers are under discussion to optimize dosing in transplant prevention; further evidence is awaited however (Anglicheau, Naesens, Essig, Gwinner, & Marquet, 2016).

CONFLICT OF INTEREST

The author has no conflicts of interest to declare.

REFERENCES

Anglicheau, D., Naesens, M., Essig, M., Gwinner, W., & Marquet, P. (2016). Establishing biomarkers in transplant medicine: A critical review of current approaches. *Transplantation, 100*(10), 2024–2038. https://doi.org/10.1097/TP.0000000000001321.

Anglicheau, D., Thervet, E., Etienne, I., Hurault De Ligny, B., Le Meur, Y., Touchard, G., et al. (2004). CYP3A5 and MDR1 genetic polymorphisms and cyclosporine pharmacokinetics after renal transplantation. *Clinical Pharmacology and Therapeutics, 75*(5), 422–433. https://doi.org/10.1016/j.clpt.2004.01.009.

Bains, R. K., Kovacevic, M., Plaster, C. A., Tarekegn, A., Bekele, E., Bradman, N. N., et al. (2013). Molecular diversity and population structure at the cytochrome P450 3A5 gene in Africa. *BMC Genetics, 14*, 34. https://doi.org/10.1186/1471-2156-14-34.

Baldelli, S., Merlini, S., Perico, N., Nicastri, A., Cortinovis, M., Gotti, E., et al. (2007). C-440T/T-331C polymorphisms in the UGT1A9 gene affect the pharmacokinetics of mycophenolic acid in kidney transplantation. *Pharmacogenomics, 8*(9), 1127–1141. https://doi.org/10.2217/14622416.8.9.1127.

Bandur, S., Petrasek, J., Hribova, P., Novotna, E., Brabcova, I., & Viklicky, O. (2008). Haplotypic structure of ABCB1/MDR1 gene modifies the risk of the acute allograft rejection in renal transplant recipients. *Transplantation, 86*(9), 1206–1213. https://doi.org/10.1097/TP.0b013e318187c4d1.

Barbarino, J. M., Staatz, C. E., Venkataramanan, R., Klein, T. E., & Altman, R. B. (2013). PharmGKB summary: Cyclosporine and tacrolimus pathways. *Pharmacogenetics and Genomics, 23*(10), 563–585. https://doi.org/10.1097/FPC.0b013e328364db84.

Barraclough, K. A., Isbel, N. M., Lee, K. J., Bergmann, T. K., Johnson, D. W., McWhinney, B. C., et al. (2012). NR1I2 polymorphisms are related to tacrolimus dose-adjusted exposure and BK viremia in adult kidney transplantation. *Transplantation, 94*(10), 1025–1032. https://doi.org/10.1097/TP.0b013e31826c3985.

Birdwell, K. A., Decker, B., Barbarino, J. M., Peterson, J. F., Stein, C. M., Sadee, W., et al. (2015). Clinical Pharmacogenetics Implementation Consortium (CPIC) guidelines for CYP3A5 genotype and tacrolimus dosing. *Clinical Pharmacology and Therapeutics, 98*(1), 19–24. https://doi.org/10.1002/cpt.113.

Bruckmueller, H., Werk, A. N., Renders, L., Feldkamp, T., Tepel, M., Borst, C., et al. (2015). Which genetic determinants should be considered for tacrolimus dose optimization in kidney transplantation? A combined analysis of genes affecting the CYP3A locus. *Therapeutic Drug Monitoring, 37*(3), 288–295. https://doi.org/10.1097/FTD.0000000000000142.

Bruhn, O., & Cascorbi, I. (2014). Polymorphisms of the drug transporters ABCB1, ABCG2, ABCC2 and ABCC3 and their impact on drug bioavailability and clinical relevance.

Expert Opinion on Drug Metabolism & Toxicology, *10*(10), 1337–1354. https://doi.org/10.1517/17425255.2014.952630.

Cascorbi, I. (2011). P-glycoprotein: Tissue distribution, substrates, and functional consequences of genetic variations. *Handbook of Experimental Pharmacolology*, *201*, 261–283. https://doi.org/10.1007/978-3-642-14541-4_6.

Cascorbi, I., & Haenisch, S. (2010). Pharmacogenetics of ATP-binding cassette transporters and clinical implications. *Methods in Molecular Biology*, *596*, 95–121. https://doi.org/10.1007/978-1-60761-416-6_6.

Chao, K., Wang, X., Cao, Q., Qian, J., Wu, K., Zhu, X., et al. (2017). Combined detection of NUDT15 variants could highly predict thiopurine-induced leukopenia in Chinese patients with inflammatory bowel disease: A multicenter analysis. *Inflammatory Bowel Diseases*, *23*(9), 1592–1599. https://doi.org/10.1097/MIB.0000000000001148.

Debette-Gratien, M., Woillard, J. B., Picard, N., Sebagh, M., Loustaud-Ratti, V., Sautereau, D., et al. (2016). Influence of donor and recipient CYP3A4, CYP3A5, and ABCB1 genotypes on clinical outcomes and nephrotoxicity in liver transplant recipients. *Transplantation*, *100*(10), 2129–2137. https://doi.org/10.1097/TP.0000000000001394.

Elens, L., Bouamar, R., Shuker, N., Hesselink, D. A., van Gelder, T., & van Schaik, R. H. (2014). Clinical implementation of pharmacogenetics in kidney transplantation: Calcineurin inhibitors in the starting blocks. *British Journal of Clinical Pharmacology*, *77*(4), 715–728. https://doi.org/10.1111/bcp.12253.

Elens, L., Capron, A., van Schaik, R. H., De Meyer, M., De Pauw, L., Eddour, D. C., et al. (2013). Impact of CYP3A4*22 allele on tacrolimus pharmacokinetics in early period after renal transplantation: Toward updated genotype-based dosage guidelines. *Therapeutic Drug Monitoring*, *35*(5), 608–616. https://doi.org/10.1097/FTD.0b013e318296045b.

Elens, L., & Haufroid, V. (2017). Genotype-based tacrolimus dosing guidelines: With or without CYP3A4*22? *Pharmacogenomics*, *18*(16), 1473–1480. https://doi.org/10.2217/pgs-2017-0131.

Elens, L., van Schaik, R. H., Panin, N., de Meyer, M., Wallemacq, P., Lison, D., et al. (2011). Effect of a new functional CYP3A4 polymorphism on calcineurin inhibitors' dose requirements and trough blood levels in stable renal transplant patients. *Pharmacogenomics*, *12*(10), 1383–1396. https://doi.org/10.2217/pgs.11.90.

Elion, G. B. (1989). The purine path to chemotherapy. *Science*, *244*(4900), 41–47.

Emoto, C., Fukuda, T., Venkatasubramanian, R., & Vinks, A. A. (2015). The impact of CYP3A5*3 polymorphism on sirolimus pharmacokinetics: Insights from predictions with a physiologically-based pharmacokinetic model. *British Journal of Clinical Pharmacology*, *80*(6), 1438–1446. https://doi.org/10.1111/bcp.12743.

Fraser, A. G., Orchard, T. R., & Jewell, D. P. (2002). The efficacy of azathioprine for the treatment of inflammatory bowel disease: A 30 year review. *Gut*, *50*(4), 485–489.

Galivan, J., Ryan, T. J., Chave, K., Rhee, M., Yao, R., & Yin, D. (2000). Glutamyl hydrolase. Pharmacological role and enzymatic characterization. *Pharmacology & Therapeutics*, *85*(3), 207–215.

Geng, F., Jiao, Z., Dao, Y. J., Qiu, X. Y., Ding, J. J., Shi, X. J., et al. (2012). The association of the UGT1A8, SLCO1B3 and ABCC2/ABCG2 genetic polymorphisms with the pharmacokinetics of mycophenolic acid and its phenolic glucuronide metabolite in Chinese individuals. *Clinica Chimica Acta*, *413*(7–8), 683–690. https://doi.org/10.1016/j.cca.2011.12.003.

Gensburger, O., Van Schaik, R. H., Picard, N., Le Meur, Y., Rousseau, A., Woillard, J. B., et al. (2010). Polymorphisms in type I and II inosine monophosphate dehydrogenase genes and association with clinical outcome in patients on mycophenolate mofetil. *Pharmacogenetics and Genomics*, *20*(9), 537–543. https://doi.org/10.1097/FPC.0b013e32833d8cf5.

Girard, H., Court, M. H., Bernard, O., Fortier, L. C., Villeneuve, L., Hao, Q., et al. (2004). Identification of common polymorphisms in the promoter of the UGT1A9 gene: Evidence that UGT1A9 protein and activity levels are strongly genetically controlled in the liver. *Pharmacogenetics*, *14*(8), 501–515.

Guo, D., Pang, L. F., Han, Y., Yang, H., Wang, G., Tan, Z. R., et al. (2013). Polymorphisms of UGT1A9 and UGT2B7 influence the pharmacokinetics of mycophenolic acid after a single oral dose in healthy Chinese volunteers. *European Journal of Clinical Pharmacology*, *69*(4), 843–849. https://doi.org/10.1007/s00228-012-1409-0.

Haenisch, S., Zimmermann, U., Dazert, E., Wruck, C. J., Dazert, P., Siegmund, W., et al. (2007). Influence of polymorphisms of ABCB1 and ABCC2 on mRNA and protein expression in normal and cancerous kidney cortex. *The Pharmacogenomics Journal*, 7(1), 56–65. https://doi.org/10.1038/sj.tpj.6500403.

Hariharan, S., Johnson, C. P., Bresnahan, B. A., Taranto, S. E., McIntosh, M. J., & Stablein, D. (2000). Improved graft survival after renal transplantation in the United States, 1988 to 1996. *The New England Journal of Medicine*, *342*(9), 605–612. https://doi.org/10.1056/NEJM200003023420901.

Hegyi, M., Arany, A., Semsei, A. F., Csordas, K., Eipel, O., Gezsi, A., et al. (2017). Pharmacogenetic analysis of high-dose methotrexate treatment in children with osteosarcoma. *Oncotarget*, *8*(6), 9388–9398. https://doi.org/10.18632/oncotarget.11543.

Hesselink, D. A., van Gelder, T., van Schaik, R. H., Balk, A. H., van der Heiden, I. P., van Dam, T., et al. (2004). Population pharmacokinetics of cyclosporine in kidney and heart transplant recipients and the influence of ethnicity and genetic polymorphisms in the MDR-1, CYP3A4, and CYP3A5 genes. *Clinical Pharmacology and Therapeutics*, *76*(6), 545–556. https://doi.org/10.1016/j.clpt.2004.08.022.

Hustert, E., Haberl, M., Burk, O., Wolbold, R., He, Y. Q., Klein, K., et al. (2001). The genetic determinants of the CYP3A5 polymorphism. *Pharmacogenetics*, *11*(9), 773–779.

Kakuta, Y., Naito, T., Onodera, M., Kuroha, M., Kimura, T., Shiga, H., et al. (2016). NUDT15 R139C causes thiopurine-induced early severe hair loss and leukopenia in Japanese patients with IBD. *The Pharmacogenomics Journal*, *16*(3), 280–285. https://doi.org/10.1038/tpj.2015.43.

Kim, J. H., Cheon, J. H., Hong, S. S., Eun, C. S., Byeon, J. S., Hong, S. Y., et al. (2010). Influences of thiopurine methyltransferase genotype and activity on thiopurine-induced leukopenia in Korean patients with inflammatory bowel disease: A retrospective cohort study. *Journal of Clinical Gastroenterology*, *44*(10), e242–248. https://doi.org/10.1097/MCG.0b013e3181d6baf5.

Klein, K., Thomas, M., Winter, S., Nussler, A. K., Niemi, M., Schwab, M., et al. (2012). PPARA: A novel genetic determinant of CYP3A4 in vitro and in vivo. *Clinical Pharmacology and Therapeutics*, *91*(6), 1044–1052. https://doi.org/10.1038/clpt.2011.336.

Kozyra, M., Ingelman-Sundberg, M., & Lauschke, V. M. (2017). Rare genetic variants in cellular transporters, metabolic enzymes, and nuclear receptors can be important determinants of interindividual differences in drug response. *Genetics in Medicine*, *19*(1), 20–29. https://doi.org/10.1038/gim.2016.33.

Kronbach, T., Fischer, V., & Meyer, U. A. (1988). Cyclosporine metabolism in human liver: Identification of a cytochrome P-450III gene family as the major cyclosporine-metabolizing enzyme explains interactions of cyclosporine with other drugs. *Clinical Pharmacology and Therapeutics*, *43*(6), 630–635.

Kuehl, P., Zhang, J., Lin, Y., Lamba, J., Assem, M., Schuetz, J., et al. (2001). Sequence diversity in CYP3A promoters and characterization of the genetic basis of polymorphic CYP3A5 expression. *Nature Genetics*, *27*(4), 383–391. https://doi.org/10.1038/86882.

Kuypers, D. R., Naesens, M., Vermeire, S., & Vanrenterghem, Y. (2005). The impact of uridine diphosphate-glucuronosyltransferase 1A9 (UGT1A9) gene promoter region single-nucleotide polymorphisms T-275A and C-2152T on early mycophenolic acid dose-interval exposure in de novo renal allograft recipients. *Clinical Pharmacology and Therapeutics*, *78*(4), 351–361. https://doi.org/10.1016/j.clpt.2005.06.007.

Laechelt, S., Turrini, E., Ruehmkorf, A., Siegmund, W., Cascorbi, I., & Haenisch, S. (2011). Impact of ABCC2 haplotypes on transcriptional and posttranscriptional gene regulation and function. *The Pharmacogenomics Journal*, *11*(1), 25–34. https://doi.org/10.1038/tpj.2010.20.

Lauschke, V. M., & Ingelman-Sundberg, M. (2016). Precision medicine and rare genetic variants. *Trends in Pharmacological Sciences*, *37*(2), 85–86. https://doi.org/10.1016/j.tips.2015.10.006.

Levesque, E., Benoit-Biancamano, M. O., Delage, R., Couture, F., & Guillemette, C. (2008). Pharmacokinetics of mycophenolate mofetil and its glucuronide metabolites in healthy volunteers. *Pharmacogenomics*, *9*(7), 869–879. https://doi.org/10.2217/14622416.9.7.869.

Liu, C., Yang, W., Pei, D., Cheng, C., Smith, C., Landier, W., et al. (2017). Genomewide approach validates thiopurine methyltransferase activity is a monogenic pharmacogenomic trait. *Clinical Pharmacology and Therapeutics*, *101*(3), 373–381. https://doi.org/10.1002/cpt.463.

Lloberas, N., Elens, L., Llaudo, I., Padulles, A., van Gelder, T., Hesselink, D. A., et al. (2017). The combination of CYP3A4*22 and CYP3A5*3 single-nucleotide polymorphisms determines tacrolimus dose requirement after kidney transplantation. *Pharmacogenetics and Genomics*, *27*(9), 313–322. https://doi.org/10.1097/FPC.0000000000000296.

Mikkelsen, T. S., Thorn, C. F., Yang, J. J., Ulrich, C. M., French, D., Zaza, G., et al. (2011). PharmGKB summary: Methotrexate pathway. *Pharmacogenetics and Genomics*, *21*(10), 679–686. https://doi.org/10.1097/FPC.0b013e328343dd93.

Miura, M., Niioka, T., Kato, S., Kagaya, H., Saito, M., Habuchi, T., et al. (2011). Monitoring of mycophenolic acid predose concentrations in the maintenance phase more than one year after renal transplantation. *Therapeutic Drug Monitoring*, *33*(3), 295–302. https://doi.org/10.1097/FTD.0b013e3182197e38.

Miura, M., Satoh, S., Inoue, K., Kagaya, H., Saito, M., Inoue, T., et al. (2007). Influence of SLCO1B1, 1B3, 2B1 and ABCC2 genetic polymorphisms on mycophenolic acid pharmacokinetics in Japanese renal transplant recipients. *European Journal of Clinical Pharmacology*, *63*(12), 1161–1169. https://doi.org/10.1007/s00228-007-0380-7.

Moriyama, T., Nishii, R., Perez-Andreu, V., Yang, W., Klussmann, F. A., Zhao, X., et al. (2016). NUDT15 polymorphisms alter thiopurine metabolism and hematopoietic toxicity. *Nature Genetics*, *48*(4), 367–373. https://doi.org/10.1038/ng.3508.

Moriyama, T., Yang, Y. L., Nishii, R., Ariffin, H., Liu, C., Lin, T. N., et al. (2017). Novel variants in NUDT15 and thiopurine intolerance in children with acute lymphoblastic leukemia from diverse ancestry. *Blood*, *130*(10), 1209–1212. https://doi.org/10.1182/blood-2017-05-782383.

Naesens, M., Kuypers, D. R., Verbeke, K., & Vanrenterghem, Y. (2006). Multidrug resistance protein 2 genetic polymorphisms influence mycophenolic acid exposure in renal allograft recipients. *Transplantation*, *82*(8), 1074–1084. https://doi.org/10.1097/01.tp.0000235533.29300.e7.

Picard, N., Bergan, S., Marquet, P., van Gelder, T., Wallemacq, P., Hesselink, D. A., et al. (2016). Pharmacogenetic biomarkers predictive of the pharmacokinetics and pharmacodynamics of immunosuppressive drugs. *Therapeutic Drug Monitoring*, *38*(Suppl. 1), S57–S69. https://doi.org/10.1097/FTD.0000000000000255.

Picard, N., Yee, S. W., Woillard, J. B., Lebranchu, Y., Le Meur, Y., Giacomini, K. M., et al. (2010). The role of organic anion-transporting polypeptides and their common genetic variants in mycophenolic acid pharmacokinetics. *Clinical Pharmacology and Therapeutics*, *87*(1), 100–108. https://doi.org/10.1038/clpt.2009.205.

Plumpton, C. O., Roberts, D., Pirmohamed, M., & Hughes, D. A. (2016). A systematic review of economic evaluations of pharmacogenetic testing for prevention of adverse drug reactions. *Pharmacoeconomics*, *34*(8), 771–793. https://doi.org/10.1007/s40273-016-0397-9.

Pouche, L., Koitka, M., Stojanova, J., Woillard, J. B., Monchaud, C., Villeneuve, C., et al. (2016). A candidate gene approach of the calcineurin pathway to identify variants associated with clinical outcomes in renal transplantation. *Pharmacogenomics*, *17*(4), 375–391. https://doi.org/10.2217/pgs.15.181.

Rau, T., Erney, B., Gores, R., Eschenhagen, T., Beck, J., & Langer, T. (2006). High-dose methotrexate in pediatric acute lymphoblastic leukemia: Impact of ABCC2 polymorphisms on plasma concentrations. *Clinical Pharmacology and Therapeutics*, *80*(5), 468–476. https://doi.org/10.1016/j.clpt.2006.08.012.

Relling, M. V., Gardner, E. E., Sandborn, W. J., Schmiegelow, K., Pui, C. H., Yee, S. W., et al. (2011). Clinical Pharmacogenetics Implementation Consortium guidelines for thiopurine methyltransferase genotype and thiopurine dosing. *Clinical Pharmacology and Therapeutics*, *89*(3), 387–391. https://doi.org/10.1038/clpt.2010.320.

Relling, M. V., Gardner, E. E., Sandborn, W. J., Schmiegelow, K., Pui, C. H., Yee, S. W., et al. (2013). Clinical Pharmacogenetics Implementation Consortium guidelines for thiopurine methyltransferase genotype and thiopurine dosing: 2013 update. *Clinical Pharmacology and Therapeutics*, *93*(4), 324–325. https://doi.org/10.1038/clpt.2013.4.

Renders, L., Frisman, M., Ufer, M., Mosyagin, I., Haenisch, S., Ott, U., et al. (2007). CYP3A5 genotype markedly influences the pharmacokinetics of tacrolimus and sirolimus in kidney transplant recipients. *Clinical Pharmacology and Therapeutics*, *81*(2), 228–234. https://doi.org/10.1038/sj.clpt.6100039.

Schaeffeler, E., Fischer, C., Brockmeier, D., Wernet, D., Moerike, K., Eichelbaum, M., et al. (2004). Comprehensive analysis of thiopurine S-methyltransferase phenotype-genotype correlation in a large population of German-Caucasians and identification of novel TPMT variants. *Pharmacogenetics*, *14*(7), 407–417.

Schwab, M., Schaffeler, E., Marx, C., Fischer, C., Lang, T., Behrens, C., et al. (2002). Azathioprine therapy and adverse drug reactions in patients with inflammatory bowel disease: Impact of thiopurine S-methyltransferase polymorphism. *Pharmacogenetics*, *12*(6), 429–436.

Staatz, C. E., Goodman, L. K., & Tett, S. E. (2010). Effect of CYP3A and ABCB1 single nucleotide polymorphisms on the pharmacokinetics and pharmacodynamics of calcineurin inhibitors: Part II. *Clinical Pharmacokinetics*, *49*(4), 207–221. https://doi.org/10.2165/11317550-000000000-00000.

Staatz, C. E., & Tett, S. E. (2004). Clinical pharmacokinetics and pharmacodynamics of tacrolimus in solid organ transplantation. *Clinical Pharmacokinetics*, *43*(10), 623–653.

Sun, B., Guo, Y., Gao, J., Shi, W., Fan, G., Li, X., et al. (2017). Influence of CYP3A and ABCB1 polymorphisms on cyclosporine concentrations in renal transplant recipients. *Pharmacogenomics*, *18*(16), 1503–1513. https://doi.org/10.2217/pgs-2017-0127.

Tao, X. R., Xia, X. Y., Zhang, J., Tong, L. Y., Zhang, W., Zhou, X., et al. (2015). CYP3A4 *18B and CYP3A5 *3 polymorphisms contribute to pharmacokinetic variability of cyclosporine among healthy Chinese subjects. *European Journal of Pharmaceutical Sciences*, *76*, 238–244. https://doi.org/10.1016/j.ejps.2015.05.011.

Teml, A., Schaeffeler, E., Herrlinger, K. R., Klotz, U., & Schwab, M. (2007). Thiopurine treatment in inflammatory bowel disease: Clinical pharmacology and implication of pharmacogenetically guided dosing. *Clinical Pharmacokinetics*, *46*(3), 187–208. https://doi.org/10.2165/00003088-200746030-00001.

Traynor, C., Conlon, P., Jr., Phelan, P. J., O'Kelly, P., Elens, L., McCormack, M., et al. (2015). Association of CYP3A variants with kidney transplant outcomes. *Renal Failure*, *37*(4), 562–566. https://doi.org/10.3109/0886022X.2015.1007013.

van Gelder, T., van Schaik, R. H., & Hesselink, D. A. (2014). Pharmacogenetics and immunosuppressive drugs in solid organ transplantation. *Nature Reviews. Nephrology*, *10*(12), 725–731. https://doi.org/10.1038/nrneph.2014.172.

van Schaik, R. H., van Agteren, M., de Fijter, J. W., Hartmann, A., Schmidt, J., Budde, K., et al. (2009). UGT1A9 -275T > A/-2152C > T polymorphisms correlate with low MPA exposure and acute rejection in MMF/tacrolimus-treated kidney transplant patients. *Clinical Pharmacology and Therapeutics*, *86*(3), 319–327. https://doi.org/10.1038/clpt.2009.83.

Wang, D., Guo, Y., Wrighton, S. A., Cooke, G. E., & Sadee, W. (2011). Intronic polymorphism in CYP3A4 affects hepatic expression and response to statin drugs. *The Pharmacogenomics Journal*, *11*(4), 274–286. https://doi.org/10.1038/tpj.2010.28.

Weinshilboum, R. M. (1992). Methylation pharmacogenetics: Thiopurine methyltransferase as a model system. *Xenobiotica*, *22*(9–10), 1055–1071.

Werk, A. N., & Cascorbi, I. (2014). Functional gene variants of CYP3A4. *Clinical Pharmacology and Therapeutics*, *96*(3), 340–348. https://doi.org/10.1038/clpt.2014.129.

Werk, A. N., Lefeldt, S., Bruckmueller, H., Hemmrich-Stanisak, G., Franke, A., Roos, M., et al. (2014). Identification and characterization of a defective CYP3A4 genotype in a kidney transplant patient with severely diminished tacrolimus clearance. *Clinical Pharmacology and Therapeutics*, *95*(4), 416–422. https://doi.org/10.1038/clpt.2013.210.

Woillard, J. B., Debord, J., Benz-de-Bretagne, I., Saint-Marcoux, F., Turlure, P., Girault, S., et al. (2017). A time-dependent model describes methotrexate elimination and supports dynamic modification of MRP2/ABCC2 activity. *Therapeutic Drug Monitoring*, *39*(2), 145–156. https://doi.org/10.1097/FTD.0000000000000381.

Woillard, J. B., Rerolle, J. P., Picard, N., Rousseau, A., Guillaudeau, A., Munteanu, E., et al. (2010). Donor P-gp polymorphisms strongly influence renal function and graft loss in a cohort of renal transplant recipients on cyclosporine therapy in a long-term follow-up. *Clinical Pharmacology and Therapeutics*, *88*(1), 95–100. https://doi.org/10.1038/clpt.2010.62.

Wu, T. Y., Peng, Y., Pelleymounter, L. L., Moon, I., Eckloff, B. W., Wieben, E. D., et al. (2010). Pharmacogenetics of the mycophenolic acid targets inosine monophosphate dehydrogenases IMPDH1 and IMPDH2: Gene sequence variation and functional genomics. *British Journal of Pharmacology*, *161*(7), 1584–1598. https://doi.org/10.1111/j.1476-5381.2010.00987.x.

Yang, S. K., Hong, M., Baek, J., Choi, H., Zhao, W., Jung, Y., et al. (2014). A common missense variant in NUDT15 confers susceptibility to thiopurine-induced leukopenia. *Nature Genetics*, *46*(9), 1017–1020. https://doi.org/10.1038/ng.3060.

Yang, J. J., Landier, W., Yang, W., Liu, C., Hageman, L., Cheng, C., et al. (2015). Inherited NUDT15 variant is a genetic determinant of mercaptopurine intolerance in children with acute lymphoblastic leukemia. *Journal of Clinical Oncology*, *33*(11), 1235–1242. https://doi.org/10.1200/JCO.2014.59.4671.

Zaza, G., Cheok, M., Krynetskaia, N., Thorn, C., Stocco, G., Hebert, J. M., et al. (2010). Thiopurine pathway. *Pharmacogenetics and Genomics*, *20*(9), 573–574. https://doi.org/10.1097/FPC.0b013e328334338f.

Zgheib, N. K., Akra-Ismail, M., Aridi, C., Mahfouz, R., Abboud, M. R., Solh, H., et al. (2014). Genetic polymorphisms in candidate genes predict increased toxicity with methotrexate therapy in Lebanese children with acute lymphoblastic leukemia. *Pharmacogenetics and Genomics*, *24*(8), 387–396. https://doi.org/10.1097/FPC.0000000000000069.

Zhang, W. X., Chen, B., Jin, Z., Yu, Z., Wang, X., Chen, H., et al. (2008). Influence of uridine diphosphate (UDP)-glucuronosyltransferases and ABCC2 genetic polymorphisms on the pharmacokinetics of mycophenolic acid and its metabolites in Chinese renal transplant recipients. *Xenobiotica*, *38*(11), 1422–1436. https://doi.org/10.1080/00498250802488585.

Zhang, J. J., Zhang, H., Ding, X. L., Ma, S., & Miao, L. Y. (2013). Effect of the P450 oxidoreductase 28 polymorphism on the pharmacokinetics of tacrolimus in Chinese healthy male volunteers. *European Journal of Clinical Pharmacology*, *69*(4), 807–812. https://doi.org/10.1007/s00228-012-1432-1.

CHAPTER TWELVE

Pharmacogenetics in Psychiatry

Filippo Corponi, Chiara Fabbri, Alessandro Serretti[1]
Department of Biomedical and Neuromotor Sciences, University of Bologna, Bologna, Italy
[1]Corresponding author: e-mail address: alessandro.serretti@unibo.it

Contents

1. Introduction 299
2. Antidepressants 301
   2.1 Candidate Genes 301
   2.2 Genome-Wide Association Studies 309
   2.3 Clinical Applications 310
3. Mood Stabilizers 311
   3.1 Candidate Genes 312
   3.2 Genome-Wide Association Studies 313
   3.3 Clinical Applications 314
4. Antipsychotics 315
   4.1 Candidate Genes 315
   4.2 Genome-Wide Association Studies 320
   4.3 Clinical Applications 322
5. Conclusion 323
References 325

Abstract

Mental illness represents a major health issue both at the individual and at the socioeconomical level. This is partly due to the current suboptimal treatment options: existing psychotropic medications, including antidepressants, antipsychotics, and mood stabilizers, are effective only in a subset of patients or produce partial response and they are often associated with debilitating side effects that discourage adherence. Pharmacogenetics is the study of how genetic information impacts on drug response/side effects with the goal to provide tailored treatments, thereby maximizing efficacy and tolerability. The first pharmacogenetic studies focused on candidate genes, previously known to be relevant to the pharmacokinetics and pharmacodynamics of psychotropic drugs. Results were mainly inconclusive, but some replicated candidates were identified and included as pharmacogenetic biomarkers in drug labeling and in some commercial kits. With the advent of the genomic revolution, it became possible to study the genetic variation on an unprecedented scale, throughout the whole genome with no need of a priori hypothesis. This may lead to the personalized prescription of existing medications and potentially to the development of innovative ones, thanks to new

Advances in Pharmacology, Volume 83
ISSN 1054-3589
https://doi.org/10.1016/bs.apha.2018.03.003

insights into the genetics of mental illness. Promising findings were obtained, but methods for the generation and analysis of genome-wide and sequencing data are still in evolution. Future pharmacogenetic tests may consist of hundreds/thousands of polymorphisms throughout the genome or selected pathways in order to take into account the complex interactions across variants in a number of genes.

ABBREVIATIONS

5-HT	serotonin
5-HTTLPR	serotonin transporter polymorphism
ABCB1	ATP-binding cassette subfamily B member 1
AIWG	antipsychotic-induced weight gain
BD	bipolar disorder
BDNF	brain-derived neurotrophic factor
CIA	clozapine-induced agranulocytosis
COMT	catechol-*O*-methyl-transferase
CPI	Clinical Pharmacogenetics Implementation Consortium
CPS1	carbamoyl phosphate synthetase 1
CRH	corticotropin-releasing hormone
CYP450	cytochrome P450
DA	dopamine
DPWG	Royal Dutch Association for the Advancement of Pharmacy—Pharmacogenetics Working Group
EMs	extensive metabolizers
EPSs	extrapyramidal symptoms
FDA	Food and Drug Administration
FGA	first-generation antipsychotic
FKBP5	FK506-binding protein 51
GR	glucocorticoid receptor
GWAS	genome-wide association studies
HCSC	Health Care Service Corporation
HLA	human leukocyte antigen
HPA axis	hypothalamic–pituitary–adrenal axis
HTR1A	serotonin receptor 1A
HTR2A	serotonin receptor 2A
IMs	intermediate metabolizers
LD	linkage disequilibrium
MAO	monoamine oxidase
MAOIs	monoamine oxidase inhibitors
MDD	major depressive disorder
ncRNAs	noncoding RNAs
NE	norepinephrine
OTC	ornithine transcarbamylase
P-gp	P-glycoprotein
PMs	poor metabolizers
PMDA	Pharmaceuticals and Medical Devices Agency
PRS	polygenic risk scores

SERT	serotonin transporter
SGA	second-generation antipsychotic
SJS	Stevens–Johnson syndrome
SNP	single nucleotide polymorphism
SNRIs	serotonin norepinephrine reuptake inhibitors
SSRIs	selective serotonin reuptake inhibitors
TCAs	tricyclic antidepressants
TD	tardive dyskinesia
TPH	tryptophan hydroxylase
UM	ultrarapid metabolizers
VNTR	variable number tandem repeat

1. INTRODUCTION

The development and introduction of psychotropic drugs in the second half of the 20th century was a major breakthrough in the treatment of mental illness and revolutionized the way in which these disorders are managed. Nevertheless, mental illness still poses a major burden on both personal well-being and socioeconomical welfare, partly as a result of the long time needed to identify the right treatment for each subject: in 2010, mental illness along with substance use disorders accounted for 10.4% of the global burden of disease and they were the leading cause of years lived with disability among all disease groups (Patel et al., 2016). In the same year the global cost of mental disorders was estimated to be approximately US$2.5 billion and by 2039 that figure is projected to increase by 240%, to US$6.0 trillion (Bloom et al., 2011). Medications are effective in only a subset of patients or produce partial response and debilitating side effects can discourage adherence. In major depressive disorder (MDD), schizophrenia, and bipolar disorder (BD), only ~1/3 of patients reach full and stable symptom remission and do not discontinue their medications (Lieberman et al., 2005; Rush et al., 2006; Thase, 2007). In consideration of such data, the prediction of response to treatment has become a crucial but daunting task for clinicians. Personalized prescription can be implemented as personalized dosing and/or drug selection and it could take into account both genetic and environmental variables (e.g., comedications, life stress events, smoking, foods, and beverages). Genetic variants were estimated to account for 20%–95% of variability in central nervous system drug disposition and pharmacodynamics (Cacabelos et al., 2012).

The greatest part of human genetic variability is explained by single nucleotide polymorphisms (SNPs) that are single base pair changes in the DNA sequence. Less common and larger variations include deletions, insertions, and copy number variations, but genetic studies of complex traits (such as drug response) are usually focused on SNPs. Pharmacogenetics is the study of how human genetic information impacts on drug response/side effects with the goal to provide personalized treatments. Insights into how genetic variation influences drug response can also provide clues relating to underlying pharmacological and pathogenic mechanisms. The first pharmacogenetic studies were focused on candidate genes selected on the base of previous knowledge about the pharmacokinetics and pharmacodynamics of psychotropic drugs. A number of studies have been performed but yielded inconclusive findings for the most part of the investigated genes. The reasons behind this disappointing result include the investigation of individual polymorphisms with small effect sizes (responsible for not more than 2%–3% of the variance in response or side effect of interest) that was often performed in underpowered sample sizes; the possible lack of any genuine association in some cases should also be considered. On the other hand, candidate gene association studies allowed the identification of polymorphisms in key genes for the mechanisms of medication action or metabolism with possible clinical applications that are discussed further on in this chapter.

The introduction of chip-based microarray technology capable of interrogating thousands of polymorphisms whining the genome has given fresh momentum to genetic association studies and ushered new design studies, namely, genome-wide association studies (GWAS). Such advances have brought in a new term, pharmacogenomics, which reflects the shift from single genes to virtually the whole genome, accurately genotyping 500,000 to over 4 million SNPs in a cost-effective manner. GWAS do not need a priori hypothesis overcoming the problem that the mechanisms of psychotropic drug action are not completely known. Further, the most significantly associated polymorphisms in behavioral GWAS were found in noncoding sequence (Zhang & Lupski, 2015) and the disruption in a gene or pathway function is due to the cumulative effect of multiple variants. GWAS are focused on the study of common polymorphisms, in line with the theory named common disease/common variant (Reich & Lander, 2001). According to this model, common disorders are influenced by genetic variations that are also common in the general population and therefore the effect size (or penetrance) for each single polymorphism is expected to be small relative to that found for rare disorders. This assumption and the heritability of common disorders imply that multiple common alleles influence disease susceptibility. This theory and GWAS have also some limitations: (1) microarrays include a limited number of preselected SNPs, while over 39 millions are currently known according to the first data release of the Haplotype Reference Consortium (McCarthy et al., 2016); (2) statistical methods for the analysis of multimarker genetic effects in large databases are not easy to develop and implement; and (3) the effect of rare and unknown genetic polymorphisms should not be overlooked since different rare variants in specific pathways may be responsible for relevant effects in common disorders. The latter hypothesis is suggested by the observation that the heritability of several common traits remains partly unexplained considering common variants only and it is usually defined missing heritability. Further, the high number of variants analyzed in a GWAS requires the application of a strict multiple testing correction, called genome-wide correction, that implies usually samples of thousands of subjects are required to have adequate statistical power and variants with small but genuine effects may not be detected.

In the following paragraphs the main findings of candidate gene studies and GWAS are described and discussed for antidepressants, antipsychotics, and mood stabilizers (primarily lithium). Ethnicity is often considered in genetic studies since the frequency of the most part of polymorphisms significantly varies across populations. Present (and possible future) clinical applications are also taken into account.

2. ANTIDEPRESSANTS

The vast majority of pharmacogenetic studies were focused on selective serotonin reuptake inhibitors (SSRIs), although several have examined serotonin norepinephrine reuptake inhibitors (SNRIs) or older drugs such as monoamine oxidase inhibitors (MAOIs) and tricyclic antidepressants (TCAs).

2.1 Candidate Genes

Candidate genes can be classified according to their relevance to either pharmacokinetic or pharmacodynamic mechanisms: the former comprises genes involved in antidepressants metabolism and transport, the latter includes genes involved in monoaminergic neurotransmission, neuroprotection and neuroplasticity, second messenger cascades, and glucocorticoid signaling (Table 1).

Table 1 Overview of the Different Methodological Approaches Applied to the Study of Psychotropic Pharmacogenetics/Pharmacogenomics, Most Interesting/Replicated Findings for Each Class of Psychotropic Medication and Existing Clinical Applications

Drug Class and Phenotype	Candidate Gene Studies	GWAS	Aggregated Tests	Clinical Applications
Antidepressant response	SCL6A4, HTR2A, ABCB1, FKBP5, BDNF, GNB3, CYP2C19, CYP2D6	AUTS2	Pathways involved in neuroplasticity, neural survival, and inflammation	SLC6A4, HTR2A, BDNF, CYP2C19, CYP2D6, COMT, ABCB1, FKBP5
Antidepressants-induced side effects	CYP2C19, CYP2D6, SCL6A4	EMID2	—	CYP2C19, CYP2D6, SCL6A4
Lithium relapse prophylaxis	INPP1, GSK-3β, NR1D1, SLC6A4, COMT, DRD1, BDNF, NTRK2	AL157359.3 AL157359.4 (two noncoding RNAs)	Glutamatergic regulatory pathway	—
Carbamazepine-induced Stevens–Johnson syndrome	HLA-B*1502 (Han Chinese ancestry), HLA-A*3101 (European ancestry)	—	—	HLA-B*1502, HLA-A*3101
Valproate-induced liver impairment and metabolic abnormalities	POLG, GNB3, CPS1, OTC	—	—	POLG, CPS1, OTC

Antipsychotics response	DRD2, DRD3, HTR2A, HTR1A, HTR2C, COMT, GNB3, BDNF, ZNF804A, CYP2D6, CYP2C19, ABCB1	DRD2, ATP1A2, PDE4D, GPR98, NR3C1, MEIS2	Polygenic overlap between schizophrenia risk and antipsychotic response	CYP2D6, CYP2C19, DRD2, HTR2A, HTR2C
Antipsychotics-induced weight gain	HTR2C, MC4R, ADRA2A, DRD2, GNB3, INSIG2	PTPRD	Pathways involved in glucosamine metabolic process, amino sugar metabolic process, and regulation of peptidyl tyrosine phosphorylation	HTR2C
Antipsychotics-induced tardive dyskinesia	CYP2D6, DRD2 HTR2A, HSPG2, SLC18A2, DPP6	ZNF202, rs17022444, and rs7669317 (intergenic SNPs)	GABA receptor signaling pathway	CYP2D6, DRD2 HTR2A
Clozapine-induced agranulocytosis	HLA-DQB1	HLA-DQB1, HLA-B, SLCO1B3, SLCO1B7, UBAP2, STARD9	—	HLA-DQB1

GWAS, genome-wide association studies.

2.1.1 Pharmacokinetics

The core processes responsible for antidepressant metabolism are catalyzed by cytochrome P450 (CYP450) enzymes (phase I reactions), while uridine 5′-diphospho-glucuronosyltransferase enzymes (phase II reactions) have a marginal role; thus, they not discussed in this chapter.

The CYP450 superfamily is a class of enzymes, encompassing over 50 isoforms, with a major role in the oxidation and reduction of both endogenous and xenobiotic substances (phase I reactions). The isoenzymes mainly involved in antidepressant metabolism are CYP2D6, CYP2C19, CYP2C9, and CYP2B6; CYP2D6 and CYP2C19 have received the greatest attention in existing studies. The genes coding for these isoforms are highly polymorphic, and alleles may show normal, partially, or totally defective activity, defining some metabolizing groups according to the allele combination, namely, poor metabolizers (PMs), lacking functional enzymes due to two copies of defective alleles; intermediate metabolizers (IMs), usually carrying one functional and one defective allele, or two partially defective alleles; extensive metabolizers (EMs), carrying two functional genes; and ultrarapid metabolizers (UMs), carrying more than two active copies of a CYP450 gene or functional polymorphisms associated with increased gene expression or protein functionality. The metabolizing group of belonging shows a demonstrated correlation with antidepressant pharmacokinetics (e.g., drug and metabolite plasma levels, plasma half-life, oral clearance), while the possible association with antidepressant response and side effects is controversial (Porcelli, Fabbri, Spina, Serretti, & De Ronchi, 2011). Some studies reported that PMs may have increased risk of antidepressant-induced side effects, while UMs may be less likely to show positive response to treatment, but others did not report any association (Porcelli, Drago, Fabbri, & Serretti, 2011; Porcelli, Fabbri, Spina, et al., 2011). Several reasons may be responsible for this inconsistency: (1) there is no clear correlation between antidepressant plasma levels and response (with the exception of TCAs), reflecting the difference between antidepressant concentration in the brain and plasma; thus, differences in response across CYP450-metabolizing groups are expected to be small at most; (2) extreme metabolizing groups, particularly PMs, are quite rare in the most part of populations (e.g., CYP2C19 PMs are ~2% in Caucasian populations) and existing studies were probably underpowered to detect differences involving extreme metabolizing groups; no meta-analysis of existing evidence has been performed.

The ATP-binding cassette subfamily B member 1 (ABCB1) gene, encoding the P-glycoprotein (P-gp), is the most relevant gene in antidepressant transport. P-gp is an ATP-dependent drug efflux pump for xenobiotic compounds which limits uptake and accumulation of some lipophilic drugs, including a number of antidepressants, into the brain. Some polymorphisms within ABCB1—rs2032582, rs1045642, rs2032583, rs2235040—were associated with altered P-gp expression or function and thus they appear of particular interest in the field of pharmacogenetics. Higher treatment efficacy was found in rs2032582 TT genotype, rs2032583 C allele, and rs2235040 A allele carriers. These variants may possibly impact on treatment response to antidepressants by affecting the transport of drugs across the brain–blood barrier with a mechanism that does not imply modification of drug plasma concentration (Fabbri, Crisafulli, Calabrò, Spina, & Serretti, 2016). There is preliminary evidence suggesting ABCB1 variants may provide valid clinical guide to antidepressant prescription (Breitenstein et al., 2014).

2.1.2 Pharmacodynamics

Antidepressants are thought to exert their therapeutic action through monoamines modulation, at least partly; thus, genes involved in monoaminergic transmission have received much attention in pharmacogenetic studies. Serotonin (5-HT) has a primary role in the regulation of mood and emotions (Nutt et al., 2007). SLC6A4 gene codes for the serotonin transporter (SERT), one of the main sites of antidepressant action; therefore, it has been the most extensively studied. An insertion/deletion functional polymorphism (5-HTTLPR) within the promoter of this gene influences transcriptional level. In detail, the 16-repeat long (L) allele produces twice the basal expression compared to the 14-repeat long (S) allele. The L allele has been associated with better antidepressant efficacy and lower risk of side effects, especially in patients of Caucasian ancestry treated with SSRIs, despite not all studies were concordant (Kato & Serretti, 2010; Porcelli, Fabbri, & Serretti, 2012). Studies in patients of Asian descent produced controversial outcomes, possibly as a consequence of: (1) different 5-HTTLPR allelic frequencies across populations (42% of Caucasians carry the S allele in comparison to 79% of Asians) and (2) genetic variants within the SLC6A4 gene or related genes which may concur to gene expression regulation. Other functional polymorphisms within the SLC6A4 gene have provided more controversial results compared to 5-HTTLPR. The rs25531

G variant in conjunction with the 5-HTTLPR L allele was reported to reduce gene expression, nullifying the protective effect of the L allele, but the most part of studies failed to demonstrate an effect on antidepressant efficacy (Fabbri, Di Girolamo, & Serretti, 2013). The 12-repeat variant in the variable number tandem repeat (VNTR) Stin2 was associated with higher gene expression and it may determine higher chances of response in patients of Asian ethnicity, but few data with high heterogeneity are available (Niitsu, Fabbri, Bentini, & Serretti, 2013).

Among serotoninergic genes, 5-HT receptors were also widely investigated, especially 5-HT receptors 2A (HTR2A) and 1A (HTR1A). HTR2A codes for the main serotoninergic postsynaptic excitatory receptor and several polymorphisms in this gene were associated with antidepressant response, mainly to SSRIs. The most studied polymorphisms were rs7997012, rs6311, and rs6313, and for the first homozygous for the A allele were reported to have an 18% reduction in absolute risk of having no response to treatment (McMahon et al., 2006). HTR2A rs6311 G allele was weakly associated with antidepressant response in Asian populations, while rs6313 yielded mainly negative findings (Niitsu et al., 2013). HTR1A codes for an autoreceptor, expressed both at postsynaptic and presynaptic level, with the role of preventing the further release of 5-HT with a negative feedback. Within the HTR1A gene, rs6295 was the most investigated polymorphism because the G allele was associated with an upregulation of the receptor, which supposedly contrasts the antidepressant action. Meta-analytic evidence showed that rs6295 may not have a role in antidepressant response (Niitsu et al., 2013), but it may modulate response only in patients with particular clinical features, i.e., melancholic depression (Baune et al., 2008).

Other genes are relevant in monoamine metabolism (synthesis and degradation), namely, tryptophan hydroxylase (TPH), catechol-O-methyltransferase (COMT), and monoamine oxidase (MAO). TPH catalyzes the limiting step in the rate of 5-HT biosynthesis. Two main TPH isoforms have been identified, TPH1 and TPH2, both are expressed in the brain, but pharmacogenetic studies were focused on the former because the functional polymorphism rs1800532 was reported within it. rs1800532 (A218C) is located in a potential GATA transcription factor-binding site (i.e., a site on DNA that regulates the binding of transcription factors) and the rarer A allele is associated with lower gene expression and decreased 5-HT synthesis. According to the monoaminergic theory of depression this may determine worse antidepressant efficacy. Pharmacogenetic studies, however, yielded heterogeneous and mostly negative results (Niitsu et al., 2013). No correlation with antidepressant-induced side effects was established either (Kato & Serretti, 2010).

In the COMT gene the functional rs4680 (Val108/158Met) has been considered particularly relevant since the Val/Val homozygote catabolizes dopamine (DA) at up to four times the rate of Met/Met homozygote, with a modulating effect on DA bioavailability in the frontal cortex. Pharmacogenetic studies mainly reported the Met variant as the favorable allele for antidepressant response, with an allele dose effect (better outcome in Met/Met carriers and intermediate outcome in Met/Val carriers), in line with the monoaminergic theory of depression (Fabbri et al., 2013). Recent meta-analytic evidence did not confirm this association (Niitsu et al., 2013).

MAO has two known isoforms, MAOA and MAOB: the former metabolizes norepinephrine (NE) and 5-HT and contributes to the breakdown of DA. An interesting functional VNTR is located within the promoter of the MAOA gene: this variant regulates the transcriptional level and is linked to variations in the enzyme activity. Consistently, it was correlated with the concentrations of 5-hydroxyindoleacetic acid (the main metabolite of 5-HT) in cerebrospinal fluid. Despite promising preclinical findings, pharmacogenetic studies mainly failed to establish any conclusive correlation with clinical outcomes (Fabbri et al., 2013).

Finally, other monoaminergic transporters were studied in addition to SERT, even if in a more marginal way. SLC6A2 codes for the NE transporter, which is among the main targets of antidepressant, especially some TCAs and SNRIs. Pharmacogenetic studies reported some evidence of association with polymorphisms within this gene (rs5569, rs2242446, rs36024), but confirmatory findings are still lacking (Fabbri, Porcelli, & Serretti, 2014). Compared to 5-HT and NE, the dopaminergic system has been less investigated in antidepressant pharmacogenetics, although both preclinical and clinical data support its involvement in the pathogenesis of MDD. Several studies supported a role of the DRD2 gene (dopamine D2 receptor) in antidepressants pharmacodynamics, leading to the hypothesis that the dopaminergic–mesolimbic pathway may represent a final common pathway in antidepressant action (Porcelli, Drago, et al., 2011). Nevertheless, pharmacogenetic studies investigating the functional polymorphism DRD2 rs1801028 (S311C) reported negative findings. Promising results were reached for rs4245147, although confirmations are still lacking (Perlis et al., 2010).

The neurotrophic hypothesis of MDD was formulated after the observation that hippocampus atrophy following stress was reversed by antidepressants in parallel to an increase in the expression of neurotrophic factors, especially brain-derived neurotrophic factor (BDNF).

The Valine66Methionine (Val66Met) SNP (rs6265) is the most investigated variant within the BDNF gene. In vitro analysis has demonstrated that the variant BDNF Met protein is less efficiently targeted by the secretory pathway than the BDNF Val protein, which implies its decreased secretion. In humans, the rs6265 Met allele has been associated with reduced hippocampal volume, reduced cognitive performance, and psychiatric disorders including mood disorders and anxiety, despite none of these associations have been consistently replicated (Glatt & Lee, 2016). Pharmacogenetic studies mainly reported better response in the heterozygote genotype, particularly in Asian populations possibly due to the considerable BDNF allele and haplotype diversity among global populations (Niitsu et al., 2013). This result can be explained by animal models showing that although BDNF exerts an antidepressant effect, BDNF overexpression may increase stress-induced plasticity in the amygdala and increase anxiety-like behaviors (Govindarajan et al., 2006).

Second messenger signaling proteins are also involved in the generation of cellular responses that are involved in neural plasticity. GNB3 encodes for guanine nucleotide-binding protein (G protein), beta polypeptide 3, that is involved in the generation of second messengers in response to a number of signals, such as neurotransmitters and hormones. The T allele of the rs5443 (C825T) polymorphism leads to a splice variant that results in altered activity of the protein. T allele carriers show better response to antidepressants, controversial results have been also reported though (Niitsu et al., 2013).

The hypothalamic–pituitary–adrenal (HPA) axis dysfunction is one of the main neuroendocrine abnormalities found in MDD. FK506-binding protein 51 (FKBP5 gene) acts as a key factor of the HPA axis by modulating glucocorticoid receptor (GR) sensitivity. When FKBP5 is bound to the receptor complex, cortisol binds with lower affinity and nuclear translocation of the receptor occurs to a less extent. FKBP5 expression is induced by GR activation, as an ultrashort feedback loop for GR sensitivity. Several polymorphisms (rs3800373, rs1360780, rs9296158, rs9470080) were associated with enhanced expression of FKBP5 and they lead to increased GR resistance and decreased efficiency of the negative feedback of the stress hormone axis; thus, they may increase the risk of MDD and influence antidepressant efficacy. The effect of rs1360780 and rs3800373 on antidepressant response was the most strongly supported (Niitsu et al., 2013) and the former has preliminary evidence of clinical usefulness in guiding antidepressant prescription (Stamm et al., 2016). Other less investigated HPA axis genes are corticotropin-releasing hormone (CRH) receptors 1 and 2 (CRHR1 and CRHR2) and GR itself, coded by the NR3C1 gene. A number of variants have been suggested to influence antidepressant response, but results are heterogeneous and need further study (Fabbri et al., 2013).

2.2 Genome-Wide Association Studies

GWAS of antidepressant response and side effects did not have great success in the identification of the individual polymorphisms influencing these traits. On the other hand, the use of aggregated tests provided some encouraging findings, since they increase the power of GWAS compared to single SNP analysis. For example, a sample size of ~2000 subjects is required in a GWAS to provide adequate power to identify individual variants associated with a binary trait with heritability ~40%. The power increase in an aggregated approach can be attributed to the reduction in the number of tests performed and the capture of the cumulative effects of a number of variants (the disruption of a gene or pathway functioning is the result of cumulative effects of variants within it) (Li, Samuels, Zhao, Shyr, & Guo, 2017). These considerations can at least partially explain the negative results found by GWAS of antidepressant response and their meta-analyses in samples of mostly Caucasian origin (GENDEP Investigators et al., 2013; Tansey et al., 2012). The scenario does not change much when considering GWAS performed in Asian samples (Biernacka et al., 2016), but one study reported some genome-wide significant signals in the AUTS2 gene (rs7785360 and rs12698828), a gene implicated in neurodevelopmental disorders including autism but also schizoaffective or bipolar affective disorders (Myung et al., 2015). The latter study applied a multistage design (i.e., the sample was split into three subsamples for focused replication of the initial findings) and this strategy may increase power. Anyway, AUTS2 signals were not replicated in other samples. GWAS results were not more successful for antidepressant-induced side effects (Adkins et al., 2012; Clark et al., 2012). The latter did report a genome-wide significant finding in an intronic SNP within EMID2 (collagen alpha-1), mediating the effects of citalopram on vision/hearing side effects. Besides the unclear clinical relevance of these side effects, the association was not replicated.

Aggregated approaches mostly consisted in pathway analysis, i.e., the analysis of all genetic variants in a group of genes functionally related to each other (e.g., a chemical process, a cellular signaling cascade, proteins contributing to particular cellular functions such as cell adhesion or migration, survival or proliferation). Thus genome-wide data are usually required for performing pathway analysis. The most strongly supported pathways in antidepressant response are involved in neuroplasticity and inflammation processes. Indeed the long-term potentiation pathway, the inorganic cation transmembrane transporter activity pathway, and the GAP43 pathway (Fabbri et al., 2015) are involved in hippocampal plasticity and neurogenesis and they were associated with antidepressant efficacy (Cocchi et al., 2016; Fabbri et al., 2015; Hunter et al., 2013). These pathways include a number of genes coding for glutamate receptors (GRM1, GRM5, GRIA1, GRIN2A, GRIN2B, GRIN2C), postsynaptic L-type voltage-dependent Ca^{2+} channels (CACNA1C, CACNA1C, CACNB1, CACNB2), regulators of GABA and glutamatergic neurotransmission (e.g., ZDHHC7, NRG1, and HOMER1), and cell adhesion processes (e.g., FN1, EFNA5, and EPHA5). Some pathways mediating inflammatory processes were also associated with antidepressant response, in detail: the KEGG B cell receptor signaling pathway, the antigen processing and presentation pathway, and the tumor necrosis factor pathway (Fabbri, Marsano, et al., 2014; Fabbri, Porcelli, & Serretti, 2014; Hunter et al., 2013).

Polygenic risk scores (PRS) are another aggregated approach that has been recently developed in order to take into account the cumulative effect of a number of variants in complex traits and the observation that single variants may not have significant effects per se but in conjunction with other variants. The most used approach consists in calculating the PRS as the sum of associated alleles, weighted by effect sizes, for polymorphisms with *P* values less than predefined thresholds in a training sample, then to test the predictive ability of the PRS in a replication or target sample. Flexibility is allowed in setting the *P* threshold, i.e., from several to thousands of *P* thresholds can be tested with the aim to improve prediction at the price of a degree of uncertainty. This approach has produced still few applications in antidepressant pharmacogenomics (GENDEP Investigators et al., 2013), but it is expected to have more spread use in the next years.

2.3 Clinical Applications

Available clinical applications are based on few candidate genes selected from the results of candidate gene association studies. A number of pharmacogenetic tests are commercialized by private companies, but they are still not recommended by clinical guidelines and they are not refunded by public health systems. The main reason is the lack of demonstration of effectiveness and favorable cost/benefit ratio independently from the producing companies, since the prediction algorithms are not publicly available.

Some of the genes included in these pharmacogenetic tests are SLC6A4, serotonin receptor genes, CYP450 isoforms, COMT, BDNF (Fabbri et al., 2016). Few genes have been tested for clinical application in guiding antidepressant treatment by academic institutions, i.e., ABCB1 and FKBP5, with preliminary positive evidence (Breitenstein et al., 2014; Stamm et al., 2016). Currently, the only polymorphisms included as pharmacogenetic biomarkers in antidepressant drug labeling are in CYP2C19 and CYP2D6 according to the Food and Drug Administration (FDA) (Center for Drug Evaluation and Research, 2017) for the possible higher risk of side effects, toxicity, drug interactions, and possible need of dose adjustments in poor metabolizers. Clinical guidelines, such as those provided by the Clinical Pharmacogenetics Implementation Consortium (CPIC) and the Royal Dutch Association for the Advancement of Pharmacy—Pharmacogenetics Working Group (DPWG), include recommendations based on CYP2C19 and CYP2D6 functional groups, similar to that included in drug labels. Currently, there are ~20 antidepressants of different classes that have pharmacogenetic biomarkers according to these guidelines, and in several cases dosing recommendations based on CYP2C19 and CYP2D6 functionality are included, for example, for some TCAs (e.g., amitriptyline, clomipramine, nortriptyline) and SSRIs (e.g., citalopram, escitalopram, paroxetine) (Whirl-Carrillo et al., 2012).

Taking into account the complex nature of antidepressant mechanisms of action and the recent development of aggregated tests, future clinical applications may include arrays designed to include a number of polymorphisms throughout the genome, in specific genes or pathways, and they may be able to classify each patient within a spectrum of risk of nonresponse or side effects.

3. MOOD STABILIZERS

Compared to the extensive literature about antidepressants, the pharmacogenetics of mood-stabilizing drugs has been less investigated (Table 1). Phenotypes of interest in bipolar disorder range from acute mania to depression, but most studies focus on relapse prevention. Relatively few studies were published and they were almost exclusively focused on lithium.

There is consolidated evidence suggesting that response to lithium is a familiar trait, making it a suitable target for genetic studies. Specifically, about one-third of lithium-treated patients are excellent responders, showing total prevention of the episodes: these patients are clinically characterized by an episodic clinical course, complete remission, a family history of bipolar disorder, no psychiatric comorbidity, and a hyperthymic temperament. Lithium-responsive bipolar disorder may then constitute a distinctive subtype of the disorder with an important genetic burden (Goes, 2016).

3.1 Candidate Genes

Candidate genes were selected on the basis of the mechanisms of action of lithium and/or the neurobiology of bipolar disorder. They are primarily related to the inositol signaling pathway, the circadian signaling system, various neurotransmitter systems, and neuroprotection. Few findings were replicated at least in two studies and involved eight genes (INPP1, GSK-3β, NR1D1, SLC6A4, COMT, DRD1, BDNF, and NTRK2).

Inositol depletion is one of the first hypotheses formulated to explain the mechanism of action of lithium. The inositol phosphate pathway is a second messenger system involved in signal transduction. Lithium directly inhibits two important enzymes of this system: inositol monophosphatase and inositol polyphosphatase, leading to a reduction of inositol levels. Based on the evidence that this inhibition is more pronounced when the substrate concentration is high, lithium has been suggested to act on this system only in case of a pathological overactivation. Although promising results from preclinical investigations support the inositol depletion hypothesis, pharmacogenetic findings were far less conclusive. An association between lithium response and a polymorphism of the inositol polyphosphate 1-phosphatase gene was reported (Budde, Degner, Brockmöller, & Schulze, 2017).

One of the most investigated targets of lithium is the glycogen synthase kinase 3 enzyme (GSK-3β), involved in synaptic plasticity, apoptosis, and the circadian cycle. Through its inhibition, lithium affects a large number of downstream targets, including several transcription factors and the Wnt signaling pathway. The −50 T/C SNP in GSK-3β, disrupting a transcription factor-binding site in the promoter and producing altered gene splicing, may be associated with lithium response; a role for this pharmacogenetics variant has been largely documented. In a network coordinating circadian rhythms, GSK-3β interacts with a number of proteins including Rev-Erbα, coded by NR1D1 gene, and a variant of NR1D1 is possibly associated with prophylactic lithium response (Pisanu, Melis, & Squassina, 2016).

Variants in genes involved in neurotransmission were hypothesized to affect lithium response, similar to antidepressants. In particular, the functional promoter polymorphism (5-HTTLPR) of the SERT gene (SLC6A4) may influence lithium response in a similar way to antidepressant response: the S allele, associated with a lower gene expression level, may predispose to lithium nonresponse; this is the most replicated pharmacogenetic finding for lithium response to date. The COMT rs4680 (Val108/158Met) variant may modulate lithium response in addition to antidepressant response, The Met allele, resulting in a lower DA catabolism, appears to be the favorable variant. Lastly, we mention the −48 A/G polymorphism in the DA receptor D1 (DRD1) gene for which G allele and G/G genotype were associated with a predisposition to bipolar illness and a poorer prophylactic effect of lithium (Pisanu, Melis, et al., 2016).

In the context of the neurotrophic hypothesis of bipolar disorders, BDNF and the TrkB receptor play an important role in lithium mechanism of action. Two polymorphisms within the BDNF gene, i.e., Val66Met and −270 C/T, could be relevant to lithium prophylactic action. The Val66Met in BDNF may interact with the SLC6A4 5-HTTLPR, having Val/Val genotype and S allele a synergic effect predisposing to lithium nonresponse (Rybakowski et al., 2007). BDNF binds to TrkB receptor, coded by the NTRK2 gene; variants in this gene may predict lithium response, but only in patient who experience euphoric mania, suggesting a genetic basis for this well-known clinical predictor of good response (Rybakowski, 2013).

Pharmacogenetics of lithium-related adverse effects was insufficiently explored. There may be an association between the C allele in the functional −50 C/T polymorphism of GSK3B and a decrease in kidney function, a very common adverse event of lithium, in long-term lithium-treated bipolar patients (Rybakowski et al., 2013).

3.2 Genome-Wide Association Studies

In the past few years, GWAS suggested several genetic variants that may be associated with lithium response (Chen et al., 2014; Perlis et al., 2009; Song et al., 2017; Squassina et al., 2011). However, most of these GWAS were limited by small sample size. Collaborative approaches such as the International Consortium on Lithium Genetics (ConLiGen) (Schulze et al., 2010) have the potential to overcome the limitations of previous studies by collecting large cohorts of patients with long-term follow-up. In 2016, the largest study on lithium response conducted to date—more than 2500 individuals, recruited from 22 ConLiGen sites—reported intriguing data supporting the role of two noncoding RNAs (ncRNAs), AL157359.3 and AL157359.4, in lithium response (Hou et al., 2016). ncRNAs are RNA molecules that are not translated into a protein acting as important regulators of gene expression; they are analytically classified as long ncRNAs (more than 100 nucleotides in length) and small ncRNAs (less than 100 nucleotides in length) according to their molecular size (Gomes, Nolasco, & Soares, 2013). The aforementioned finding was also replicated in a small, independent sample of bipolar patients prospectively evaluated for lithium response (Pisanu, Papadima, Del Zompo, & Squassina, 2016). In the future, valuable results will be available through ongoing initiatives, such as the Pharmacogenomics of Bipolar Disorder study, a prospective nonrandomized open trial of lithium monotherapy (Oedegaard et al., 2016).

Using an aggregated approach it was possible to identify a glutamatergic regulatory pathway, expressed in the same brain regions subject to tissue volume loss in bipolar disorder, that mediates lithium response in individuals of European ancestry. This network comprises a number of genes coding for transcription factors (ARNTL, CREB1, NR1D1), calcium channels subunits (CACNG2, CACNA1C), proteins for glutamate synaptic transmission (SLC1A2, GRIA2), regulators of sodium channel activity (ANK3) and chromatin remodeling (CDKN1A), and the above mentioned GSK3B gene (Higgins, Allyn-Feuer, Barbour, & Athey, 2015).

3.3 Clinical Applications

Carbamazepine, lamotrigine, and valproic acid are commonly used mood stabilizers, but they were investigated in a relatively lower number of pharmacogenetics studies compared to lithium. However, findings led up to some clinical applications.

The most relevant discovery regards a rare, but potentially fatal, adverse effect known as toxic epidermal necrolysis or Stevens–Johnson syndrome (SJS). Patients of Han Chinese ancestry who carry the human leukocyte antigen (HLA) marker known as HLA-B*1502 are more likely to develop SJS when exposed to carbamazepine. Clinical testing for this marker, which is also present in other Asian populations, has been included as a "boxed warning" in the labeling of carbamazepine by the FDA (Chung et al., 2004). In populations of European descent HLA-B*1502 is uncommon but in this group carriers of HLA-A*3101 allele were reported to have similar increased risk of developing the SJS. This last variant is a risk factor for adverse cutaneous reaction among Asians too, although rarer in this ethnic group (McCormack et al., 2011).

Some genes have been associated with valproate-induced side effects and they have been included in drug labels according to several regulatory agencies. Valproate-induced liver impairment was related to mitochondrial DNA depletion and mutations in the POLG gene that codes for the mitochondrial DNA polymerase gamma in pediatric patients (Pronicka et al., 2011; Saneto et al., 2010). Thus, POLG gene testing has been recommended by the US FDA in children/adolescents since they are particularly at risk of developing valproate-induced liver toxicity (PharmGKB, 2018). Variants in the genes coding for carbamoyl phosphate synthetase 1 (CPS1) and ornithine transcarbamylase (OTC) impact on the risk of hyperammonemia via impairment of urea cycle in valproate-treated patients. In a small study, the rs1047891A (4217C > A) polymorphism of CPS1 was associated with an increased risk of hyperammonemia when receiving combined treatment of valproate with two or more other antiepileptics (Yagi et al., 2010). This SNP is also associated with lower CPS1 activity (Summar et al., 2004). Finally, OTC deficiency, an X-linked semidominant disorder, is the most common inherited defect in ureagenesis resulting in hyperammonemia (Choi et al., 2015). Detrimental variants in CPS1 or OTC contraindicate valproate treatment according to drug labels provided by Pharmaceuticals and Medical Devices Agency (PMDA) and Health Care Service Corporation (HCSC) (Whirl-Carrillo et al., 2012).

4. ANTIPSYCHOTICS

Second-generation antipsychotics (SGAs) pharmacogenetics has been more investigated compared to first-generation antipsychotics (FGAs). Antipsychotics are routinely used in the treatment of not only schizophrenia and related spectrum disorders but also for mood disorders and various other conditions, such as obsessive–compulsive disorder, eating disorders, or behavioral disturbances. However, the investigated phenotypes mainly relate to schizophrenia spectrum disorders and include response in acute disease, long-term prophylaxis, and liability to side effects (Table 1).

4.1 Candidate Genes

Similar to antidepressants and mood stabilizers, candidate genes investigated as predictors of antipsychotic treatment outcomes are involved in either pharmacokinetics or pharmacodynamics of these drugs. In the case of antipsychotics, special attention has been directed to dynamic and kinetic mechanisms relevant to side effects. Harmful side effects of antipsychotic treatment are indeed one of the strongest predictors of noncompliance reported by first episode schizophrenia patients, with an estimated noncompliance rate of 42% (Cramer & Rosenheck, 1998). Antipsychotic-induced weight gain (AIWG), tardive dyskinesia (TD), and clozapine-induced agranulocytosis (CIA) have been particularly investigated.

4.1.1 Pharmacokinetics

Candidate genes relevant to the pharmacokinetics of antipsychotics are essentially the same involved in antidepressant metabolism, i.e., isoenzymes of the CYP450 superfamily and the ABCB1 gene.

As we previously outlined, functional polymorphisms in CYP450 genes lead to decreased or increased catalytic activity, thereby distinguishing different metabolizing groups. Approximately 40% of antipsychotics are major substrates of CYP2D6, 23% of CYP3A4, and 18% of CYP1A2 (Cacabelos, Cacabelos, & Aliev, 2013). CYP2D6 is not inducible and genotype strongly affects the bioavailability of many antipsychotics. CYP2D6-poor metabolizers were reported to have higher dose-corrected levels of risperidone, haloperidol, aripiprazole, and perphenazine following antipsychotic treatment. However, genetic variation in CYP2D6 seems to exert a stronger influence on the occurrence of adverse effects than on medication response, most likely because plasma levels of antipsychotics often do not correlate with treatment response (Sim & Ingelman-Sundberg, 2010). Specifically, CYP2D6-poor or -intermediate metabolizers probably have greater risk and severity of TD compared to extensive metabolizers. TD is a specific extrapyramidal symptom (EPS) characterized by repetitive and involuntary movements such as grimacing, rapid eye blinking, and lip smacking. It is a potentially irreversible side effect experienced by an estimated 25% of patients treated long-term with FGAs (MacNeil & Müller, 2016). CYP2D6-poor metabolizers were also demonstrated to have higher risk of proarrhythmic effects when treated with pimozide, one of the highest-risk antipsychotic regarding this type of side effect. Thus, CYP2D6 genotyping is now recommended in the pimozide US product label before exceeding 4 mg of pimozide daily in adults or 0.05 mg/kg/day in children (Rogers et al., 2012). CYP3A4 is the most abundant CYP450 isoform in the human liver; it is inducible, and its activity can be altered by medications. Available studies suggested no effect of CYP3A4 genotype on antipsychotic plasma levels (clozapine (Jaquenoud Sirot et al., 2009) and risperidone (Du et al., 2010)), although the decreased activity of the CYP3A4*1G allele was associated with greater improvement in psychotic symptoms (Du et al., 2010). The CYP1A2 enzyme is inducible, but genetics is responsible for a large proportion of variability in its activity. It accounts for up to 70% of clozapine and 60% of olanzapine metabolism. Individuals with CYP1A2 ultrarapid phenotypes tend to experience delay or lack of response to these two antipsychotics (Arranz & Kapur, 2008).

P-glycoprotein or P-gp (coded by the ABCB1 gene) mediates the transport of many antipsychotics through the blood–brain barrier, including amisulpride, aripiprazole, olanzapine, and risperidone. Three polymorphisms (rs1045642, rs2032582, and rs1128503) in ABCB1 have been investigated in association with antipsychotic efficacy with positive results, despite the risk genotypes/alleles are partially inconsistent. These SNPs form a haplotype block (i.e., they are usually inherited together) that has been associated with ABCB1 gene expression as well as P-gp activity and substrate specificity (Moons, de Roo, Claes, & Dom, 2011).

4.1.2 Pharmacodynamics

Genes belonging to the dopaminergic and serotonergic neurotransmitter systems have been particularly studied since their central role in both antipsychotic efficacy and liability to side effects.

The block of DA receptors, particularly D2 receptors, is considered the main mechanism of antipsychotic action. Therefore, genetic variants in DA receptors influencing receptor density, expression, and activity may be essential regulators of individual treatment response. The del allele of the −141C ins/del polymorphism in the DRD2 promoter region (rs1799732) is associated with reduced D2 density and activity and it may predispose to poorer outcome and to AIWG (Zhang, Lencz, & Malhotra, 2010; Zhang et al., 2016). The Taq1A (rs1800497) polymorphism of DRD2 has also been extensively studied: the A1 allele is associated with reduced gene expression compared to the A2 allele. It does not appear to have a significant impact on antipsychotic response (Zhang et al., 2010), but it is robustly associated with TD: A2 carriers showed significantly greater odds of developing TD compared to non-A2 carriers (Zhang et al., 2016). The D3 receptor is another important target for some antipsychotics. rs6280 is a nonsynonymous variant (i.e., it leads to the substitution of one amino acid) in the first exon of DRD3, associated with changes in receptor density. The variant allele (C) may predict improved response to clozapine, olanzapine, and possibly other SGAs in Caucasian populations (Vehof et al., 2012).

SGAs, compared to FGAs, show higher affinity for 5-HT receptors. 5-HT2A antagonism is hypothesized to contribute to their reduced propensity to cause EPS/hyperprolactinemia and greater efficacy on negative symptoms (Schmidt, Sorensen, Kehne, Carr, & Palfreyman, 1995). Three polymorphisms within HTR2A have been extensively studied. rs6313 (T102C) is a synonymous polymorphism within the coding region. Methylation is thought to be responsible for the functional effect of this SNP, since the C allele was associated with lower HTR2A expression. This polymorphism is weakly predictive of antipsychotic response particularly for SGAs (better response in T allele carriers), but there is strong support for its involvement in susceptibility to TD, with the C allele conferring increased risk of developing TD (MacNeil & Müller, 2016). The rs6311 (A1438G) polymorphism, located in the promoter region of HTR2A, is in linkage disequilibrium (LD) with rs6313 and it may be associated with antipsychotic response, although results are inconsistent regarding the risk allele. Finally, the missense rs6314 (His452Tyr) polymorphism was repeatedly associated with antipsychotic response. The His allele confers increased signaling efficacy and binding affinity of HTR2A and it was associated with better response to antipsychotics. Of interest, imprinting effects modulate transcription of HTR2A in males; thus, it is monoallelic or biallelic depending on the individual. This could complicate the interpretation of HTR2A polymorphisms in pharmacogenetic studies, making difficult to ascertain whether observed associations are the result of genotype or expression profile due to imprinting (Pouget & Müller, 2014).

The 5-HT1A receptor (HTR1A gene) may influence antipsychotic drug response, particularly in terms of negative and cognitive symptoms. The rs6295 (C1019G) polymorphism has shown consistent association with antipsychotic response, particularly for SGAs, with G allele carriers showing lower improvement of negative symptoms. This polymorphism is located in the promoter region of HTR1A and it affects a transcription factor-binding site; thus, the G allele is associated with increased gene expression (Pouget & Müller, 2014).

HTR2C, coding 5-HT2C receptor, showed the most consistent association with AIWG. Weight gain is a common and serious side effect of antipsychotic treatment, particularly with SGAs, with up to 30% of patients gaining $\geq$7% of their baseline weight. Antagonists at 5-HT2C receptor, including many antipsychotics, may increase food intake, despite satiety, causing weight gain. The most studied SNP in HTR2C, rs3813929, is located in the promoter region of the gene and it may play a role in regulating gene expression. T allele is associated with increased transcriptional of the gene, compared to the C allele, and it seems to be protective against antipsychotic-related weight gain, perhaps by enhancing gene expression of HTR2C, which partially counterbalances the 5-HT2C antagonistic antipsychotic effect (Zhang et al., 2016). Another gene that has convincing evidence for its association with AIWG is MC4R, coding melanocortin-4 receptor. MC4R mutations have been linked to extreme early-onset obesity and MC4R knockout mice develop obesity. AA homozygotes at rs489693 are at significantly greater risk of AIWG than C carriers, with a moderate effect size (Zhang et al., 2016). Other genes for which there is moderate evidence supporting the association with AIWG are ADRA2A (adrenoreceptor alpha-2A), DRD2, GNB3, and INSIG2 (insulin-induced gene 2) (Zhang et al., 2016).

Other candidate genes that may influence treatment response have not been studied as thoroughly as the above mentioned and results have often been divergent. The role of the rs4680 (Val108/158Met) SNP in the COMT gene is not fully understood and deserves further study, despite its potential relevance as a consequence of its functional impact on enzyme activity. The product of the GNB3 gene is involved in dopaminergic and serotonergic receptors signal transduction. GNB3 rs5443 (C825T) may have a weak association with overall symptom improvement during antipsychotic treatment. The T allele produces a splice variant that confers enhanced activation of the coded G protein and it may predict worse response. Growing evidence support the role of BDNF in antipsychotic response and the Met allele of the rs6265 (Val66Met) polymorphism may be associated with poorer treatment response (Brandl, Kennedy, & Müller, 2014). Lastly, ZNF804A, a zinc finger domain-containing protein, playing a role in neurodevelopment, has recently been related to the risk for schizophrenia and to antipsychotics response. The rs1344706 A allele leads to increased protein expression and it may be associated with lower improvement in positive symptoms (Mössner et al., 2012).

CIA deserves a special mention since this serious adverse effect mandates great caution in patients on clozapine: this antipsychotic is the most effective medication for treatment-resistant schizophrenia, but it is associated with the highest incidence of agranulocytosis (up to 2%), which limits its usage. A number of classical HLA alleles have shown association with clozapine-induced agranulocytosis in small samples, but these results have not yet been replicated. Importantly, the HLA-DQB1 variant G6672C (rs113332494) showed strong association with clozapine-induced agranulocytosis across two independent samples (Sriretnakumar, Huang, & Müller, 2015).

4.2 Genome-Wide Association Studies

The strongest associations observed in GWAS have been in previously uninvestigated genes or intergenic regions, providing new insights into genetic factors regulating antipsychotic response. Although intergenic findings may reflect the effects of regulatory processes, GWAS usually interpreted results in terms of the closest gene and they deprioritized genes that have not previously been implicated in antipsychotic response or neuropsychiatric diseases. Unlike many previous candidate gene studies, GWAS for the most part have investigated drug-specific response and little evidence was found that a given genetic variant impacts on response to more than one drug. Despite the promise of GWAS, however, there is poor replication and functional validation of the plethora of results generated, particularly with regard to noncoding variants (Pouget & Müller, 2014).

Treatment response has been investigated in relation to specific symptom domains. Besides intergenic regions, genome-wide significant findings pointed to variants in some pharmacodynamic genes in populations of Caucasian descent, such as DRD2 (rs11214606) for working memory improvement with olanzapine. Despite rs11214606 is in LD with both the Taq1A variant (rs1800497) and the DRD2-241A/G (rs1799978) variant, these results should be interpreted cautiously since no other SNP in the region showed highly significant associations (McClay et al., 2011). Variants in the ATP1A2 and PDE4D genes were associated with global severity improvement during treatment with olanzapine and quetiapine, respectively. The former encodes a subunit of a sodium/potassium transporting ATPase (involved in electrical conductance of nerve impulses), the latter a cyclic AMP-specific phosphodiesterase expressed in the brain (presumably involved in dopamine D1 receptor signaling) (Clark et al., 2013). Other GWAS reported associations with genes involved in glutamatergic neurotransmission (GRM7 (Sacchetti et al., 2017), GRIA4 (Lavedan et al., 2009)).

The aggregated analysis of genome-wide loci associated with schizophrenia demonstrated that they have a significant overlap with targets of antipsychotic drugs. Interestingly, patients with treatment-resistant schizophrenia show an excess of rare disruptive variants in gene targets of antipsychotics and in genes with evidence for a role in antipsychotic efficacy. This finding is consistent with the polygenic nature of antipsychotic response and it suggests that the identification of antipsychotics with alternative mechanisms of action would be beneficial. Further, the identification of patients carrying these disruptive variants may guide the early prescription of clozapine (Ruderfer et al., 2016).

Concerning antipsychotic-induced side effects, interesting results emerged in relation to metabolic side effects. Findings suggested that variants in genes that impact on the general metabolic status may influence susceptibility to AIWG: GPR98 (rs1967256 and rs11954387), NR3C1 (rs17100498 and rs17100506), MC4R (rs489693), and MEIS2 (rs1568679) are indeed genes implicated in metabolic phenotypes in the general population that reached genome-wide significance for association with AIWG. Most of the whole genome significant findings for SGAs, however, were in SNPs within intergenic region (Adkins et al., 2011). PTPRD gene (coding protein tyrosine phosphatase, receptor type D) is a receptor-type protein tyrosine phosphatase expressed in particular brain regions (e.g., hippocampal CA2 and CA3), in B lymphocytes, and in the thymic medulla and it is also related to metabolic regulation in the general population, specifically liability to type II diabetes. Two SNPs within an intron of the PTPRD gene (rs10977144, rs10977154) reached genome-wide significant association with AIWG in a recent GWAS. A pathway analysis conducted on the same sample indicated that multiple genes in metabolic processes might jointly contribute to AIWG, such as glucosamine metabolic process, amino sugar metabolic process, and regulation of peptidyl tyrosine phosphorylation. These results further confirmed the earlier observation that metabolic pathways were involved in AIWG in schizophrenia (Yu et al., 2016).

Lastly, preliminary GWAS findings suggested an association between EPS and three SNPs: two intergenic (rs17022444 and rs7669317) and one (rs2126709) within the ZNF202 gene, which encodes a transcriptional repressor controlling, among other genes, PLP1, which is the major protein in myelin (Åberg et al., 2010). Further, the GABA receptor signaling pathway may be involved in genetic susceptibility to treatment-resistant TD, as found in a cohort of Japanese patients (Inada et al., 2008).

GWAS investigating CIA confirmed a role for HLA antigens (HLA-DQB1 and HLA-B, specifically) and they identified a novel association with rs149104283, an intronic variant within SLCO1B3 and SLCO1B7, members of a family of hepatic transporter genes previously implicated in adverse drug reactions. Other signals were identified within STARD9, a mitotic kinesin, and UBAP2, whose function is still undetermined but which appears to be widely expressed across tissues including bone marrow (Goldstein et al., 2014; Legge et al., 2016).

4.3 Clinical Applications

Similar to antidepressant drugs, some commercial pharmacogenetic tests have already been developed and commercialized. However, insufficient validation of the clinical benefit of these pharmacogenetics tests has delayed the development of clinical guidelines for their use and interpretation. The lack of clinical expert consensus guidelines about pharmacogenetics tests in schizophrenia has contributed to poor clinical uptake and inconsistent patient reimbursement for testing.

Polymorphisms in CYP2D6 are the only pharmacokinetic variants with a well-replicated role and a probable clinical utility for guiding treatment with SGAs. CYP2D6-metabolizing activity impacts on drug dose requirement; thus, CYP2D6 genotyping is included in all commercialized tests. It is recommended by DPWG and variants of this gene are included in drug labels for a number of antipsychotics (e.g., aripiprazole, clozapine, olanzapine, risperidone) according to several regulatory agencies such as FDA (Whirl-Carrillo et al., 2012). However, genetic variation in CYP450 genes seems to exert a stronger influence on the risk of adverse effects than medication response. The first FDA-approved pharmacogenetic test, the AmpliChip™ CYP450 Test, genotypes up to 33 alleles in CYP2D6 and 3 alleles in CYP2C19 associated with different metabolizing phenotypes. The intended use of the chip cleared by the FDA is very general and does not refer to any specific drug.

A number of pharmacodynamic variants have replicated associations with both antipsychotic response and some adverse effects, and they may be useful in predicting efficacy and tolerability. In particular, variants in DRD2 and HTR2A were associated with antipsychotic efficacy. Variants in HTR2C were robustly associated with antipsychotics-induced weight gain, while variants in DRD2 and HTR2A showed association with susceptibility to TD. These variants are generally underrepresented in commercially available pharmacogenetics tests, which have typically focused on CYP450 genes, although GeneSight® and Genecept™ include some pharmacodynamic markers. Finally, the G6672C polymorphism in HLA-DQB1 was strongly associated with clozapine-induced agranulocytosis and it can be genotyped by a specific kit (PGxPredict:CLOZAPINE®)

which has reportedly 21% sensitivity and 98% specificity (Pouget & Müller, 2014). The very low sensitivity clearly makes it not adequate for clinical application.

Recently, approaches that combine clinical and genetic variables using cluster analysis or machine learning were applied to identify sets of predictors with adequate performance. Preliminary evidence demonstrated that ziprasidone response may be predicted with sensitivity 0.75, specificity 0.74, and accuracy 0.74 using 13 SNPs and 53 baseline clinical variables (Lee et al., 2017).

5. CONCLUSION

The use of pharmacogenetics to personalize psychotropic treatments may dramatically improve health care in psychiatry. Results of candidate gene studies were mostly inconclusive, but some replicated genes were identified and included in pharmacogenetic tests, which in some cases demonstrated preliminary evidence of clinical usefulness and potential cost savings. Some pharmacogenetic biomarkers were demonstrated to be valuable for side effects prevention and they are recommended in clinical practice: HLA-B*1502 predicts liability to SJS in patients of Han Chinese ancestry treated with carbamazepine, and CYP2D6-poor metabolizers have higher risk of proarrhythmic effects when treated with pimozide. Pharmacokinetic variants, mainly polymorphisms in isoenzymes of the CYP450 superfamily, were associated with plasma drugs concentration and they are the variants most commonly included in pharmacogenetic tests. Plasma levels, however, seem to exert a stronger influence on the occurrence of adverse effects than on medication response, most likely because plasma concentration of psychotropic drugs does not necessarily reflect drug concentration in the brain. Among pharmacodynamic markers the most replicated finding to date is the association between the 5-HTTLPR polymorphism in the SERT gene, antidepressant response, and lithium prophylaxis. The results of candidate gene studies were valuable for discovering some relevant associations and producing some useful clinical applications, but response and side effects to psychotropic medications are complex phenotypes that are affected by multiple nonindependent variants throughout the genome.

The genomics revolution has provided an unprecedented technological improvement to pursue the goals of pharmacogenetics. It is likely that future pharmacogenetic tests will consist of hundreds/thousands of polymorphisms throughout the genome or selected pathways in order to take into account the complex interactions among variants in a number of genes rather than focus on polymorphisms in relatively few candidate genes. Considerable progress has been made since the advent of GWAS, but there are still unsolved issues. One important limitation of GWAS has been the use of underpowered sample sizes. The development of consortia aims to meet the need for larger cohorts of patients with adequate power. The use of aggregated tests, such as pathway analysis and PRS, increases the power of GWAS compared to single SNP analysis. The reduction in the number of tests performed and the capture of the cumulative effects of a number of variants (the disruption of a gene or pathway functioning is the result of cumulative effects of variants within it) are responsible for the power increase provided by aggregated approaches. Another issue probably responsible for the poor replication of previous results is the inconsistent definition of response or adverse events. The development of consensus phenotype definitions could increase the replication of findings and facilitate meta-analysis. Lastly, psychiatric diseases are clinically heterogeneous and classical nosography has been repeatedly discussed, since diagnostic categories based on clinical consensus often fail to align with findings emerging from clinical neuroscience and genetics. For this reason, the US National Institute of Mental Health (NIMH) has launched the Research Domain Criteria (RDoC) project to create a framework for research on pathophysiology. RDoC classification assumes that mental diseases are the consequence of the dysfunction in neural circuits and this can be identified with the tools of clinical neuroscience. Thus, genetics and clinical neuroscience will yield biosignatures that will augment clinical symptoms and signs for clinical management. Examples where clinically relevant models of circuitry–behavior relationships may be translated in future clinical use include fear/extinction, reward, executive function, and impulse control. For example, the practitioner of the future could supplement a clinical evaluation of what we now call MDD with data from functional or structural imaging and genomic sequencing to determine prognosis and appropriate treatment, analogous to what is done routinely today in many other areas of medicine (Insel et al., 2010).

CONFLICT OF INTEREST

Prof. A. Serretti is/has been consultant/speaker for: Abbott, Abbvie, Angelini, Astra Zeneca, Clinical Data, Boheringer, Bristol Myers Squibb, Eli Lilly, GlaxoSmithKline, Innovapharma, Italfarmaco, Janssen, Lundbeck, Naurex, Pfizer, Polifarma, Sanofi, Servier. The other authors declare no potential conflict of interest.

REFERENCES

Åberg, K., Adkins, D. E., Bukszár, J., Webb, B. T., Caroff, S. N., Miller, D. D., et al. (2010). Genome-wide association study of movement-related adverse antipsychotic effects. *Biological Psychiatry*, *67*(3), 279–282. https://doi.org/10.1016/j.biopsych.2009.08.036.

Adkins, D. E., Aberg, K., McClay, J. L., Bukszár, J., Zhao, Z., Jia, P., et al. (2011). Genome-wide pharmacogenomic study of metabolic side effects to antipsychotic drugs. *Molecular Psychiatry*, *16*(3), 321–332. https://doi.org/10.1038/mp.2010.14.

Adkins, D. E., Clark, S. L., Åberg, K., Hettema, J. M., Bukszár, J., McClay, J. L., et al. (2012). Genome-wide pharmacogenomic study of citalopram-induced side effects in STAR*D. *Translational Psychiatry*, *2*(7), e129. https://doi.org/10.1038/tp.2012.57.

Arranz, M. J., & Kapur, S. (2008). Pharmacogenetics in psychiatry: Are we ready for widespread clinical use? *Schizophrenia Bulletin*, *34*(6), 1130–1144. https://doi.org/10.1093/schbul/sbn114.

Baune, B. T., Hohoff, C., Roehrs, T., Deckert, J., Arolt, V., & Domschke, K. (2008). Serotonin receptor 1A − 1019C/G variant: Impact on antidepressant pharmacoresponse in melancholic depression? *Neuroscience Letters*, *436*(2), 111–115. https://doi.org/10.1016/j.neulet.2008.03.001.

Biernacka, J. M., Sangkuhl, K., Jenkins, G., Whaley, R. M., Barman, P., Batzler, A., et al. (2016). The International SSRI Pharmacogenomics Consortium (ISPC): A genome-wide association study of antidepressant treatment response. *Translational Psychiatry*, *6*(11), e937. https://doi.org/10.1038/tp.2016.187.

Bloom, D. E., Cafiero, E. T., Jané-Llopis, E., Abrahams-Gessel, S., Bloom, L. R., Fathima, S., et al. (2011). *The global economic burden of non-communicable diseases*. Geneva: World Economic Forum. Retrieved from http://www3.weforum.org/docs/WEF_Harvard_HE_GlobalEconomicBurdenNonCommunicableDiseases_2011.pdf.

Brandl, E. J., Kennedy, J. L., & Müller, D. J. (2014). Pharmacogenetics of antipsychotics. *The Canadian Journal of Psychiatry*, *59*(2), 76–88. https://doi.org/10.1177/070674371405900203.

Breitenstein, B., Scheuer, S., Pfister, H., Uhr, M., Lucae, S., Holsboer, F., et al. (2014). The clinical application of ABCB1 genotyping in antidepressant treatment: A pilot study. *CNS Spectrums*, *19*(2), 165–175. https://doi.org/10.1017/S1092852913000436.

Budde, M., Degner, D., Brockmöller, J., & Schulze, T. G. (2017). Pharmacogenomic aspects of bipolar disorder: An update. *European Neuropsychopharmacology: The Journal of the European College of Neuropsychopharmacology*, *27*(6), 599–609. https://doi.org/10.1016/j.euroneuro.2017.02.001.

Cacabelos, R., Cacabelos, P., & Aliev, G. (2013). Genomics of schizophrenia and pharmacogenomics of antipsychotic drugs. *Open Journal of Psychiatry*, *3*(1), 46–139. https://doi.org/10.4236/ojpsych.2013.31008.

Cacabelos, R., Martinez-Bouza, R., Carril, J. C., Fernandez-Novoa, L., Lombardi, V., Carrera, I., et al. (2012). Genomics and pharmacogenomics of brain disorders. *Current Pharmaceutical Biotechnology*, *13*(5), 674–725. Retrieved from http://www.ncbi.nlm.nih.gov/pubmed/22122480.

Center for Drug Evaluation and Research. (2017). *Genomics—Table of pharmacogenomic biomarkers in drug labeling*. Retrieved from https://www.fda.gov/drugs/scienceresearch/researchareas/pharmacogenetics/ucm083378.htm.

Chen, C.-H., Lee, C.-S., Lee, M.-T. M., Ouyang, W.-C., Chen, C.-C., Chong, M.-Y., et al. (2014). Variant GADL1 and response to lithium therapy in bipolar I disorder. *The New England Journal of Medicine*, *370*(2), 119–128. https://doi.org/10.1056/NEJMoa1212444.

Choi, J.-H., Lee, B. H., Kim, J. H., Kim, G.-H., Kim, Y.-M., Cho, J., et al. (2015). Clinical outcomes and the mutation spectrum of the OTC gene in patients with ornithine transcarbamylase deficiency. *Journal of Human Genetics*, *60*(9), 501–507. https://doi.org/10.1038/jhg.2015.54.

Chung, W.-H., Hung, S.-I., Hong, H.-S., Hsih, M.-S., Yang, L.-C., Ho, H.-C., et al. (2004). Medical genetics: A marker for Stevens-Johnson syndrome. *Nature, 428*(6982), 486. https://doi.org/10.1038/428486a.

Clark, S. L., Adkins, D. E., Aberg, K., Hettema, J. M., McClay, J. L., Souza, R. P., et al. (2012). Pharmacogenomic study of side-effects for antidepressant treatment options in STAR*D. *Psychological Medicine, 42*(6), 1151–1162. https://doi.org/10.1017/S003329171100239X.

Clark, S. L., Souza, R. P., Adkins, D. E., Aberg, K., Bukszár, J., McClay, J. L., et al. (2013). Genome-wide association study of patient-rated and clinician-rated global impression of severity during antipsychotic treatment. *Pharmacogenetics and Genomics, 23*(2), 69–77. https://doi.org/10.1097/FPC.0b013e32835ca260.

Cocchi, E., Fabbri, C., Han, C., Lee, S.-J., Patkar, A. A., Masand, P. S., et al. (2016). Genome-wide association study of antidepressant response: Involvement of the inorganic cation transmembrane transporter activity pathway. *BMC Psychiatry, 16*(1), 106. https://doi.org/10.1186/s12888-016-0813-x.

Cramer, J. A., & Rosenheck, R. (1998). Compliance with medication regimens for mental and physical disorders. *Psychiatric Services, 49*(2), 196–201. https://doi.org/10.1176/ps.49.2.196.

Du, J., Zhang, A., Wang, L., Xuan, J., Yu, L., Che, R., et al. (2010). Relationship between response to risperidone, plasma concentrations of risperidone and *CYP3A4* polymorphisms in schizophrenia patients. *Journal of Psychopharmacology, 24*(7), 1115–1120. https://doi.org/10.1177/0269881109104932.

Fabbri, C., Crisafulli, C., Calabrò, M., Spina, E., & Serretti, A. (2016). Progress and prospects in pharmacogenetics of antidepressant drugs. *Expert Opinion on Drug Metabolism & Toxicology, 12*(10), 1157–1168. https://doi.org/10.1080/17425255.2016.1202237.

Fabbri, C., Crisafulli, C., Gurwitz, D., Stingl, J., Calati, R., Albani, D., et al. (2015). Neuronal cell adhesion genes and antidepressant response in three independent samples. *The Pharmacogenomics Journal, 15*(6), 538–548. https://doi.org/10.1038/tpj.2015.15.

Fabbri, C., Di Girolamo, G., & Serretti, A. (2013). Pharmacogenetics of antidepressant drugs: An update after almost 20 years of research. *American Journal of Medical Genetics Part B: Neuropsychiatric Genetics, 162*(6), 487–520. https://doi.org/10.1002/ajmg.b.32184.

Fabbri, C., Marsano, A., Albani, D., Chierchia, A., Calati, R., Drago, A., et al. (2014). PPP3CC gene: A putative modulator of antidepressant response through the B-cell receptor signaling pathway. *The Pharmacogenomics Journal, 14*(5), 463–472. https://doi.org/10.1038/tpj.2014.15.

Fabbri, C., Porcelli, S., & Serretti, A. (2014). From pharmacogenetics to pharmacogenomics: The way toward the personalization of antidepressant treatment. *Canadian Journal of Psychiatry. Revue Canadienne de Psychiatrie, 59*(2), 62–75. https://doi.org/10.1177/070674371405900202.

GENDEP Investigators, MARS Investigators, STAR*D Investigators, Wolfgang, M., Mors, O., Hauser, J., et al. (2013). Common genetic variation and antidepressant efficacy in major depressive disorder: A meta-analysis of three genome-wide pharmacogenetic studies. *The American Journal of Psychiatry, 170*(2), 207–217. https://doi.org/10.1176/appi.ajp.2012.12020237.

Glatt, C. E., & Lee, F. S. (2016). Common polymorphisms in the age of research domain criteria (RDoC): Integration and translation. *Biological Psychiatry, 79*(1), 25–31. https://doi.org/10.1016/j.biopsych.2014.12.020.

Goes, F. S. (2016). Genetics of bipolar disorder. *Psychiatric Clinics of North America, 39*(1), 139–155. https://doi.org/10.1016/j.psc.2015.10.004.

Goldstein, J. I., Fredrik Jarskog, L., Hilliard, C., Alfirevic, A., Duncan, L., Fourches, D., et al. (2014). Clozapine-induced agranulocytosis is associated with rare HLA-DQB1 and HLA-B alleles. *Nature Communications, 5*, 4757. https://doi.org/10.1038/ncomms5757.

Gomes, A. Q., Nolasco, S., & Soares, H. (2013). Non-coding RNAs: Multi-tasking molecules in the cell. *International Journal of Molecular Sciences*, *14*(8), 16010–16039. https://doi.org/10.3390/ijms140816010.

Govindarajan, A., Rao, B. S. S., Nair, D., Trinh, M., Mawjee, N., Tonegawa, S., et al. (2006). Transgenic brain-derived neurotrophic factor expression causes both anxiogenic and antidepressant effects. *Proceedings of the National Academy of Sciences of the United States of America*, *103*(35), 13208–13213. https://doi.org/10.1073/pnas.0605180103.

Higgins, G. A., Allyn-Feuer, A., Barbour, E., & Athey, B. D. (2015). A glutamatergic network mediates lithium response in bipolar disorder as defined by epigenome pathway analysis. *Pharmacogenomics*, *16*(14), 1547–1563. https://doi.org/10.2217/pgs.15.106.

Hou, L., Heilbronner, U., Degenhardt, F., Adli, M., Akiyama, K., Akula, N., et al. (2016). Genetic variants associated with response to lithium treatment in bipolar disorder: A genome-wide association study. *The Lancet*, *387*(10023), 1085–1093. https://doi.org/10.1016/S0140-6736(16)00143-4.

Hunter, A. M., Leuchter, A. F., Power, R. A., Muthén, B., McGrath, P. J., Lewis, C. M., et al. (2013). A genome-wide association study of a sustained pattern of antidepressant response. *Journal of Psychiatric Research*, *47*(9), 1157–1165. https://doi.org/10.1016/j.jpsychires.2013.05.002.

Inada, T., Koga, M., Ishiguro, H., Horiuchi, Y., Syu, A., Yoshio, T., et al. (2008). Pathway-based association analysis of genome-wide screening data suggest that genes associated with the gamma-aminobutyric acid receptor signaling pathway are involved in neuroleptic-induced, treatment-resistant tardive dyskinesia. *Pharmacogenetics and Genomics*, *18*(4), 317–323. https://doi.org/10.1097/FPC.0b013e3282f70492.

Insel, T., Cuthbert, B., Garvey, M., Heinssen, R., Pine, D. S., Quinn, K., et al. (2010). Research domain criteria (RDoC): Toward a new classification framework for research on mental disorders. *The American Journal of Psychiatry*, *167*(7), 748–751. https://doi.org/10.1176/appi.ajp.2010.09091379.

Jaquenoud Sirot, E., Knezevic, B., Morena, G. P., Harenberg, S., Oneda, B., Crettol, S., et al. (2009). ABCB1 and cytochrome P450 polymorphisms. *Journal of Clinical Psychopharmacology*, *29*(4), 319–326. https://doi.org/10.1097/JCP.0b013e3181acc372.

Kato, M., & Serretti, A. (2010). Review and meta-analysis of antidepressant pharmacogenetic findings in major depressive disorder. *Molecular Psychiatry*, *15*(5), 473–500. https://doi.org/10.1038/mp.2008.116.

Lavedan, C., Licamele, L., Volpi, S., Hamilton, J., Heaton, C., Mack, K., et al. (2009). Association of the NPAS3 gene and five other loci with response to the antipsychotic iloperidone identified in a whole genome association study. *Molecular Psychiatry*, *14*(8), 804–819. https://doi.org/10.1038/mp.2008.56.

Lee, B. S., McIntyre, R. S., Gentle, J. E., Park, N. S., Chiriboga, D. A., Lee, Y., et al. (2017). A computational algorithm for personalized medicine in schizophrenia. *Schizophrenia Research*, *192*, 131–136. https://doi.org/10.1016/j.schres.2017.05.001.

Legge, S. E., Hamshere, M. L., Ripke, S., Pardinas, A. F., Goldstein, J. I., Rees, E., et al. (2016). Genome-wide common and rare variant analysis provides novel insights into clozapine-associated neutropenia. *Molecular Psychiatry*, *22*, 1502–1508. https://doi.org/10.1038/mp.2016.97.

Li, C.-I., Samuels, D. C., Zhao, Y.-Y., Shyr, Y., & Guo, Y. (2017). Power and sample size calculations for high-throughput sequencing-based experiments. *Briefings in Bioinformatics*. https://doi.org/10.1093/bib/bbx061. Epub ahead of print.

Lieberman, J. A., Stroup, T. S., McEvoy, J. P., Swartz, M. S., Rosenheck, R. A., Perkins, D. O., et al. (2005). Effectiveness of antipsychotic drugs in patients with chronic schizophrenia. *The New England Journal of Medicine*, *353*(12), 1209–1223. https://doi.org/10.1056/NEJMoa051688.

MacNeil, R. R., & Müller, D. J. (2016). Genetics of common antipsychotic-induced adverse effects. *Molecular Neuropsychiatry*, *2*(2), 61–78. https://doi.org/10.1159/000445802.

McCarthy, S., Das, S., Kretzschmar, W., Delaneau, O., Wood, A. R., Teumer, A., et al. (2016). A reference panel of 64,976 haplotypes for genotype imputation. *Nature Genetics*, *48*(10), 1279–1283. https://doi.org/10.1038/ng.3643.

McClay, J. L., Adkins, D. E., Åberg, K., Bukszár, J., Khachane, A. N., Keefe, R. S. E., et al. (2011). Genome-wide pharmacogenomic study of neurocognition as an indicator of antipsychotic treatment response in schizophrenia. *Neuropsychopharmacology*, *36*(3), 616–626. https://doi.org/10.1038/npp.2010.193.

McCormack, M., Alfirevic, A., Bourgeois, S., Farrell, J. J., Kasperavičiūtė, D., Carrington, M., et al. (2011). HLA-A*3101 and carbamazepine-induced hypersensitivity reactions in Europeans. *The New England Journal of Medicine*, *364*(12), 1134–1143. https://doi.org/10.1056/NEJMoa1013297.

McMahon, F. J., Buervenich, S., Charney, D., Lipsky, R., Rush, A. J., Wilson, A. F., et al. (2006). Variation in the gene encoding the serotonin 2A receptor is associated with outcome of antidepressant treatment. *American Journal of Human Genetics*, *78*(5), 804–814. https://doi.org/10.1086/503820.

Moons, T., de Roo, M., Claes, S., & Dom, G. (2011). Relationship between P-glycoprotein and second-generation antipsychotics. *Pharmacogenomics*, *12*(8), 1193–1211. https://doi.org/10.2217/pgs.11.55.

Mössner, R., Schuhmacher, A., Wagner, M., Lennertz, L., Steinbrecher, A., Quednow, B. B., et al. (2012). The schizophrenia risk gene ZNF804A influences the antipsychotic response of positive schizophrenia symptoms. *European Archives of Psychiatry and Clinical Neuroscience*, *262*(3), 193–197. https://doi.org/10.1007/s00406-011-0235-1.

Myung, W., Kim, J., Lim, S.-W., Shim, S., Won, H.-H., Kim, S., et al. (2015). A genome-wide association study of antidepressant response in Koreans. *Translational Psychiatry*, *5*(11), e672. https://doi.org/10.1038/tp.2015.173.

Niitsu, T., Fabbri, C., Bentini, F., & Serretti, A. (2013). Pharmacogenetics in major depression: A comprehensive meta-analysis. *Progress in Neuro-Psychopharmacology & Biological Psychiatry*, *45*, 183–194. https://doi.org/10.1016/j.pnpbp.2013.05.011.

Nutt, D., Demyttenaere, K., Janka, Z., Aarre, T., Bourin, M., Canonico, P. L., et al. (2007). The other face of depression, reduced positive affect: The role of catecholamines in causation and cure. *Journal of Psychopharmacology (Oxford, England)*, *21*(5), 461–471. https://doi.org/10.1177/0269881106069938.

Oedegaard, K. J., Alda, M., Anand, A., Andreassen, O. A., Balaraman, Y., Berrettini, W. H., et al. (2016). The Pharmacogenomics of Bipolar Disorder study (PGBD): Identification of genes for lithium response in a prospective sample. *BMC Psychiatry*, *16*(1), 129. https://doi.org/10.1186/s12888-016-0732-x.

Patel, V., Chisholm, D., Parikh, R., Charlson, F. J., Degenhardt, L., Dua, T., et al. (2016). Addressing the burden of mental, neurological, and substance use disorders: Key messages from disease control priorities, 3rd edition. *The Lancet*, *387*(10028), 1672–1685. https://doi.org/10.1016/S0140-6736(15)00390-6.

Perlis, R. H., Adams, D. H., Fijal, B., Sutton, V. K., Farmen, M., Breier, A., et al. (2010). Genetic association study of treatment response with olanzapine/fluoxetine combination or lamotrigine in bipolar I depression. *The Journal of Clinical Psychiatry*, *71*(5), 599–605. https://doi.org/10.4088/JCP.08m04632gre.

Perlis, R. H., Smoller, J. W., Ferreira, M. A. R., McQuillin, A., Bass, N., Lawrence, J., et al. (2009). A genomewide association study of response to lithium for prevention of recurrence in bipolar disorder. *The American Journal of Psychiatry*, *166*(6), 718–725. https://doi.org/10.1176/appi.ajp.2009.08111633.

PharmGKB. (2018). *Annotation of FDA label for valproic acid and ABL2,ASL,ASS1,CPS1, NAGS,OTC,POLG*. Retrieved August 7, 2017, from https://www.pharmgkb.org/label/PA166104825.

Pisanu, C., Melis, C., & Squassina, A. (2016). Lithium pharmacogenetics: Where do we stand? *Drug Development Research*, 77(7), 368–373. https://doi.org/10.1002/ddr.21341.

Pisanu, C., Papadima, E. M., Del Zompo, M., & Squassina, A. (2016). Understanding the molecular mechanisms underlying mood stabilizer treatments in bipolar disorder: Potential involvement of epigenetics. *Neuroscience Letters*, *669*, 24–31. https://doi.org/10.1016/j.neulet.2016.06.045.

Porcelli, S., Drago, A., Fabbri, C., & Serretti, A. (2011). Mechanisms of antidepressant action: An integrated dopaminergic perspective. *Progress in Neuro-Psychopharmacology & Biological Psychiatry*, *35*(7), 1532–1543. https://doi.org/10.1016/j.pnpbp.2011.03.005.

Porcelli, S., Fabbri, C., & Serretti, A. (2012). Meta-analysis of serotonin transporter gene promoter polymorphism (5-HTTLPR) association with antidepressant efficacy. *European Neuropsychopharmacology: The Journal of the European College of Neuropsychopharmacology*, *22*(4), 239–258. https://doi.org/10.1016/j.euroneuro.2011.10.003.

Porcelli, S., Fabbri, C., Spina, E., Serretti, A., & De Ronchi, D. (2011). Genetic polymorphisms of cytochrome P450 enzymes and antidepressant metabolism. *Expert Opinion on Drug Metabolism & Toxicology*, 7(9), 1101–1115. https://doi.org/10.1517/17425255.2011.597740.

Pouget, J. G., & Müller, D. J. (2014). Pharmacogenetics of antipsychotic treatment in schizophrenia. *Methods in Molecular Biology (Clifton, N.J.)*, *1175*, 557–587. https://doi.org/10.1007/978-1-4939-0956-8_14.

Pronicka, E., Weglewska-Jurkiewicz, A., Pronicki, M., Sykut-Cegielska, J., Kowalski, P., Pajdowska, M., et al. (2011). Drug-resistant epilepsia and fulminant valproate liver toxicity. Alpers-Huttenlocher syndrome in two children confirmed post mortem by identification of p.W748S mutation in POLG gene. *Medical Science Monitor: International Medical Journal of Experimental and Clinical Research*, 17(4), CR203–9. Retrieved from http://www.ncbi.nlm.nih.gov/pubmed/21455106.

Reich, D. E., & Lander, E. S. (2001). On the allelic spectrum of human disease. *Trends in Genetics: TIG*, *17*(9), 502–510. Retrieved from http://www.ncbi.nlm.nih.gov/pubmed/11525833.

Rogers, H. L., Bhattaram, A., Zineh, I., Gobburu, J., Mathis, M., Laughren, T. P., et al. (2012). CYP2D6 genotype information to guide pimozide treatment in adult and pediatric patients: Basis for the U.S. Food and Drug Administration's new dosing recommendations. *The Journal of Clinical Psychiatry*, *73*(9), 1187–1190. https://doi.org/10.4088/JCP.11m07572.

Ruderfer, D. M., Charney, A. W., Readhead, B., Kidd, B. A., Kähler, A. K., Kenny, P. J., et al. (2016). Polygenic overlap between schizophrenia risk and antipsychotic response: A genomic medicine approach. *The Lancet Psychiatry*, *3*(4), 350–357. https://doi.org/10.1016/S2215-0366(15)00553-2.

Rush, A. J., Trivedi, M. H., Wisniewski, S. R., Nierenberg, A. A., Stewart, J. W., Warden, D., et al. (2006). Acute and longer-term outcomes in depressed outpatients requiring one or several treatment steps: A STAR*D report. *The American Journal of Psychiatry*, *163*(11), 1905–1917. https://doi.org/10.1176/ajp.2006.163.11.1905.

Rybakowski, J. K. (2013). Genetic influences on response to mood stabilizers in bipolar disorder: Current status of knowledge. *CNS Drugs*, *27*(3), 165–173. https://doi.org/10.1007/s40263-013-0040-7.

Rybakowski, J. K., Abramowicz, M., Szczepankiewicz, A., Michalak, M., Hauser, J., & Czekalski, S. (2013). The association of glycogen synthase kinase-3beta (GSK-3β) gene polymorphism with kidney function in long-term lithium-treated bipolar patients. *International Journal of Bipolar Disorders*, *1*(1), 8. https://doi.org/10.1186/2194-7511-1-8.

Rybakowski, J. K., Suwalska, A., Skibinska, M., Dmitrzak-Weglarz, M., Leszczynska-Rodziewicz, A., & Hauser, J. (2007). Response to lithium prophylaxis: Interaction between serotonin transporter and BDNF genes. *American Journal of Medical Genetics*.

Part B, Neuropsychiatric Genetics: The Official Publication of the International Society of Psychiatric Genetics, 144B(6), 820–823. https://doi.org/10.1002/ajmg.b.30420.

Sacchetti, E., Magri, C., Minelli, A., Valsecchi, P., Traversa, M., Calza, S., et al. (2017). The GRM7 gene, early response to risperidone, and schizophrenia: A genome-wide association study and a confirmatory pharmacogenetic analysis. *The Pharmacogenomics Journal, 17*(2), 146–154. https://doi.org/10.1038/tpj.2015.90.

Saneto, R. P., Lee, I.-C., Koenig, M. K., Bao, X., Weng, S.-W., Naviaux, R. K., et al. (2010). POLG DNA testing as an emerging standard of care before instituting valproic acid therapy for pediatric seizure disorders. *Seizure, 19*(3), 140–146. https://doi.org/10.1016/j.seizure.2010.01.002.

Schmidt, C. J., Sorensen, S. M., Kehne, J. H., Carr, A. A., & Palfreyman, M. G. (1995). The role of 5-HT2A receptors in antipsychotic activity. *Life Sciences, 56*(25), 2209–2222. Retrieved from http://www.ncbi.nlm.nih.gov/pubmed/7791509.

Schulze, T. G., Alda, M., Adli, M., Akula, N., Ardau, R., Bui, E. T., et al. (2010). The International Consortium on Lithium Genetics (ConLiGen): An initiative by the NIMH and IGSLI to study the genetic basis of response to lithium treatment. *Neuropsychobiology, 62*(1), 72–78. https://doi.org/10.1159/000314708.

Sim, S. C., & Ingelman-Sundberg, M. (2010). The human cytochrome P450 (CYP) allele nomenclature website: A peer-reviewed database of CYP variants and their associated effects. *Human Genomics, 4*(4), 278–281. Retrieved from http://www.ncbi.nlm.nih.gov/pubmed/20511141.

Song, J., Bergen, S. E., Di Florio, A., Karlsson, R., Charney, A., Ruderfer, D. M., et al. (2017). Genome-wide association study identifies SESTD1 as a novel risk gene for lithium-responsive bipolar disorder. *Molecular Psychiatry, 22*(8), 1223. https://doi.org/10.1038/mp.2016.246.

Squassina, A., Manchia, M., Borg, J., Congiu, D., Costa, M., Georgitsi, M., et al. (2011). Evidence for association of an ACCN1 gene variant with response to lithium treatment in Sardinian patients with bipolar disorder. *Pharmacogenomics, 12*(11), 1559–1569. https://doi.org/10.2217/pgs.11.102.

Sriretnakumar, V., Huang, E., & Müller, D. J. (2015). Pharmacogenetics of clozapine treatment response and side-effects in schizophrenia: An update. *Expert Opinion on Drug Metabolism & Toxicology, 11*(11), 1709–1731. https://doi.org/10.1517/17425255.2015.1075003.

Stamm, T. J., Rampp, C., Wiethoff, K., Stingl, J., Mössner, R., O Malley, G., et al. (2016). The FKBP5 polymorphism rs1360780 influences the effect of an algorithm-based antidepressant treatment and is associated with remission in patients with major depression. *Journal of Psychopharmacology (Oxford, England), 30*(1), 40–47. https://doi.org/10.1177/0269881115620459.

Summar, M. L., Gainer, J. V., Pretorius, M., Malave, H., Harris, S., Hall, L. D., et al. (2004). Relationship between carbamoyl-phosphate synthetase genotype and systemic vascular function. *Hypertension (Dallas, Tex.: 1979), 43*(2), 186–191. https://doi.org/10.1161/01.HYP.0000112424.06921.52.

Tansey, K. E., Guipponi, M., Perroud, N., Bondolfi, G., Domenici, E., Evans, D., et al. (2012). Genetic predictors of response to serotonergic and noradrenergic antidepressants in major depressive disorder: A genome-wide analysis of individual-level data and a meta-analysis. *PLoS Medicine, 9*(10), e1001326. https://doi.org/10.1371/journal.pmed.1001326.

Thase, M. E. (2007). STEP-BD and bipolar depression: What have we learned? *Current Psychiatry Reports, 9*(6), 497–503. Retrieved from http://www.ncbi.nlm.nih.gov/pubmed/18221631.

Vehof, J., Burger, H., Wilffert, B., Al Hadithy, A., Alizadeh, B. Z., Snieder, H., et al. (2012). Clinical response to antipsychotic drug treatment: Association study of polymorphisms in six candidate genes. *European Neuropsychopharmacology*, *22*(9), 625–631. https://doi.org/10.1016/j.euroneuro.2012.01.006.

Whirl-Carrillo, M., McDonagh, E. M., Hebert, J. M., Gong, L., Sangkuhl, K., Thorn, C. F., et al. (2012). Pharmacogenomics knowledge for personalized medicine. *Clinical Pharmacology and Therapeutics*, *92*(4), 414–417. https://doi.org/10.1038/clpt.2012.96.

Yagi, M., Nakamura, T., Okizuka, Y., Oyazato, Y., Kawasaki, Y., Tsuneishi, S., et al. (2010). Effect of CPS14217C > A genotype on valproic-acid-induced hyperammonemia. *Pediatrics International*, *52*(5), 744–748. https://doi.org/10.1111/j.1442-200X.2010.03157.x.

Yu, H., Wang, L., Lv, L., Ma, C., Du, B., Lu, T., et al. (2016). Genome-wide association study suggested the PTPRD polymorphisms were associated with weight gain effects of atypical antipsychotic medications. *Schizophrenia Bulletin*, *42*(3), 814–823. https://doi.org/10.1093/schbul/sbv179.

Zhang, J.-P., Lencz, T., & Malhotra, A. K. (2010). D_2 receptor genetic variation and clinical response to antipsychotic drug treatment: A meta-analysis. *American Journal of Psychiatry*, *167*(7), 763–772. https://doi.org/10.1176/appi.ajp.2009.09040598.

Zhang, J.-P., Lencz, T., Zhang, R. X., Nitta, M., Maayan, L., John, M., et al. (2016). Pharmacogenetic associations of antipsychotic drug-related weight gain: A systematic review and meta-analysis. *Schizophrenia Bulletin*, *42*(6), 1418–1437. https://doi.org/10.1093/schbul/sbw058.

Zhang, F., & Lupski, J. R. (2015). Non-coding genetic variants in human disease. *Human Molecular Genetics*, *24*(R1), R102–R110. https://doi.org/10.1093/hmg/ddv259.

CHAPTER THIRTEEN

Pharmacogenetics in Cardiovascular Medicine

Peter E. Weeke[1]

Department of Cardiology, Copenhagen University Hospital, Bispebjerg and Frederiksberg, Denmark

[1]Corresponding author: e-mail address: peterweeke@gmail.com

Contents

1. Introduction 334
2. Cardiovascular-Specific Drug Responses 336
   2.1 Clopidogrel 336
   2.2 Warfarin 338
   2.3 Statins 343
   2.4 β-Blockers and Drug Responses 345
3. Drug-Induced Long QT Syndrome 346
4. Implementation Challenges 347
5. Conclusion 349
References 350
Further Reading 360

Abstract

Considerable interindividual variability in response to cardiovascular pharmacotherapy exists with drug responses varying from being efficacious to inadequate to induce severe adverse events. Fueled by advancements and multidisciplinary collaboration across disciplines such as genetics, bioinformatics, and basic research, the vision of personalized medicine, rather than a one-size-fits-all approach, may be within reach. Pharmacogenetics offers the potential to optimize the benefit–risk profile of drugs by tailoring diagnostic and treatment strategies according to the individual patient. To date, a multitude of studies has tried to delineate the effects of gene–drug interactions for drugs commonly used to treat cardiovascular-related disease. The focus of this review is on how genetic variability may modify drug responsiveness and patient outcomes following therapy with commonly used cardiovascular drugs including clopidogrel, warfarin, statins, and β-blockers. Also included are examples of how genetic studies can be used to guide drug discovery and examples of how genetic information may be deployed in clinical decision making.

Advances in Pharmacology, Volume 83
ISSN 1054-3589
https://doi.org/10.1016/bs.apha.2018.04.002

ABBREVIATIONS

ADP	adenosine diphosphate
CI	95% confidence interval
CPIC	the Clinical Pharmacogenetic Implementation Consortium
CYP2C9	cytochrome P450 2C9
FDA	the US Food and Drug Administration
GIFT	genetic informatics trial
GWAS	genome-wide association study
HMGCR	3-hydroxy-3-methylglutaryl HMG-CoA reductase
HR	hazard ratio
MACE	major adverse cardiovascular events
MI	myocardial infarction
NOAC	nonvitamin K antagonist oral anticoagulants
PREDICT	the Vanderbilt Pharmacogenomics Resource for Enhanced Decisions in Care and Treatment
SNP	single-nucleotide polymorphism
VKAs	vitamin K antagonists
VKORC1	vitamin K epoxide reductase multiprotein complex, subunit 1

1. INTRODUCTION

The ability to incorporate genomics-based knowledge into clinical practice to accurately predict drug responsiveness has been proposed as one of the "grand challenges" in the future of genomics research (Collins, 2004). Rather than a one-size-fits-all approach, personalized medicine holds the promise of delivering tailored diagnostic and treatment strategies aiming to improve clinical outcomes and the benefit–risk profile of drugs. That is, identifying patients with an efficacious drug response, patients who fail to elicit an adequate drug response or patients who have an adverse drug response. However, predicting a drug response is multifaceted and relies not only on individual factors such as physiological factors (e.g., weight or kidney function), environmental factors (e.g., smoking or concomitant drug therapy), or genomic factors (e.g., race) but also on the interplay between them. Over the last decade, advances across multiple disciplines (e.g., genomics, proteomics, and bioinformatics) have led not only to novel drug discoveries (e.g., *PCSK9* inhibitors) but also to improved understanding of drug variability, which ultimately may see the enormous potential of personalized medicine being fulfilled.

Interindividual drug variability is commonly influenced by pharmacokinetic and pharmacodynamic properties. The pharmacokinetic properties of a given drug are typically altered when there are changes in the function of organs associated with absorption, distribution, metabolism, or elimination. By contrast, the pharmacodynamic properties of a drug are altered by changes in the molecular target of the drug. Thus, genetic variability in drug-metabolizing enzymes and transporters, directly or indirectly involved in drug metabolism, may modulate drug responsiveness. Most drug development programs perform extensive pharmacokinetic and pharmacodynamic studies in order to delineate drug metabolism properties in the setting of, e.g., abnormal renal function or concomitant pharmacotherapy.

One example of how adverse drug effects may arise following modulation of pharmacokinetic properties is the nonselective antihistamine, terfenadine. Terfenadine is administered as a prodrug and requires biotransformation by *CYP3A4* to generate the active isoform, fexofenadine. However, the enzymatic activity of *CYP3A4* can be modulated by genetic variation but also by other agents ranging from commonly prescribed antibiotics to grapefruit juice. For example, inhibition of *CYP3A4* activity in the setting of concomitant terfenadine treatment will lead to a significant increase in systemic exposure of terfenadine that may translate into adverse cardiovascular events; besides blocking the H1-receptor, terfenadine can also block the potassium channel *KCNH2* that is involved in cardiac repolarization, which can lead to the development of malignant ventricular arrhythmias. Terfenadine has subsequently been removed from the market (Leurs, Church, & Taglialatela, 2002; Woosley, Chen, Freiman, & Gillis, 1993).

In recent years, the role of gene–drug interactions has been increasingly appreciated. To date, the Clinical Pharmacogenetics Implementation Consortium (CPIC) has published more than 30 consensus guidelines calling for genotype-guided therapy (https://cpicpgx.org/). Highlighting the potential for gene–drug interactions was an analysis of ~10,000 patients from the Vanderbilt Pharmacogenomics Resource for Enhanced Decisions in Care and Treatment (PREDICT) program which saw more than 91% of patients harboring a clinical actionable variant in a subset of five well-established gene–drug interactions (clopidogrel [*CYP2C19*], simvastatin [*SLCO1B1*], warfarin [*CYP2C9* and *VKORC1*], thiopurines [*TPMT*], and tacrolimus [*CYP3A5*]) (Pulley et al., 2012; Van Driest et al., 2014).

This review will summarize the current state of knowledge in cardiovascular pharmacogenetics and describe how this information may help guide drug therapy for the treatment of cardiovascular disease.

2. CARDIOVASCULAR-SPECIFIC DRUG RESPONSES

2.1 Clopidogrel

Clopidogrel is an antiplatelet drug, approved in the late 1990s, commonly used to prevent thromboembolic complications including acute coronary syndrome, myocardial infarction (MI), stroke, or in the setting of percutaneous coronary intervention (PCI). Clopidogrel, a thienopyridine prodrug, is rapidly absorbed from the intestine via an efflux pump, encoded by *ABCB1,* with peak plasma concentrations occurring within 1 h after oral administration (Close, 2012). Approximately 85% of the absorbed clopidogrel is metabolized by ubiquitous carboxylesterases (CES) into inactive metabolites. The remaining ~15% undergoes hepatic bioactivation via different isoforms of the human cytochrome P450 (CYP450) enzymatic complex, predominantly cytochrome P450 2C19 (CYP2C19), to form the pharmacologically active thiol metabolite that irreversibly inhibits the $P2Y_{12}$ adenosine diphosphate (ADP) receptor on platelets. This way platelet aggregation is prevented (Kazui et al., 2010). While clopidogrel has been associated with favorable outcomes, considerable interindividual variability in platelet function following clopidogrel exposure has been identified (Gurbel, Bliden, Hiatt, & O'Connor, 2003).

In 2006, Hulot et al. demonstrated how genetic variability in the CYP2C19 enzymatic complex, particularly the common loss-of-function single-nucleotide polymorphism (SNP) *2 for *CYP2C19* (681 G>A, rs4244285), was critical for bioactivation and clopidogrel responsiveness (Hulot et al., 2006). The *CYP2C19*2* encodes an aberrant splice variant with no apparent enzymatic activity (Goldstein, 2001). In 2009, Shuldiner et al. performed a genome-wide association study (GWAS) among 429 Amish individuals where they identified variants associated with CYP2C19 to be the major genetic determinants of differences in response to clopidogrel; *CYP2C19*2* was identified as being the strongest genetic loci associated with diminished platelet response to clopidogrel treatment (Shuldiner et al., 2009). While the study concluded that ~73% of the diminished platelet response to clopidogrel treatment was heritable, the contribution of *CYP2C19*2* and clinical characteristics (i.e., age and gender) only accounted ~12% and ~10% of overall heritability, respectively (Shuldiner et al., 2009). Thus, much of the overall heritability remains unaccounted for. Resequencing of CYP2C19 has subsequently identified a multitude of rare, and to some extent uncharacterized, nonsynonymous variants which may also contribute to clopidogrel responsiveness. In addition, variants in other loci including *ABCB1* (Mega, Close, et al., 2010) and *PON1* (Bouman et al., 2011) have also been spuriously implicated with clopidogrel responsiveness and outcomes, but have failed to replicate in the majority of studies.

The *CYP2C19**2* is the most common loss-of-function allele in *CYP2C19* (c.681G>A; rs4244285), with reported frequencies of ~12% in Caucasians, ~15% in Africans, and 29%–35% in Asians (Scott et al., 2012). The greatest functional consequences of *CYP2C19* variability are seen in individuals homozygous for the loss-of-function variants (i.e., "poor metabolizers"), whereas heterozygotes are less affected (i.e., "intermediate metabolizers"). The most common combination of loss-of-function variants in *CYP2C19* is *CYP2C19**2* and *CYP2C19**3* (rs4986893, Gly636Ala) and makes up for ~90% of all *CYP2C19* "poor metabolizers" (Ingelman-Sundberg, Sim, Gomez, & Rodriguez-Antona, 2007; Pare et al., 2010). Other less common *CYP2C19* loss-of-function alleles include *4 (rs28399504), *5 (rs56337013), *6 (rs72552267), *7 (rs72558186), and *8 (rs41291556). To put this into a clinical context, 2%–5% of all Caucasians and Africans are homozygous for a loss-of-function allele, whereas up to 15% of Asians are homozygous for a loss-of-function allele (Yasmina, de Boer, Klungel, & Deneer, 2014). Conversely, gain-of-function alleles in *CYP2C19* (e.g., *CYP2C19**17*) are associated with increased *CYP2C19* expression and enzymatic activity. The *CYP2C19**17* allele has been associated increased bleeding risk (Sibbing et al., 2010).

Over the past decade, several studies have linked the common loss-of-function *CYP2C19**2* polymorphism with decreased antiplatelet activity (Brandt et al., 2007; Fontana, Hulot, De Moerloose, & Gaussem, 2007; Frere et al., 2008; Kim, Park, Hong, & Park, 2008; Shuldiner et al., 2009) and risk of adverse thromboembolic events including death, MI, and stroke (Collet et al., 2009; Delaney et al., 2012; Mega et al., 2009; Mega, Simon, et al., 2010; Simon et al., 2009; Trenk et al., 2008; Wang et al., 2016). The conflicting evidence implicating *CYP2C19* with clopidogrel responsiveness has since fueled a series of meta-analyses of major adverse cardiovascular events (MACE) by *CYP2C19**2* genotype (Holmes, Perel, Shah, Hingorani, & Casas, 2011; Hulot et al., 2010; Mega, Simon, et al., 2010). One meta-analysis utilizing data from a total of 9685 patients from 9 studies, of which 8847 (91.3%) underwent PCI, support the association between *CYP2C19* loss-of-function alleles and increased risk of MACE (heterozygous CYP2C19*2 status: hazard ratio (HR) = 1.55, 95% confidence interval

(CI): 1.11–2.17; homozygous carrier status: HR = 1.76, CI: 1.24–2.50) and in-stent thrombosis among patients having undergone PCI (HR = 2.67, CI: 1.69–4.22; homozygous carrier status: HR = 3.97, CI: 1.75–9.02). Notably, the *CYP2C19* clopidogrel gene–drug interaction was strongest among patients undergoing in-stent thrombosis. It has since been hypothesized that the effect of clopidogrel is greatest among "vulnerable" patients such as those undergoing PCI, which makes the impact of genomic variation in *CYP2C19* stronger and hereby detectable (Johnson et al., 2012). The confirmatory findings on loss-of-function *CYP2C19* alleles, clopidogrel, and in-stent thrombosis compared with the more conflicting findings regarding loss-of-function alleles in CYP2C19, clopidogrel, and MACE among patients with medically managed CAD support this hypothesis (Holmes et al., 2011).

Based on the level of evidence implicating loss-of-function variants in *CYP2C19* with reduced clopidogrel responsiveness and adverse outcomes, the US Food and Drug Administration (FDA) included a "boxed warning" in the drug label highlighting the potential for reduced clopidogrel responsiveness (increased adverse cardiovascular outcomes) based on *CYP2C19* genotype; the warning was limited to "poor metabolizers" and focused on patients undergoing PCI. Despite the "boxed warning" issued by the FDA, the American College of Cardiology and American Heart Association formed a taskforce who decided not to recommend routine *CYP2C19* testing based on the absence of outcomes data from prospective, randomized, genotype-directed clinical trials (Holmes et al., 2010) Thus, the results from ongoing genotype-directed randomized clinical trials (RCTs) are greatly awaited. Recognizing that genetic tests are becoming increasingly widespread CPIC provides peer-reviewed guidelines aiding to facilitate the translation of genetic test results into clinical decision making. For patients undergoing PCI who are also carriers of the *CYP2C19* loss-of-function alleles, the CPIC recommends use of alternative therapies such as prasugrel or ticagrelor (Scott et al., 2011).

2.2 Warfarin

Despite the introduction of nonvitamin K antagonist oral anticoagulants (NOAC) in 2010, warfarin, a vitamin K antagonist, remains one of the most commonly used anticoagulants to control and prevent thromboembolic events worldwide (Huisman et al., 2017). Although more than 60 years of experience with warfarin has been accumulated, it still remains one of the most difficult drugs to manage due to a narrow therapeutic index, food and drug interactions, and genetic effects which translates into effective therapeutic doses ranging from 1 to 20 mg per day (Johnson et al., 2011). Unsurprisingly, warfarin-related adverse drug reactions are one of the most common causes for hospitalizations and emergency department visits (Budnitz, Lovegrove, Shehab, & Richards, 2011).

To date, more than 30 genes have been identified as having potential effects on the anticoagulative properties of warfarin; however, only two genes have been directly implicated with warfarin dosing variability: vitamin K epoxide reductase multiprotein complex, subunit 1 (*VKORC1*) and cytochrome P450 2C9 (CYP2C9) (Johnson et al., 2011; Jonas & McLeod, 2009). Warfarin is administered as a mix of enantiomers, S-warfarin and R-warfarin, with the more potent enantiomer S-warfarin being metabolized by *CYP2C9* in the liver. *CYP2C9*2* (rs1799853) and *CYP2C9*3* (rs1057910) are two relatively common loss-of-function SNPs in *CYP2C9* that have been shown to reduce enzymatic activity and ability to metabolize warfarin by ~30% and ~90% in Caucasians, respectively, compared to the wild-type allele (Rettie, Haining, Bajpai, & Levy, 1999). Additionally, lower warfarin dosing requirements and increased bleeding risk have been observed among patients harboring the CYP2C9*2 and CYP2C9*3 alleles (Aithal, Day, Kesteven, & Daly, 1999; Cooper et al., 2008; Lindh, Holm, Andersson, & Rane, 2009).

The pharmacological target of warfarin is *VKORC1*. *VKORC1* is the rate-limiting enzyme that controls the formation of vitamin K-dependent clotting factors clotting factors II, VII, IX, and X (Schalekamp & de Boer, 2010). *VKORC1* was first implicated with warfarin dosing variability in 2004 where a rare cause of familial warfarin resistance identified causative genetic variants within the coding regions of *VKORC1* (Rost et al., 2004). Studies have since identified multiple common genetic variants in the promoter region of *VKORC1* that modulate warfarin steady-state dosing requirement. Particularly two SNPs, rs9923231 (−1639G>A) and rs9934438 (−1173C>T), located in the promoter region of *VKORC1* and in high linkage disequilibrium in Caucasians, have been shown to reduce hepatic *VKORC1* mRNA transcript abundance and protein expression which means that lower warfarin dosage requirements are needed to achieve sufficient anticoagulation (Rieder et al., 2005). Conversely, carriers of SNPs leading to greater *VKORC1* protein expression require greater warfarin dosages (Wang et al., 2008). Aside confirming the *CYP2C9* and *VKORC1* loci as modulators of warfarin dosing requirements, GWAS analysis conditioned on these specific loci, have since implicated variants in *CYP2F4* with warfarin variability (Cooper et al., 2008; Takeuchi et al., 2009). CYP4F2 acts as a counterpart to *VKORC1* in limiting excessive accumulation of vitamin K by catalyzing the metabolism of reduced vitamin K by removing vitamin K from the vitamin K cycle (Danese et al., 2012).

Among individuals of Caucasian ancestry, genetic variants in *CYP2C9* and *VKORC1 account* for ~50% of the variance in warfarin steady-state dose. Taken together with clinical covariates (10%–20%) and concomitant pharmacotherapy (5%–10%), ~60%–70% of the variability in warfarin dosing can be accounted for among Caucasians (Gage et al., 2008; Jonas & McLeod, 2009; Wadelius et al., 2009). By contrast, less of the variability is accounted for in other ethnic groups including Africans and Asians (Cavallari et al., 2010). Among individuals of African descent, the prevalence of increased function *VKORC1* promoter variants is more common, whereas it is lower among Asians which translates into higher and lower steady-state dosage requirements, respectively. Moreover, the *CYP2C9*2* and *CYP2C9*3* variants are less common among individuals of African ancestry. Yet other *CYP2C9* SNPs (*CYP2C9*5*, **6*, **8*, and **11*), mostly absent among Caucasians, may also contribute to warfarin variability in these individuals (Allabi, Gala, & Horsmans, 2005). In 2013, a GWAS performed among Africans implicated an unknown locus close to the *CYP2C9* locus (Perera et al., 2013).

Based on the level of evidence implicating pharmacogenetic loci in *CYP2C9* and *VKORC1* with warfarin responsiveness, the FDA updated the warfarin label to also include a dosing table based on the genotypic profile of *CYP2C9* and *VKORC1* alleles; according to carrier status, patients can be normal, sensitive, or highly sensitive responders to warfarin. Based on the updated warfarin dosing table, a prespecified genetic subanalysis among warfarin-exposed subjects in the ENGAGE TIMI-48 randomized double-blinded clinical trial confirmed the utility of using *CYP2C9* and *VKORC1* genotypes to identify at risk patients for warfarin-related adverse bleeding events. Compared with normal responders, sensitive or highly sensitive responders were at greater risk of adverse bleeding events (HR=1.31, 95% CI, 1.05–1.64 and HR=2.66, 1.69–4.19, respectively) (Mega et al., 2015). The CPIC guidelines also recommend using genotype-driven warfarin dosing, if available (Johnson et al., 2011).

In 2013, three RCTs, the clarification of optimal anticoagulation through genetics (COAG) (Kimmel et al., 2013) trial and two European pharmacogenetics of anticoagulant therapy (EU-PACT) trials (Pirmohamed et al., 2013; Verhoef et al., 2013), sought to test if prospective genotype-guided warfarin treatment performed better than nongenotype-driven treatment in terms of achieving and maintaining time in therapeutic range (TTR) (INR 2–3) (Kimmel et al., 2013; Pirmohamed et al., 2013; Verhoef et al., 2013). Two of the studies, the COAG trial and the EU-PACT trial of other vitamin K antagonists (VKAs) (Verhoef et al., 2013), used clinical algorithms and compared these to combined clinical and genetic algorithms. No significant difference in TTR was identified in either study, although improvements in TTR in the genetic arm of the EU-PACT study of other VKAs were seen within the first 4 weeks of treatment (Kimmel et al., 2013; Verhoef et al., 2013). The third study, the EU-PACT trial, compared an empiric loading algorithm with a combined clinical and genetic algorithm; a significant difference of TTR was demonstrated in favor of the combined algorithm (Pirmohamed et al., 2013). Unfortunately, neither of the studies was powered to evaluate clinical end points. In the largest of the studies, the COAG trial, only 14 warfarin-related major bleeding events among 1015 patients were recorded.

In trying to understand the diverging results of these trials, it is important to evaluate differences in study designs. First, the studies used different dosing algorithms. The COAG trial and the EU-PACT trial of other VKAs used clinical algorithms as the comparator, whereas the EU-PACT trial used an empiric dosing algorithm. Thus, given the established superiority of a clinical dosing algorithm compared with an empiric dosing algorithm, the findings in the EU-PACT may not be too surprising. Second, the composition of patients included in the studies differed with the EU-PACT trials being predominantly of Caucasian ancestry, whereas the COAG trial consisted of ~30% African Americans which could have influenced the study findings. Moreover, the genotypes included in the COAG trial (i.e., *VKORC1* − 1639G > A, *CYP2C9*2*, and *CYP2C9*3*) were not ancestry specific. That is, only ~6% of African Americans carry the *CYP2C9*2* or *CYP2C9*3* allele, whereas ~20% have at least one *CYP2C9*5*, *CYP2C9*6*, *CYP2C9*8*, or *CYP2C9*11* allele that are also known to modify warfarin responsiveness. Thus, much of the population-specific genetic variability was not accounted for. This is of interest given that there were indications of adverse events among African Americans in the COAG trial. Third, genotypes were only available for 45% of patients in the COAG trial at the time of first warfarin dose compared with 100% in the EU-PACT trials. Not having the genotypes at hand when starting treatment could potentially bias the study toward null. Fourth, the patients enrolled in COAG were younger (mean age was 53 years in African Americans and

59 years in non-Africans Americans), compared with the EU-PACT trials (mean age 67 years) (Johnson & Cavallari, 2015). In sum, although there were differences in the three study designs, which has since been a topic of debate, it may be concluded that genotype-driven warfarin treatment algorithms are of limited usefulness regarding achieving and maintaining TTR in the very early phases of warfarin treatment (30 and 90 days). However, no conclusions could be drawn regarding clinical outcomes.

By contrast, the recently published randomized clinical genetic informatics trial (GIFT) of warfarin to prevent deep vein thrombosis trial did evaluate clinical outcomes (i.e., major bleeding, INR $\geq$4, venous thromboembolism, and death) among 1597 patients undergoing elective hip or knee arthroplasty who were assigned to genotype-guided perioperative warfarin therapy vs clinically perioperative-guided warfarin therapy. The genetic variants that were included in the study were *VKORC1−1639-G>A*, *CYP2C9*2*, *CYP2C9*3*, and *CYP4F2 V433M*. In the GIFT trial, genotype-guided warfarin therapy significantly reduced the risk of the composite endpoint comprised of major bleeding events, INR $\geq$ 4, venous thromboembolism, and death (relative rate = 0.73; 95% confidence interval 0.56–0.95). Moreover, patients who were in the genotype-guided group also experienced a significantly higher TTR than did patients in the clinical group (54.7% vs 51.3%, respectively). No deaths were recorded (Gage et al., 2017).

In summary, aside being one of the first pharmacogenetic RCTs evaluating clinical outcomes, the findings from GIFT are uplifting and suggest that genotype-driven warfarin treatment does improve outcomes among patients undergoing elective hip or knee arthroplasty in terms of reducing drug-induced adverse events (Gage et al., 2017). However, the generalizability of the results needs to be explored in subsequent studies and aspects of cost-effectiveness also need to be addressed, as 26 patients would need genotyping to prevent 1 composite event according to the findings from GIFT.

Since NOACs were approved in 2010, a substantial increase in its usage compared to VKA has been observed (Staerk et al., 2016). While NOACs do not seem to share the same pharmacogenomic profile as VKA, reports of gene–drug interactions have been reported. A common variant in carboxylesterase 1 (*CES1*, rs2244613) has been associated with bleeding risk following dabigatran treatment (Pare et al., 2013). Whether similar gene–drug interactions exist for other NOACs (e.g., rivaroxaban or apixaban) remains to be determined.

2.3 Statins

Statins are one of the cornerstones for treatment and prevention of atherosclerotic cardiovascular disease. Statins lower systemic cholesterol levels, particularly low-density lipoprotein cholesterol (LDL-C), through an inhibition of 3-hydroxy-3-methylglutaryl HMG-CoA reductase (HMGCR) which results in an upregulation of hepatocyte LDL-C receptors, increased LDL-C clearance, and attenuated intrahepatic cholesterol synthesis. While studies have shown a ~20% risk reduction of major cardiovascular events per 1 mmol/L LDL-C decrease, substantial interindividual variability in statin response exists with up to one-third of patients not obtaining clinically desired LDL-C levels (Baigent et al., 2005; Davidson et al., 2005). Moreover, an estimated 7%–29% of patients experience statin-induced muscle-related symptoms, which may be accompanied by an increase in plasma creatinine kinase levels (Stroes et al., 2015). While statin-induced rhabdomyolysis is rare, it is potentially fatal (~10% mortality rate) (Law & Rudnicka, 2006; Thompson, Clarkson, & Karas, 2003). To date, a multitude of factors influencing statin outcomes and responsiveness have been identified including genetic variability (Mangravite, Thorn, & Krauss, 2006).

Early efforts aimed to delineate the effects of genetic variability on statin responsiveness were mainly focused on genes involved in lipid and statin metabolism including *ApoE* (a protein that interacts with the LDL receptor), *CYP3A4* (a key drug-metabolizing enzyme), and *ABCB1* and *ABCG2* (drug transporters) (Pasanen, Neuvonen, Neuvonen, & Niemi, 2006; Wilke, Moore, & Burmester, 2005). Genetic variants in both *CYP3A4* and *CYP3A5* have also inconsistently been associated with statin pharmacokinetics and dynamics. *CYP3A5**3 (rs776746) and *CYP3A4**22 (rs35599367) are polymorphisms associated with decreased enzymatic activity which translates into higher simvastatin bioavailability compared to wild type (Kitzmiller, Luzum, Baldassarre, Krauss, & Medina, 2014; Tsamandouras et al., 2014). One study by Wang et al. identified *CYP3A4**22 variant carriers to require 20%–60% lower statin dose to achieve optimal lipid concentrations compared to noncarriers (Wang, Guo, Wrighton, Cooke, & Sadee, 2011). By contrast, Ragia et al. were unable to identify a significant gene–drug interaction among 209 patients who received 10–40 mg simvastatin daily for a 6-month period (Ragia et al., 2015).

The kinesin-like protein 6 (*KIF6*) is involved in intracellular molecular transport and early studies identified carriers of a missense SNP (Trp719Arg, rs20455) to have greater risk of adverse cardiovascular outcomes (Iakoubova et al., 2010), but greater benefit from statin therapy compared to wild type

(Iakoubova et al., 2008). The association between KIF6 and statin response (Ridker, MacFadyen, Glynn, & Chasman, 2011) and cardiovascular outcomes has not been validated in subsequent analysis including a large meta-analysis comprised of more than 144,000 patients (Assimes et al., 2010).

Genetic variation in *HMGCR* has also been associated with variable statin response. The H7 haplotype is comprised of three intronic variants (rs17244841, rs3846662, and rs17238540) and has been shown to attenuate statin-induced lipid-lowering response by ~20% in one study (Krauss et al., 2008), whereas as other studies have been unable to validate these findings (Donnelly et al., 2008; Thompson et al., 2009). The proposed mechanism of action is attributable to an alternatively spliced HMGCR that is less sensitive simvastatin (Medina, Gao, Ruan, Rotter, & Krauss, 2008).

The gene *SLCO1B1* encodes the polypeptide organic anion transporter OATP1B1 and is involved in hepatic statin uptake, except for fluvastatin (Law & Rudnicka, 2006). However, despite its direct effects on hepatic statin uptake, variants in *SLCO1B1* seem to induce only minor effects on the overall lipid variability (<5%) for patients treated with simvastatin, lovastatin, pravastatin, or atorvastatin (Peters et al., 2010). In 2008, a GWAS comprised of 175 individuals who received simvastatin 80 mg daily identified a strong association between the common variant rs4363657, in close vicinity of *SLCO1B1*, and statin-induced myopathy (Link et al., 2008). Notably, the rs4363657 is in near-perfect disequilibrium ($R^2 = 0.97$) with a previously studied nonsynonymous variant in *SLCO1B1* (SLCO1B1*5, rs4149056, V174A) which suggest a reduced ability to transport simvastatin into hepatocytes which in turn leads to increased systemic simvastatin concentrations and risk of myopathy among variant carriers. Compared to wild type, heterozygote and homozygote carriers of the *SLCO1B1* loss-of-function variant (24.7% and 2.1%, respectively) were 4.5 and 16.9 times more likely to develop myopathy following treatment with 80 mg simvastatin daily. A similar dose–response pattern was replicated in patients from the heart protection study who received simvastatin 40 mg daily. Approximately 60% of all patients with simvastatin-induced myopathy (80 mg daily) were found to be *SLCO1B1*5* carriers compared with ~15% of the overall study population (Link et al., 2008). These findings were also confirmed in the Genetics of Diabetes Audit and Research in Tayside Scotland database (GO-DARTS) ($n = 4340$) where homozygous carriers of the rs4363657 variant had a threefold increased risk of being statin intolerant compared to wild type (Donnelly et al., 2011). Interestingly, *SLCO1B1*5* has also been associated with CK levels three times greater than the upper limit of normal and reduced statin adherence (simvastatin and atorvastatin), which may be attributable to statin-induced myopathy (Voora et al., 2009). The Rotterdam Study also identified carriers of the *SLCO1B1*5* variant to be more likely to require simvastatin dose decreases and drug switching which could be suggestive of statin-induced adverse effects (de Keyser et al., 2014). A recent pilot study in primary care patients tested *SLCO1B1*5* genotype-guided statin therapy ($n = 59$) compared with nongenotype-guided therapy ($n = 58$) and identified improved patient statin perception, adherence, and cholesterol-lowering effects among patients who received genotype-guided therapy (Li et al., 2014). However, routine screening of *SLCO1B1*5* prior to statin treatment is not recommended, but if genotype information is available, then the CPIC has released consensus guidelines calling for genotype-guided therapy (Wilke et al., 2012). Other genes associated with statin-induced adverse events include *GATM, COQ2, RYR, ABCB1*, but results have been conflicting.

Rare variants in *PCSK9* and *NPC1L1* have also been shown to be associated with decreased cholesterol levels and coronary disease, and both proteins have been targeted for cholesterol-lowering agents (Cannon et al., 2015; Myocardial Infarction Genetics Consortium et al., 2014; Sabatine et al., 2017).

2.4 β-Blockers and Drug Responses

Beta-adrenergic antagonists (β-blockers) are associated with improved outcomes among patients with hypertension, angina pectoris, MI, and cardiac arrhythmias. To date, several genes have been implicated with variable β-blocker response including *CYP2D6*, the beta-1-adrenergic receptor (*ADBR1*), the beta-2-adrenergic receptor (*ADBR2*), and *GRK5*.

The greatest level of evidence for β-blocker gene interaction includes two nonsynonymous variants in *ADRB1* (S49G [rs1801252] and R389G [rs1801253]) (Muthumala, Drenos, Elliott, & Humphries, 2008). One study found carriers of the R389 genotype who were in treatment with carvedilol or metoprolol to experience greater improvements in left ventricular ejection fraction than other genotypes (Chen et al., 2007). These findings have since been validated in one study for carvedilol, but not for metoprolol (Petersen et al., 2011). In the β-blocker evaluation of survival trial (BEST), a study of heart failure patients treated with bucindolol, patients homozygous for R389 had improved contractility and survival (Bristow et al., 2010; Liggett et al., 2006). Consequently, the effect of bucindolol is now being evaluated specifically in patients with the *ADRB1* Arg389Arg genotype.

Common polymorphisms in *ADRB2* (R16G [rs1042713] and Q27G [rs1042714]) have been shown to be resistant to agonist-mediated downregulation (Green, Turki, Innis, & Liggett, 1994), but the translational importance of these polymorphisms on cardiovascular outcomes has been conflicting (de Groote et al., 2005; Small, Wagoner, Levin, Kardia, & Liggett, 2002).

Genetic variability in *CYP2D6* has also been associated with variable metoprolol responsiveness; *CYP2D6* is the primary enzyme involved in the oxidation of metoprolol. Approximately 8% of individuals of European and 2% of "other" ancestry lack activity of *CYP2D6* and will at recommended metoprolol doses experience increased β-blockade compared with extensive metabolizers. Similar findings have been made in patients in concomitant treatment with drugs that inhibit *CYP2D6* (Blaus et al., 2015).

Atrial fibrillation (AF) is one of the most common cardiac arrhythmias encountered in a clinical setting, and rate-limiting therapy with β-blockers is commonly indicated. While various risk factors (e.g., hypertension and diabetes) have been linked to the development of AF, the genetic underpinnings for the development of AF are both strong and polygenic (Christophersen et al., 2017; Weeke et al., 2015; Weeke, Muhammad, et al., 2014). The strongest genetic correlation for development of AF is reported for a common SNP in the chromosome 4q25 locus (rs10033464) in *Pitx2* in near proximity. *Pitx2* encodes a gene with regulatory properties for cardiac development and right–left differentiation of the embryonic heart, thorax, and aorta (Chinchilla et al., 2011; Mommersteeg et al., 2007). Clinical studies have suggested that polymorphisms at the chromosome 4q25 locus response to antiarrhythmic drug therapy. One study saw carriers of the rs10033464 to be less able to maintain sinus rhythm in response to antiarrhythmic pharmacotherapy compared to noncarriers (Parvez, Chopra, et al., 2012; Parvez, Vaglio, et al., 2012). Patients with low levels of *pitx2* mRNA and AF have also been shown to have improved effectiveness of sodium channel blocker therapy (Syeda et al., 2016). Moreover, carriers of the chromosome 4q25 locus variant, rs10033464, have also been associated with variable response to cardioversion and radiofrequency ablation for AF (Parvez et al., 2013; Shoemaker et al., 2015).

3. DRUG-INDUCED LONG QT SYNDROME

Drug-induced long QT syndrome (diLQTS) phenocopies the congenital long QT syndrome (cLQTS) and is associated with QT prolongation and torsade de pointes ventricular tachycardia (TdP) that have resulted in drug withdrawals (e.g., terfenadine). To date, >150 drugs are listed on CredibleMeds.org as being associated with QT prolongation and/or TdP. "Reduced repolarization reserve", as was originally proposed, (Roden, 2004) suggests that patients remain asymptomatic until multiple hits (e.g., hypokalemia, bradycardia, or exposure to a drug, typically a block of the potassium current [I_{kr}] encoded by *KCNH2*) unmask the extreme drug response phenotype (i.e., QT prolongation) that can lead to the development of fatal arrhythmias.

To date, several studies have tried to identify the underlying genetic architecture predisposing patients to diLQTS (Behr et al., 2013; Kaab et al., 2012; Paulussen et al., 2004; Weeke, Mosley, et al., 2014). One candidate gene study evaluated the genetic predisposition to diLQTS among 176 cases and 1044 controls and identified a nonsynonymous variant in *KCNE1* (rs1805128, D85N) that conferred risk of diLQTS (OR=9.0) (Kaab et al., 2012). In an exome sequencing study of 65 diLQTS cases and 148 controls, a significant excess of rare variants in *KCNE1* and *ACN9* was identified. Moreover, 37% of diLQTS cases were also carriers of a rare variant in potassium channel genes compared with 21% of controls (Weeke, Mosley, et al., 2014). While a previous GWAS did not implicate common variants with diLQTS at a genome-wide level (Behr et al., 2013), Strauss et al. recently demonstrated that a polygenic risk score comprised of 61 variants previously associated with baseline QT interval at genome-wide level was also associated with drug-induced QT prolongation and was a significant predictor of drug-induced TdP (Strauss et al., 2017). These studies highlight the importance of individualized treatment and risk stratification in the setting of adverse drug reactions.

4. IMPLEMENTATION CHALLENGES

While genotype-guided therapy has the potential to greatly benefit patients by enabling personalized medication management, improving drug effectiveness, and decreasing the risk of adverse drug effects, several challenges need to be addressed before the full potential of precision medicine can be fulfilled. One issue that has been debated is the level of evidence needed for implementing pharmacogenetic findings into clinical practice. To date, several common variants with large pharmacogenomic effect sizes and a clear underlying biology have been identified and replicated (Daly, 2010). However, deciding when a pharmacogenetic variant has sufficient evidence to be "clinically actionable" and should be used to guide drug treatment is less clear. Today, RCTs are commonly considered as the "gold standard" to establish new treatment regimens (Mrazek & Lerman, 2011). However, in the setting of pharmacogenomic research, RCTs can be hard to perform, considering the study size requirements needed to prove a clinical benefit in patient "subgroups" (i.e., based on genotype) as well the need for replication studies. Thus, considering the complexity and sometimes rarity of the traits studied (e.g., serious adverse drug reactions), performing an RCT can be troublesome. The CPIC and the Evaluation of Genomic Applications in Practice and Prevention (EGAPP) aim to evaluate the level of evidence needed for implementation of genetic findings into clinical practice (Relling & Klein, 2011; Teutsch et al., 2009).

Incorporating genetic information to predict drug responsiveness or optimize dosing algorithms at the "point of care" is one approach by which pharmacogenetic information may be used to individualize treatment. Naturally, having the genotype result at hand before treatment is initiated is imperative, but may take days or even weeks (Scott, 2013). Thus, genotype-guided therapy is of limited use if drug treatment is initiated before the genotype results are available. However, some point-of-care tests do exist, but may take over 60 min to process (Roberts et al., 2012). An alternate approach, known as preemptive genotyping, focuses on identifying patients who are likely to receive a given drug with known gene–drug interactions (e.g., clopidogrel and *CYP2C19*) before the drug is actually prescribed. The genetic information is subsequently embedded into an electronic medical record and available to the clinicians before it is actually needed (Schildcrout et al., 2012). The Vanderbilt PREDICT Project, the National Institutes of Health Funded Implementing Genomics in Practice (IGNITE) Network, and the National Human Genome Research Institutes Electronic Medical Records and Genomics Networks (eMERGE) are examples of genomic information which is being embedded into electronic medical records, hereby providing decision-based support on pharmacogenetic variants with the strongest levels of evidence in a cost-effective manner (Bell et al., 2014; Bielinski et al., 2014; Bowton et al., 2014; Pulley et al., 2012).

Educating clinicians is also vital as they will be at the forefront of implementation. In a recent survey, ~98% of the US physicians who responded to the survey believed that genetic variability could influence drug responsiveness, but only a minority of respondents (~10%) felt sufficiently informed about pharmacogenetic testing (Stanek et al., 2012). Thus, ensuring a sufficient and easy interpretable information flow to clinicians is key

(Haga, Burke, Ginsburg, Mills, & Agans, 2012; Peterson et al., 2016). Other operational challenges that should also be considered include large multidisciplinary collaborative efforts between, e.g., clinical leaders, laboratory technicians, pharmacists, bioinformaticians, and administrative staff (Karnes et al., 2014; Levy et al., 2014). Ethical challenges should also be considered including aspects of informed consent, confidentiality and data privacy, and handling of incidental findings (e.g., which results are considered "actionable" and how are these delivered to the patient) (Bredenoord, Kroes, Cuppen, Parker, & van Delden, 2011; Fullerton et al., 2012).

5. CONCLUSION

There is a rapidly growing level of evidence implicating genetic variability with drug responsiveness. One major hope is that we in the near future will see molecular advances within the field of cardiovascular disease and therapeutics translating into new and more efficient drug therapies being developed. That is, moving research findings more efficiently from "bench-to-bedside." While cardiovascular-related morbidity and mortality is one of the leading causes of death and disability worldwide, the development of drugs aimed to combat cardiovascular disease has remained stagnant compared to other specialties (Berggren, Moller, Moss, Poda, & Smietana, 2012). For example, within the field of oncology, extensive collaboration between basic researchers, clinicians, and industry has generated numerous new compounds with enhanced efficacy and decreased toxicity. Possible explanations to such stagnancy within the field of cardiology relate in part to a failure to adopt contemporary drug development approaches and a "traditional focus" on systemic therapies centering on large populations. Examples of how applying human genetics with detailed functional analysis in individuals with extreme phenotypes can lead to novel therapies include the discovery and development of *PCSK9* inhibitors, alirocumab and evolocumab, that lower LDL-C and reduce the risk of cardiovascular disease (Abifadel et al., 2003; Cohen, Boerwinkle, Mosley, & Hobbs, 2006; Sabatine et al., 2017). Another example of applied human genetics with functional analysis is the development of ivacaftor for patients with cystic fibrosis that harbor specific mutations in the CFTR disease gene that leads to gating defects in the encoded chloride channel (Ramsey et al., 2011). Combinational therapy with lumacaftor (a cell traffic potentiator) and ivacaftor corrects the CFTR mutational-induced abnormal gating and has been approved for treatment among patients with specific mutations in *CFTR* (Wainwright et al., 2015).

Collectively, the experience and outcomes from health care systems such as those outlined above alongside ongoing clinical trials and phenotype–genotype studies will provide important information on how to best use genetic information in a clinical setting to ultimately improve patient outcomes.

CONFLICT OF INTEREST

The author has no conflict of interest to declare.

REFERENCES

Abifadel, M., Varret, M., Rabes, J. P., Allard, D., Ouguerram, K., Devillers, M., et al. (2003). Mutations in PCSK9 cause autosomal dominant hypercholesterolemia. *Nature Genetics*, *34*(2), 154–156. https://doi.org/10.1038/ng1161.

Aithal, G. P., Day, C. P., Kesteven, P. J., & Daly, A. K. (1999). Association of polymorphisms in the cytochrome P450 CYP2C9 with warfarin dose requirement and risk of bleeding complications. *Lancet*, *353*(9154), 717–719. https://doi.org/10.1016/S0140-6736(98)04474-2.

Allabi, A. C., Gala, J. L., & Horsmans, Y. (2005). CYP2C9, CYP2C19, ABCB1 (MDR1) genetic polymorphisms and phenytoin metabolism in a Black Beninese population. *Pharmacogenetics and Genomics*, *15*(11), 779–786.

Assimes, T. L., Holm, H., Kathiresan, S., Reilly, M. P., Thorleifsson, G., Voight, B. F., et al. (2010). Lack of association between the Trp719Arg polymorphism in kinesin-like protein-6 and coronary artery disease in 19 case-control studies. *Journal of the American College of Cardiology*, *56*(19), 1552–1563. https://doi.org/10.1016/j.jacc.2010.06.022.

Baigent, C., Keech, A., Kearney, P. M., Blackwell, L., Buck, G., Pollicino, C., et al. (2005). Efficacy and safety of cholesterol-lowering treatment: Prospective meta-analysis of data from 90,056 participants in 14 randomised trials of statins. *Lancet (London, England)*, *366*(9493), 1267–1278. https://doi.org/10.1016/S0140-6736(05)67394-1.

Behr, E. R., Ritchie, M. D., Tanaka, T., Kaab, S., Crawford, D. C., Nicoletti, P., et al. (2013). Genome wide analysis of drug-induced torsades de pointes: Lack of common variants with large effect sizes. *PLoS One*, *8*(11), e78511. https://doi.org/10.1371/journal.pone.0078511.

Bell, G. C., Crews, K. R., Wilkinson, M. R., Haidar, C. E., Hicks, J. K., Baker, D. K., et al. (2014). Development and use of active clinical decision support for preemptive pharmacogenomics. *Journal of the American Medical Informatics Association*, *21*(e1), e93–99. https://doi.org/10.1136/amiajnl-2013-001993.

Berggren, R., Moller, M., Moss, R., Poda, P., & Smietana, K. (2012). Outlook for the next 5 years in drug innovation. *Nature Reviews. Drug Discovery*, *11*(6), 435–436. https://doi.org/10.1038/nrd3744.

Bielinski, S. J., Olson, J. E., Pathak, J., Weinshilboum, R. M., Wang, L., Lyke, K. J., et al. (2014). Preemptive genotyping for personalized medicine: Design of the right drug, right dose, right time-using genomic data to individualize treatment protocol. *Mayo Clinic Proceedings*, *89*(1), 25–33. https://doi.org/10.1016/j.mayocp.2013.10.021.

Blaus, A., Madabushi, R., Pacanowski, M., Rose, M., Schuck, R. N., Stockbridge, N., et al. (2015). Personalized cardiovascular medicine today: A food and drug administration/center for drug evaluation and research perspective. *Circulation*, *132*(15), 1425–1432. https://doi.org/10.1161/CIRCULATIONAHA.114.009761.

Bouman, H. J., Schomig, E., van Werkum, J. W., Velder, J., Hackeng, C. M., Hirschhauser, C., et al. (2011). Paraoxonase-1 is a major determinant of clopidogrel efficacy. *Nature Medicine*, *17*(1), 110–116. https://doi.org/10.1038/nm.2281.

Bowton, E., Field, J. R., Wang, S., Schildcrout, J. S., Van Driest, S. L., Delaney, J. T., et al. (2014). Biobanks and electronic medical records: Enabling cost-effective research. *Science Translational Medicine*, *6*(234), 234cm233. https://doi.org/10.1126/scitranslmed.3008604.

Brandt, J. T., Close, S. L., Iturria, S. J., Payne, C. D., Farid, N. A., Ernest, C. S., 2nd, et al. (2007). Common polymorphisms of CYP2C19 and CYP2C9 affect the pharmacokinetic and pharmacodynamic response to clopidogrel but not prasugrel. *Journal of Thrombosis and Haemostasis*, *5*(12), 2429–2436. https://doi.org/10.1111/j.1538-7836.2007.02775.x.

Bredenoord, A. L., Kroes, H. Y., Cuppen, E., Parker, M., & van Delden, J. J. (2011). Disclosure of individual genetic data to research participants: The debate reconsidered. *Trends in Genetics*, *27*(2), 41–47. https://doi.org/10.1016/j.tig.2010.11.004.

Bristow, M. R., Murphy, G. A., Krause-Steinrauf, H., Anderson, J. L., Carlquist, J. F., Thaneemit-Chen, S., et al. (2010). An alpha2C-adrenergic receptor polymorphism alters the norepinephrine-lowering effects and therapeutic response of the beta-blocker bucindolol in chronic heart failure. *Circulation. Heart Failure*, *3*(1), 21–28. https://doi.org/10.1161/CIRCHEARTFAILURE.109.885962.

Budnitz, D. S., Lovegrove, M. C., Shehab, N., & Richards, C. L. (2011). Emergency hospitalizations for adverse drug events in older Americans. *The New England Journal of Medicine*, *365*(21), 2002–2012. https://doi.org/10.1056/NEJMsa1103053.

Cannon, C. P., Blazing, M. A., Giugliano, R. P., McCagg, A., White, J. A., Theroux, P., et al. (2015). Ezetimibe added to statin therapy after acute coronary syndromes. *The New England Journal of Medicine*, *372*(25), 2387–2397. https://doi.org/10.1056/NEJMoa1410489.

Cavallari, L. H., Langaee, T. Y., Momary, K. M., Shapiro, N. L., Nutescu, E. A., Coty, W. A., et al. (2010). Genetic and clinical predictors of warfarin dose requirements in African Americans. *Clinical Pharmacology and Therapeutics*, *87*(4), 459–464. https://doi.org/10.1038/clpt.2009.223.

Chen, L., Meyers, D., Javorsky, G., Burstow, D., Lolekha, P., Lucas, M., et al. (2007). Arg389Gly-beta1-adrenergic receptors determine improvement in left ventricular systolic function in nonischemic cardiomyopathy patients with heart failure after chronic treatment with carvedilol. *Pharmacogenetics and Genomics*, *17*(11), 941–949. https://doi.org/10.1097/FPC.0b013e3282ef7354.

Chinchilla, A., Daimi, H., Lozano-Velasco, E., Dominguez, J. N., Caballero, R., Delpon, E., et al. (2011). PITX2 insufficiency leads to atrial electrical and structural remodeling linked to arrhythmogenesis. *Circulation. Cardiovascular Genetics*, *4*(3), 269–279. https://doi.org/10.1161/CIRCGENETICS.110.958116.

Christophersen, I. E., Rienstra, M., Roselli, C., Yin, X., Geelhoed, B., Barnard, J., et al. (2017). Large-scale analyses of common and rare variants identify 12 new loci associated with atrial fibrillation. *Nature Genetics*, *49*(6), 946–952. https://doi.org/10.1038/ng.3843.

Close, S. L. (2012). Pharmacogenetics and pharmacogenomics of thienopyridines: Clinically relevant? *Fundamental & Clinical Pharmacology*, *26*(1), 19–26. https://doi.org/10.1111/j.1472-8206.2011.00983.x.

Cohen, J. C., Boerwinkle, E., Mosley, T. H., Jr., & Hobbs, H. H. (2006). Sequence variations in PCSK9, low LDL, and protection against coronary heart disease. *The New England Journal of Medicine*, *354*(12), 1264–1272. https://doi.org/10.1056/NEJMoa054013.

Collet, J. P., Hulot, J. S., Pena, A., Villard, E., Esteve, J. B., Silvain, J., et al. (2009). Cytochrome P450 2C19 polymorphism in young patients treated with clopidogrel after myocardial infarction: A cohort study. *Lancet*, *373*(9660), 309–317. https://doi.org/10.1016/S0140-6736(08)61845-0.

Collins, F. S. (2004). The case for a US prospective cohort study of genes and environment. *Nature*, *429*(6990), 475–477. https://doi.org/10.1038/nature02628.

Cooper, G. M., Johnson, J. A., Langaee, T. Y., Feng, H., Stanaway, I. B., Schwarz, U. I., et al. (2008). A genome-wide scan for common genetic variants with a large influence on warfarin maintenance dose. *Blood*, *112*(4), 1022–1027. https://doi.org/10.1182/blood-2008-01-134247.

Daly, A. K. (2010). Genome-wide association studies in pharmacogenomics. *Nature Reviews. Genetics*, *11*(4), 241–246. https://doi.org/10.1038/nrg2751.

Danese, E., Montagnana, M., Johnson, J. A., Rettie, A. E., Zambon, C. F., Lubitz, S. A., et al. (2012). Impact of the CYP4F2 p.V433M polymorphism on coumarin dose requirement: Systematic review and meta-analysis. *Clinical Pharmacology and Therapeutics*, *92*(6), 746–756. https://doi.org/10.1038/clpt.2012.184.

Davidson, M. H., Maki, K. C., Pearson, T. A., Pasternak, R. C., Deedwania, P. C., McKenney, J. M., et al. (2005). Results of the national cholesterol education (NCEP) program evaluation ProjecT utilizing novel E-technology (NEPTUNE) II survey and implications for treatment under the recent NCEP writing group recommendations. *The American Journal of Cardiology*, *96*(4), 556–563. https://doi.org/10.1016/j.amjcard.2005.04.019.

de Groote, P., Helbecque, N., Lamblin, N., Hermant, X., Mc Fadden, E., Foucher-Hossein, C., et al. (2005). Association between beta-1 and beta-2 adrenergic receptor gene polymorphisms and the response to beta-blockade in patients with stable congestive heart failure. *Pharmacogenetics and Genomics*, *15*(3), 137–142.

de Keyser, C. E., Peters, B. J., Becker, M. L., Visser, L. E., Uitterlinden, A. G., Klungel, O. H., et al. (2014). The SLCO1B1 c.521T>C polymorphism is associated with dose decrease or switching during statin therapy in the Rotterdam Study. *Pharmacogenetics and Genomics*, *24*(1), 43–51. https://doi.org/10.1097/FPC.0000000000000018.

Delaney, J. T., Ramirez, A. H., Bowton, E., Pulley, J. M., Basford, M. A., Schildcrout, J. S., et al. (2012). Predicting clopidogrel response using DNA samples linked to an electronic health record. *Clinical Pharmacology and Therapeutics*, *91*(2), 257–263. https://doi.org/10.1038/clpt.2011.221.

Donnelly, L. A., Doney, A. S., Dannfald, J., Whitley, A. L., Lang, C. C., Morris, A. D., et al. (2008). A paucimorphic variant in the HMG-CoA reductase gene is associated with lipid-lowering response to statin treatment in diabetes: A GoDARTS study. *Pharmacogenetics and Genomics*, *18*(12), 1021–1026. https://doi.org/10.1097/FPC.0b013e3283106071.

Donnelly, L. A., Doney, A. S., Tavendale, R., Lang, C. C., Pearson, E. R., Colhoun, H. M., et al. (2011). Common nonsynonymous substitutions in SLCO1B1 predispose to statin intolerance in routinely treated individuals with type 2 diabetes: A go-DARTS study. *Clinical Pharmacology and Therapeutics*, *89*(2), 210–216. https://doi.org/10.1038/clpt.2010.255.

Fontana, P., Hulot, J. S., De Moerloose, P., & Gaussem, P. (2007). Influence of CYP2C19 and CYP3A4 gene polymorphisms on clopidogrel responsiveness in healthy subjects. *Journal of Thrombosis and Haemostasis*, *5*(10), 2153–2155. https://doi.org/10.1111/j.1538-7836.2007.02722.x.

Frere, C., Cuisset, T., Morange, P. E., Quilici, J., Camoin-Jau, L., Saut, N., et al. (2008). Effect of cytochrome p450 polymorphisms on platelet reactivity after treatment with clopidogrel in acute coronary syndrome. *The American Journal of Cardiology*, *101*(8), 1088–1093. https://doi.org/10.1016/j.amjcard.2007.11.065.

Fullerton, S. M., Wolf, W. A., Brothers, K. B., Clayton, E. W., Crawford, D. C., Denny, J. C., et al. (2012). Return of individual research results from genome-wide association studies: Experience of the electronic medical records and genomics (eMERGE) network. *Genetics in Medicine*, *14*(4), 424–431. https://doi.org/10.1038/gim.2012.15.

Gage, B. F., Bass, A. R., Lin, H., Woller, S. C., Stevens, S. M., Al-Hammadi, N., et al. (2017). Effect of genotype-guided warfarin dosing on clinical events and anticoagulation control among patients undergoing hip or knee arthroplasty: The GIFT randomized clinical trial. *JAMA*, *318*(12), 1115–1124. https://doi.org/10.1001/jama.2017.11469.

Gage, B. F., Eby, C., Johnson, J. A., Deych, E., Rieder, M. J., Ridker, P. M., et al. (2008). Use of pharmacogenetic and clinical factors to predict the therapeutic dose of warfarin. *Clinical Pharmacology and Therapeutics*, *84*(3), 326–331. https://doi.org/10.1038/clpt.2008.10.

Goldstein, J. A. (2001). Clinical relevance of genetic polymorphisms in the human CYP2C subfamily. *British Journal of Clinical Pharmacology*, *52*(4), 349–355.

Green, S. A., Turki, J., Innis, M., & Liggett, S. B. (1994). Amino-terminal polymorphisms of the human beta 2-adrenergic receptor impart distinct agonist-promoted regulatory properties. *Biochemistry*, *33*(32), 9414–9419.

Gurbel, P. A., Bliden, K. P., Hiatt, B. L., & O'Connor, C. M. (2003). Clopidogrel for coronary stenting: Response variability, drug resistance, and the effect of pretreatment platelet reactivity. *Circulation*, *107*(23), 2908–2913. https://doi.org/10.1161/01.CIR.0000072771.11429.83.

Haga, S. B., Burke, W., Ginsburg, G. S., Mills, R., & Agans, R. (2012). Primary care physicians' knowledge of and experience with pharmacogenetic testing. *Clinical Genetics*, *82*(4), 388–394. https://doi.org/10.1111/j.1399-0004.2012.01908.x.

Holmes, D. R., Jr., Dehmer, G. J., Kaul, S., Leifer, D., O'Gara, P. T., & Stein, C. M. (2010). ACCF/AHA clopidogrel clinical alert: Approaches to the FDA "boxed warning": A report of the American College of Cardiology Foundation task force on clinical expert consensus documents and the American Heart Association. *Circulation*, *122*(5), 537–557. https://doi.org/10.1161/CIR.0b013e3181ee08ed.

Holmes, M. V., Perel, P., Shah, T., Hingorani, A. D., & Casas, J. P. (2011). CYP2C19 genotype, clopidogrel metabolism, platelet function, and cardiovascular events: A systematic review and meta-analysis. *JAMA: The Journal of the American Medical Association*, *306*(24), 2704–2714. https://doi.org/10.1001/jama.2011.1880.

Huisman, M. V., Rothman, K. J., Paquette, M., Teutsch, C., Diener, H. C., Dubner, S. J., et al. (2017). The changing landscape for stroke prevention in AF: Findings from the GLORIA-AF registry phase 2. *Journal of the American College of Cardiology*, *69*(7), 777–785. https://doi.org/10.1016/j.jacc.2016.11.061.

Hulot, J. S., Bura, A., Villard, E., Azizi, M., Remones, V., Goyenvalle, C., et al. (2006). Cytochrome P450 2C19 loss-of-function polymorphism is a major determinant of clopidogrel responsiveness in healthy subjects. *Blood*, *108*(7), 2244–2247. https://doi.org/10.1182/blood-2006-04-013052.

Hulot, J. S., Collet, J. P., Silvain, J., Pena, A., Bellemain-Appaix, A., Barthelemy, O., et al. (2010). Cardiovascular risk in clopidogrel-treated patients according to cytochrome P450 2C19*2 loss-of-function allele or proton pump inhibitor coadministration: A systematic meta-analysis. *Journal of the American College of Cardiology*, *56*(2), 134–143. https://doi.org/10.1016/j.jacc.2009.12.071.

Iakoubova, O. A., Robertson, M., Tong, C. H., Rowland, C. M., Catanese, J. J., Blauw, G. J., et al. (2010). KIF6 Trp719Arg polymorphism and the effect of statin therapy in elderly patients: Results from the PROSPER study. *European Journal of Cardiovascular Prevention and Rehabilitation: Official Journal of the European Society of Cardiology, Working Groups on Epidemiology & Prevention and Cardiac Rehabilitation and Exercise Physiology*, *17*(4), 455–461. https://doi.org/10.1097/HJR.0b013e328336a0dd.

Iakoubova, O. A., Sabatine, M. S., Rowland, C. M., Tong, C. H., Catanese, J. J., Ranade, K., et al. (2008). Polymorphism in KIF6 gene and benefit from statins after acute coronary syndromes: Results from the PROVE IT-TIMI 22 study. *Journal of the American College of Cardiology*, *51*(4), 449–455. https://doi.org/10.1016/j.jacc.2007.10.017.

Ingelman-Sundberg, M., Sim, S. C., Gomez, A., & Rodriguez-Antona, C. (2007). Influence of cytochrome P450 polymorphisms on drug therapies: Pharmacogenetic, pharmacoepigenetic and clinical aspects. *Pharmacology & Therapeutics*, *116*(3), 496–526. https://doi.org/10.1016/j.pharmthera.2007.09.004.

Johnson, J. A., & Cavallari, L. H. (2015). Warfarin pharmacogenetics. *Trends in Cardiovascular Medicine*, *25*(1), 33–41. https://doi.org/10.1016/j.tcm.2014.09.001.

Johnson, J. A., Gong, L., Whirl-Carrillo, M., Gage, B. F., Scott, S. A., Stein, C. M., et al. (2011). Clinical pharmacogenetics implementation consortium guidelines for CYP2C9 and VKORC1 genotypes and warfarin dosing. *Clinical Pharmacology and Therapeutics*, *90*(4), 625–629. https://doi.org/10.1038/clpt.2011.185.

Johnson, J. A., Roden, D. M., Lesko, L. J., Ashley, E., Klein, T. E., & Shuldiner, A. R. (2012). Clopidogrel: A case for indication-specific pharmacogenetics. *Clinical Pharmacology and Therapeutics*, *91*(5), 774–776. https://doi.org/10.1038/clpt.2012.21.

Jonas, D. E., & McLeod, H. L. (2009). Genetic and clinical factors relating to warfarin dosing. *Trends in Pharmacological Sciences*, *30*(7), 375–386. https://doi.org/10.1016/j.tips.2009.05.001.

Kaab, S., Crawford, D. C., Sinner, M. F., Behr, E. R., Kannankeril, P. J., Wilde, A. A., et al. (2012). A large candidate gene survey identifies the KCNE1 D85N polymorphism as a possible modulator of drug-induced torsades de pointes. *Circulation. Cardiovascular Genetics*, *5*(1), 91–99. https://doi.org/10.1161/CIRCGENETICS.111.960930.

Karnes, J. H., Van Driest, S., Bowton, E. A., Weeke, P. E., Mosley, J. D., Peterson, J. F., et al. (2014). Using systems approaches to address challenges for clinical implementation of pharmacogenomics. *Wiley Interdisciplinary Reviews. Systems Biology and Medicine*, *6*(2), 125–135. https://doi.org/10.1002/wsbm.1255.

Kazui, M., Nishiya, Y., Ishizuka, T., Hagihara, K., Farid, N. A., Okazaki, O., et al. (2010). Identification of the human cytochrome P450 enzymes involved in the two oxidative steps in the bioactivation of clopidogrel to its pharmacologically active metabolite. *Drug Metabolism and Disposition: The Biological Fate of Chemicals*, *38*(1), 92–99. https://doi.org/10.1124/dmd.109.029132.

Kim, K. A., Park, P. W., Hong, S. J., & Park, J. Y. (2008). The effect of CYP2C19 polymorphism on the pharmacokinetics and pharmacodynamics of clopidogrel: A possible mechanism for clopidogrel resistance. *Clinical Pharmacology and Therapeutics*, *84*(2), 236–242. https://doi.org/10.1038/clpt.2008.20.

Kimmel, S. E., French, B., Kasner, S. E., Johnson, J. A., Anderson, J. L., Gage, B. F., et al. (2013). A pharmacogenetic versus a clinical algorithm for warfarin dosing. *The New England Journal of Medicine*, *369*(24), 2283–2293. https://doi.org/10.1056/NEJMoa1310669.

Kitzmiller, J. P., Luzum, J. A., Baldassarre, D., Krauss, R. M., & Medina, M. W. (2014). CYP3A4*22 and CYP3A5*3 are associated with increased levels of plasma simvastatin concentrations in the cholesterol and pharmacogenetics study cohort. *Pharmacogenetics and Genomics*, *24*(10), 486–491. https://doi.org/10.1097/FPC.0000000000000079.

Krauss, R. M., Mangravite, L. M., Smith, J. D., Medina, M. W., Wang, D., Guo, X., et al. (2008). Variation in the 3-hydroxyl-3-methylglutaryl coenzyme a reductase gene is associated with racial differences in low-density lipoprotein cholesterol response to simvastatin treatment. *Circulation*, *117*(12), 1537–1544. https://doi.org/10.1161/CIRCULATIONAHA.107.708388.

Law, M., & Rudnicka, A. R. (2006). Statin safety: A systematic review. *The American Journal of Cardiology*, *97*(8A), 52C–60C. https://doi.org/10.1016/j.amjcard.2005.12.010.

Leurs, R., Church, M. K., & Taglialatela, M. (2002). H1-antihistamines: Inverse agonism, anti-inflammatory actions and cardiac effects. *Clinical and Experimental Allergy*, *32*(4), 489–498.

Levy, K. D., Decker, B. S., Carpenter, J. S., Flockhart, D. A., Dexter, P. R., Desta, Z., et al. (2014). Prerequisites to implementing a pharmacogenomics program in a large health-care system. *Clinical Pharmacology and Therapeutics*, *96*(3), 307–309. https://doi.org/10.1038/clpt.2014.101.

Li, J. H., Joy, S. V., Haga, S. B., Orlando, L. A., Kraus, W. E., Ginsburg, G. S., et al. (2014). Genetically guided statin therapy on statin perceptions, adherence, and cholesterol lowering: A pilot implementation study in primary care patients. *Journal of Personalized Medicine*, *4*(2), 147–162. https://doi.org/10.3390/jpm4020147.

Liggett, S. B., Mialet-Perez, J., Thaneemit-Chen, S., Weber, S. A., Greene, S. M., Hodne, D., et al. (2006). A polymorphism within a conserved beta(1)-adrenergic receptor motif alters cardiac function and beta-blocker response in human heart failure. *Proceedings of the National Academy of Sciences of the United States of America*, *103*(30), 11288–11293. https://doi.org/10.1073/pnas.0509937103.

Lindh, J. D., Holm, L., Andersson, M. L., & Rane, A. (2009). Influence of CYP2C9 genotype on warfarin dose requirements—A systematic review and meta-analysis. *European Journal of Clinical Pharmacology*, *65*(4), 365–375. https://doi.org/10.1007/s00228-008-0584-5.

Link, E., Parish, S., Armitage, J., Bowman, L., Heath, S., Matsuda, F., et al. (2008). SLCO1B1 variants and statin-induced myopathy—A genomewide study. *The New England Journal of Medicine*, *359*(8), 789–799. https://doi.org/10.1056/NEJMoa0801936.

Mangravite, L. M., Thorn, C. F., & Krauss, R. M. (2006). Clinical implications of pharmacogenomics of statin treatment. *The Pharmacogenomics Journal*, *6*(6), 360–374. https://doi.org/10.1038/sj.tpj.6500384.

Medina, M. W., Gao, F., Ruan, W., Rotter, J. I., & Krauss, R. M. (2008). Alternative splicing of 3-hydroxy-3-methylglutaryl coenzyme A reductase is associated with plasma low-density lipoprotein cholesterol response to simvastatin. *Circulation*, *118*(4), 355–362. https://doi.org/10.1161/CIRCULATIONAHA.108.773267.

Mega, J. L., Close, S. L., Wiviott, S. D., Shen, L., Hockett, R. D., Brandt, J. T., et al. (2009). Cytochrome p-450 polymorphisms and response to clopidogrel. *The New England Journal of Medicine*, *360*(4), 354–362. https://doi.org/10.1056/NEJMoa0809171.

Mega, J. L., Close, S. L., Wiviott, S. D., Shen, L., Walker, J. R., Simon, T., et al. (2010). Genetic variants in ABCB1 and CYP2C19 and cardiovascular outcomes after treatment with clopidogrel and prasugrel in the TRITON-TIMI 38 trial: A pharmacogenetic analysis. *Lancet*, *376*(9749), 1312–1319. https://doi.org/10.1016/S0140-6736(10)61273-1.

Mega, J. L., Simon, T., Collet, J. P., Anderson, J. L., Antman, E. M., Bliden, K., et al. (2010). Reduced-function CYP2C19 genotype and risk of adverse clinical outcomes among patients treated with clopidogrel predominantly for PCI: A meta-analysis. *JAMA: The Journal of the American Medical Association*, *304*(16), 1821–1830. https://doi.org/10.1001/jama.2010.1543.

Mega, J. L., Walker, J. R., Ruff, C. T., Vandell, A. G., Nordio, F., Deenadayalu, N., et al. (2015). Genetics and the clinical response to warfarin and edoxaban: Findings from the randomised, double-blind ENGAGE AF-TIMI 48 trial. *Lancet*, *385*(9984), 2280–2287. https://doi.org/10.1016/S0140-6736(14)61994-2.

Mommersteeg, M. T., Brown, N. A., Prall, O. W., de Gier-de Vries, C., Harvey, R. P., Moorman, A. F., et al. (2007). Pitx2c and Nkx2-5 are required for the formation and identity of the pulmonary myocardium. *Circulation Research*, *101*(9), 902–909. https://doi.org/10.1161/CIRCRESAHA.107.161182.

Mrazek, D. A., & Lerman, C. (2011). Facilitating clinical implementation of pharmacogenomics. *JAMA*, *306*(3), 304–305. https://doi.org/10.1001/jama.2011.1010.

Muthumala, A., Drenos, F., Elliott, P. M., & Humphries, S. E. (2008). Role of beta adrenergic receptor polymorphisms in heart failure: Systematic review and meta-analysis. *European Journal of Heart Failure, 10*(1), 3–13. https://doi.org/10.1016/j.ejheart.2007.11.008.

Myocardial Infarction Genetics Consortium, Investigators, Stitziel, N. O., Won, H. H., Morrison, A. C., Peloso, G. M., Do, R., et al. (2014). Inactivating mutations in NPC1L1 and protection from coronary heart disease. *The New England Journal of Medicine, 371*(22), 2072–2082. https://doi.org/10.1056/NEJMoa1405386.

Pare, G., Eriksson, N., Lehr, T., Connolly, S., Eikelboom, J., Ezekowitz, M. D., et al. (2013). Genetic determinants of dabigatran plasma levels and their relation to bleeding. *Circulation, 127*(13), 1404–1412. https://doi.org/10.1161/CIRCULATIONAHA.112.001233.

Pare, G., Mehta, S. R., Yusuf, S., Anand, S. S., Connolly, S. J., Hirsh, J., et al. (2010). Effects of CYP2C19 genotype on outcomes of clopidogrel treatment. *The New England Journal of Medicine, 363*(18), 1704–1714. https://doi.org/10.1056/NEJMoa1008410.

Parvez, B., Chopra, N., Rowan, S., Vaglio, J. C., Muhammad, R., Roden, D. M., et al. (2012). A common beta1-adrenergic receptor polymorphism predicts favorable response to rate-control therapy in atrial fibrillation. *Journal of the American College of Cardiology, 59*(1), 49–56. https://doi.org/10.1016/j.jacc.2011.08.061.

Parvez, B., Shoemaker, M. B., Muhammad, R., Richardson, R., Jiang, L., Blair, M. A., et al. (2013). Common genetic polymorphism at 4q25 locus predicts atrial fibrillation recurrence after successful cardioversion. *Heart Rhythm, 10*(6), 849–855. https://doi.org/10.1016/j.hrthm.2013.02.018.

Parvez, B., Vaglio, J., Rowan, S., Muhammad, R., Kucera, G., Stubblefield, T., et al. (2012). Symptomatic response to antiarrhythmic drug therapy is modulated by a common single nucleotide polymorphism in atrial fibrillation. *Journal of the American College of Cardiology, 60*(6), 539–545. https://doi.org/10.1016/j.jacc.2012.01.070.

Pasanen, M. K., Neuvonen, M., Neuvonen, P. J., & Niemi, M. (2006). SLCO1B1 polymorphism markedly affects the pharmacokinetics of simvastatin acid. *Pharmacogenetics and Genomics, 16*(12), 873–879. https://doi.org/10.1097/01.fpc.0000230416.82349.90.

Paulussen, A. D., Gilissen, R. A., Armstrong, M., Doevendans, P. A., Verhasselt, P., Smeets, H. J., et al. (2004). Genetic variations of KCNQ1, KCNH2, SCN5A, KCNE1, and KCNE2 in drug-induced long QT syndrome patients. *Journal of Molecular Medicine, 82*(3), 182–188. https://doi.org/10.1007/s00109-003-0522-z.

Perera, M. A., Cavallari, L. H., Limdi, N. A., Gamazon, E. R., Konkashbaev, A., Daneshjou, R., et al. (2013). Genetic variants associated with warfarin dose in African-American individuals: A genome-wide association study. *Lancet, 382*(9894), 790–796. https://doi.org/10.1016/S0140-6736(13)60681-9.

Peters, B. J., Rodin, A. S., Klungel, O. H., van Duijn, C. M., Stricker, B. H., van't Slot, R., et al. (2010). Pharmacogenetic interactions between ABCB1 and SLCO1B1 tagging SNPs and the effectiveness of statins in the prevention of myocardial infarction. *Pharmacogenomics, 11*(8), 1065–1076. https://doi.org/10.2217/pgs.10.81.

Petersen, M., Andersen, J. T., Hjelvang, B. R., Broedbaek, K., Afzal, S., Nyegaard, M., et al. (2011). Association of beta-adrenergic receptor polymorphisms and mortality in carvedilol-treated chronic heart-failure patients. *British Journal of Clinical Pharmacology, 71*(4), 556–565. https://doi.org/10.1111/j.1365-2125.2010.03868.x.

Peterson, J. F., Field, J. R., Unertl, K. M., Schildcrout, J. S., Johnson, D. C., Shi, Y., et al. (2016). Physician response to implementation of genotype-tailored antiplatelet therapy. *Clinical Pharmacology and Therapeutics, 100*(1), 67–74. https://doi.org/10.1002/cpt.331.

Pirmohamed, M., Burnside, G., Eriksson, N., Jorgensen, A. L., Toh, C. H., Nicholson, T., et al. (2013). A randomized trial of genotype-guided dosing of warfarin. *The New England Journal of Medicine, 369*(24), 2294–2303. https://doi.org/10.1056/NEJMoa1311386.

Pulley, J. M., Denny, J. C., Peterson, J. F., Bernard, G. R., Vnencak-Jones, C. L., Ramirez, A. H., et al. (2012). Operational implementation of prospective genotyping for personalized medicine: The design of the Vanderbilt PREDICT project. *Clinical Pharmacology and Therapeutics*, *92*(1), 87–95. https://doi.org/10.1038/clpt.2011.371.

Ragia, G., Kolovou, V., Tavridou, A., Elens, L., Tselepis, A. D., Elisaf, M., et al. (2015). No effect of CYP3A4 intron 6 C>T polymorphism (CYP3A4*22) on lipid-lowering response to statins in Greek patients with primary hypercholesterolemia. *Drug Metabolism and Personalized Therapy*, *30*(1), 43–48. https://doi.org/10.1515/dmdi-2014-0021.

Ramsey, B. W., Davies, J., McElvaney, N. G., Tullis, E., Bell, S. C., Drevinek, P., et al. (2011). A CFTR potentiator in patients with cystic fibrosis and the G551D mutation. *The New England Journal of Medicine*, *365*(18), 1663–1672. https://doi.org/10.1056/NEJMoa1105185.

Relling, M. V., & Klein, T. E. (2011). CPIC: Clinical pharmacogenetics implementation consortium of the pharmacogenomics research network. *Clinical Pharmacology and Therapeutics*, *89*(3), 464–467. https://doi.org/10.1038/clpt.2010.279.

Rettie, A. E., Haining, R. L., Bajpai, M., & Levy, R. H. (1999). A common genetic basis for idiosyncratic toxicity of warfarin and phenytoin. *Epilepsy Research*, *35*(3), 253–255.

Ridker, P. M., MacFadyen, J. G., Glynn, R. J., & Chasman, D. I. (2011). Kinesin-like protein 6 (KIF6) polymorphism and the efficacy of rosuvastatin in primary prevention. *Circulation. Cardiovascular Genetics*, *4*(3), 312–317. https://doi.org/10.1161/CIRCGENETICS.110.959353.

Rieder, M. J., Reiner, A. P., Gage, B. F., Nickerson, D. A., Eby, C. S., McLeod, H. L., et al. (2005). Effect of VKORC1 haplotypes on transcriptional regulation and warfarin dose. *The New England Journal of Medicine*, *352*(22), 2285–2293. https://doi.org/10.1056/NEJMoa044503.

Roberts, J. D., Wells, G. A., Le May, M. R., Labinaz, M., Glover, C., Froeschl, M., et al. (2012). Point-of-care genetic testing for personalisation of antiplatelet treatment (RAPID GENE): A prospective, randomised, proof-of-concept trial. *Lancet*, *379*(9827), 1705–1711. https://doi.org/10.1016/S0140-6736(12)60161-5.

Roden, D. M. (2004). Drug-induced prolongation of the QT interval. *The New England Journal of Medicine*, *350*(10), 1013–1022. https://doi.org/10.1056/NEJMra032426.

Rost, S., Fregin, A., Ivaskevicius, V., Conzelmann, E., Hortnagel, K., Pelz, H. J., et al. (2004). Mutations in VKORC1 cause warfarin resistance and multiple coagulation factor deficiency type 2. *Nature*, *427*(6974), 537–541. https://doi.org/10.1038/nature02214.

Sabatine, M. S., Giugliano, R. P., Keech, A. C., Honarpour, N., Wiviott, S. D., Murphy, S. A., et al. (2017). Evolocumab and clinical outcomes in patients with cardiovascular disease. *The New England Journal of Medicine*, *376*(18), 1713–1722. https://doi.org/10.1056/NEJMoa1615664.

Schalekamp, T., & de Boer, A. (2010). Pharmacogenetics of oral anticoagulant therapy. *Current Pharmaceutical Design*, *16*(2), 187–203.

Schildcrout, J. S., Denny, J. C., Bowton, E., Gregg, W., Pulley, J. M., Basford, M. A., et al. (2012). Optimizing drug outcomes through pharmacogenetics: A case for preemptive genotyping. *Clinical Pharmacology and Therapeutics*, *92*(2), 235–242. https://doi.org/10.1038/clpt.2012.66.

Scott, S. A. (2013). Clinical pharmacogenomics: Opportunities and challenges at point of care. *Clinical Pharmacology and Therapeutics*, *93*(1), 33–35. https://doi.org/10.1038/clpt.2012.196.

Scott, S. A., Sangkuhl, K., Gardner, E. E., Stein, C. M., Hulot, J. S., Johnson, J. A., et al. (2011). Clinical pharmacogenetics implementation consortium guidelines for cytochrome P450-2C19 (CYP2C19) genotype and clopidogrel therapy. *Clinical Pharmacology and Therapeutics*, *90*(2), 328–332. https://doi.org/10.1038/clpt.2011.132.

Scott, S. A., Sangkuhl, K., Shuldiner, A. R., Hulot, J. S., Thorn, C. F., Altman, R. B., et al. (2012). PharmGKB summary: Very important pharmacogene information for cytochrome P450, family 2, subfamily C, polypeptide 19. *Pharmacogenetics and Genomics*, *22*(2), 159–165. https://doi.org/10.1097/FPC.0b013e32834d4962.

Shoemaker, M. B., Bollmann, A., Lubitz, S. A., Ueberham, L., Saini, H., Montgomery, J., et al. (2015). Common genetic variants and response to atrial fibrillation ablation. *Circulation. Arrhythmia and Electrophysiology*, *8*(2), 296–302. https://doi.org/10.1161/CIRCEP.114.001909.

Shuldiner, A. R., O'Connell, J. R., Bliden, K. P., Gandhi, A., Ryan, K., Horenstein, R. B., et al. (2009). Association of cytochrome P450 2C19 genotype with the antiplatelet effect and clinical efficacy of clopidogrel therapy. *JAMA: The Journal of the American Medical Association*, *302*(8), 849–857. https://doi.org/10.1001/jama.2009.1232.

Sibbing, D., Koch, W., Gebhard, D., Schuster, T., Braun, S., Stegherr, J., et al. (2010). Cytochrome 2C19*17 allelic variant, platelet aggregation, bleeding events, and stent thrombosis in clopidogrel-treated patients with coronary stent placement. *Circulation*, *121*(4), 512–518. https://doi.org/10.1161/CIRCULATIONAHA.109.885194.

Simon, T., Verstuyft, C., Mary-Krause, M., Quteineh, L., Drouet, E., Meneveau, N., et al. (2009). Genetic determinants of response to clopidogrel and cardiovascular events. *The New England Journal of Medicine*, *360*(4), 363–375. https://doi.org/10.1056/NEJMoa0808227.

Small, K. M., Wagoner, L. E., Levin, A. M., Kardia, S. L., & Liggett, S. B. (2002). Synergistic polymorphisms of beta1- and alpha2C-adrenergic receptors and the risk of congestive heart failure. *The New England Journal of Medicine*, *347*(15), 1135–1142. https://doi.org/10.1056/NEJMoa020803.

Staerk, L., Fosbol, E. L., Gadsboll, K., Sindet-Pedersen, C., Pallisgaard, J. L., Lamberts, M., et al. (2016). Non-vitamin K antagonist oral anticoagulation usage according to age among patients with atrial fibrillation: Temporal trends 2011-2015 in Denmark. *Scientific Reports*, *6*, 31477. https://doi.org/10.1038/srep31477.

Stanek, E. J., Sanders, C. L., Taber, K. A., Khalid, M., Patel, A., Verbrugge, R. R., et al. (2012). Adoption of pharmacogenomic testing by US physicians: Results of a nationwide survey. *Clinical Pharmacology and Therapeutics*, *91*(3), 450–458. https://doi.org/10.1038/clpt.2011.306.

Strauss, D. G., Vicente, J., Johannesen, L., Blinova, K., Mason, J. W., Weeke, P., et al. (2017). Common genetic variant risk score is associated with drug-induced QT prolongation and torsade de pointes risk: A pilot study. *Circulation*, *135*(14), 1300–1310. https://doi.org/10.1161/CIRCULATIONAHA.116.023980.

Stroes, E. S., Thompson, P. D., Corsini, A., Vladutiu, G. D., Raal, F. J., Ray, K. K., et al. (2015). Statin-associated muscle symptoms: Impact on statin therapy-European atherosclerosis society consensus panel statement on assessment, aetiology and management. *European Heart Journal*, *36*(17), 1012–1022. https://doi.org/10.1093/eurheartj/ehv043.

Syeda, F., Holmes, A. P., Yu, T. Y., Tull, S., Kuhlmann, S. M., Pavlovic, D., et al. (2016). PITX2 modulates atrial membrane potential and the antiarrhythmic effects of sodium-channel blockers. *Journal of the American College of Cardiology*, *68*(17), 1881–1894. https://doi.org/10.1016/j.jacc.2016.07.766.

Takeuchi, F., McGinnis, R., Bourgeois, S., Barnes, C., Eriksson, N., Soranzo, N., et al. (2009). A genome-wide association study confirms VKORC1, CYP2C9, and CYP4F2 as principal genetic determinants of warfarin dose. *PLoS Genetics*, *5*(3), e1000433. https://doi.org/10.1371/journal.pgen.1000433.

Teutsch, S. M., Bradley, L. A., Palomaki, G. E., Haddow, J. E., Piper, M., Calonge, N., et al. (2009). The evaluation of genomic applications in practice and prevention (EGAPP) initiative: Methods of the EGAPP working group. *Genetics in Medicine*, *11*(1), 3–14. https://doi.org/10.1097/GIM.0b013e318184137c.

Thompson, P. D., Clarkson, P., & Karas, R. H. (2003). Statin-associated myopathy. *JAMA: The Journal of the American Medical Association, 289*(13), 1681–1690. https://doi.org/10.1001/jama.289.13.1681.

Thompson, J. F., Hyde, C. L., Wood, L. S., Paciga, S. A., Hinds, D. A., Cox, D. R., et al. (2009). Comprehensive whole-genome and candidate gene analysis for response to statin therapy in the treating to new targets (TNT) cohort. *Circulation. Cardiovascular Genetics, 2*(2), 173–181. https://doi.org/10.1161/CIRCGENETICS.108.818062.

Trenk, D., Hochholzer, W., Fromm, M. F., Chialda, L. E., Pahl, A., Valina, C. M., et al. (2008). Cytochrome P450 2C19 681G>A polymorphism and high on-clopidogrel platelet reactivity associated with adverse 1-year clinical outcome of elective percutaneous coronary intervention with drug-eluting or bare-metal stents. *Journal of the American College of Cardiology, 51*(20), 1925–1934. https://doi.org/10.1016/j.jacc.2007.12.056.

Tsamandouras, N., Dickinson, G., Guo, Y., Hall, S., Rostami-Hodjegan, A., Galetin, A., et al. (2014). Identification of the effect of multiple polymorphisms on the pharmacokinetics of simvastatin and simvastatin acid using a population-modeling approach. *Clinical Pharmacology and Therapeutics, 96*(1), 90–100. https://doi.org/10.1038/clpt.2014.55.

Van Driest, S. L., Shi, Y., Bowton, E. A., Schildcrout, J. S., Peterson, J. F., Pulley, J., et al. (2014). Clinically actionable genotypes among 10,000 patients with preemptive pharmacogenomic testing. *Clinical Pharmacology and Therapeutics, 95*(4), 423–431. https://doi.org/10.1038/clpt.2013.229.

Verhoef, T. I., Ragia, G., de Boer, A., Barallon, R., Kolovou, G., Kolovou, V., et al. (2013). A randomized trial of genotype-guided dosing of acenocoumarol and phenprocoumon. *The New England Journal of Medicine, 369*(24), 2304–2312. https://doi.org/10.1056/NEJMoa1311388.

Voora, D., Shah, S. H., Spasojevic, I., Ali, S., Reed, C. R., Salisbury, B. A., et al. (2009). The SLCO1B1*5 genetic variant is associated with statin-induced side effects. *Journal of the American College of Cardiology, 54*(17), 1609–1616. https://doi.org/10.1016/j.jacc.2009.04.053.

Wadelius, M., Chen, L. Y., Lindh, J. D., Eriksson, N., Ghori, M. J., Bumpstead, S., et al. (2009). The largest prospective warfarin-treated cohort supports genetic forecasting. *Blood, 113*(4), 784–792. https://doi.org/10.1182/blood-2008-04-149070.

Wainwright, C. E., Elborn, J. S., Ramsey, B. W., Marigowda, G., Huang, X., Cipolli, M., et al. (2015). Lumacaftor-ivacaftor in patients with cystic fibrosis homozygous for Phe508del CFTR. *The New England Journal of Medicine, 373*(3), 220–231. https://doi.org/10.1056/NEJMoa1409547.

Wang, D., Chen, H., Momary, K. M., Cavallari, L. H., Johnson, J. A., & Sadee, W. (2008). Regulatory polymorphism in vitamin K epoxide reductase complex subunit 1 (VKORC1) affects gene expression and warfarin dose requirement. *Blood, 112*(4), 1013–1021. https://doi.org/10.1182/blood-2008-03-144899.

Wang, D., Guo, Y., Wrighton, S. A., Cooke, G. E., & Sadee, W. (2011). Intronic polymorphism in CYP3A4 affects hepatic expression and response to statin drugs. *The Pharmacogenomics Journal, 11*(4), 274–286. https://doi.org/10.1038/tpj.2010.28.

Wang, Y., Zhao, X., Lin, J., Li, H., Johnston, S. C., Lin, Y., et al. (2016). Association between CYP2C19 loss-of-function allele status and efficacy of clopidogrel for risk reduction among patients with minor stroke or transient ischemic attack. *JAMA, 316*(1), 70–78. https://doi.org/10.1001/jama.2016.8662.

Weeke, P., Denny, J. C., Basterache, L., Shaffer, C., Bowton, E., Ingram, C., et al. (2015). Examining rare and low-frequency genetic variants previously associated with lone or familial forms of atrial fibrillation in an electronic medical record system: A cautionary note. *Circulation. Cardiovascular Genetics, 8*(1), 58–63. https://doi.org/10.1161/CIRCGENETICS.114.000718.

Weeke, P., Mosley, J. D., Hanna, D., Delaney, J. T., Shaffer, C., Wells, Q. S., et al. (2014). Exome sequencing implicates an increased burden of rare potassium channel variants in the risk of drug-induced long QT interval syndrome. *Journal of the American College of Cardiology*, *63*(14), 1430–1437. https://doi.org/10.1016/j.jacc.2014.01.031.

Weeke, P., Muhammad, R., Delaney, J. T., Shaffer, C., Mosley, J. D., Blair, M., et al. (2014). Whole-exome sequencing in familial atrial fibrillation. *European Heart Journal*, *35*(36), 2477–2483. https://doi.org/10.1093/eurheartj/ehu156.

Wilke, R. A., Moore, J. H., & Burmester, J. K. (2005). Relative impact of CYP3A genotype and concomitant medication on the severity of atorvastatin-induced muscle damage. *Pharmacogenetics and Genomics*, *15*(6), 415–421.

Wilke, R. A., Ramsey, L. B., Johnson, S. G., Maxwell, W. D., McLeod, H. L., Voora, D., et al. (2012). The clinical pharmacogenomics implementation consortium: CPIC guideline for SLCO1B1 and simvastatin-induced myopathy. *Clinical Pharmacology and Therapeutics*, *92*(1), 112–117. https://doi.org/10.1038/clpt.2012.57.

Woosley, R. L., Chen, Y., Freiman, J. P., & Gillis, R. A. (1993). Mechanism of the cardiotoxic actions of terfenadine. *JAMA*, *269*(12), 1532–1536.

Yasmina, A., de Boer, A., Klungel, O. H., & Deneer, V. H. (2014). Pharmacogenomics of oral antiplatelet drugs. *Pharmacogenomics*, *15*(4), 509–528. https://doi.org/10.2217/pgs.14.16.

FURTHER READING

Bergstrom, R. F., Peyton, A. L., & Lemberger, L. (1992). Quantification and mechanism of the fluoxetine and tricyclic antidepressant interaction. *Clinical Pharmacology and Therapeutics*, *51*(3), 239–248.

Do, E. J., Lenzini, P., Eby, C. S., Bass, A. R., McMillin, G. A., Stevens, S. M., et al. (2012). Genetics informatics trial (GIFT) of warfarin to prevent deep vein thrombosis (DVT): Rationale and study design. *The Pharmacogenomics Journal*, *12*(5), 417–424. https://doi.org/10.1038/tpj.2011.18.

CHAPTER FOURTEEN

Pharmacogenetics of Antidiabetic Drugs

Shylaja Srinivasan[*,†], **Sook Wah Yee**[*], **Kathleen M. Giacomini**[*,1]
[*]Department of Bioengineering and Therapeutic Sciences, University of California, San Francisco, San Francisco, CA, United States
[†]Division of Pediatric Endocrinology and Diabetes, University of California, San Francisco, San Francisco, CA, United States
[1]Corresponding author: e-mail address: kathy.giacomini@ucsf.edu

Contents

1. Introduction 362
2. Discovery of Genetic Loci Related to Metformin Response Through Genome-Wide Approaches 362
3. Genome-Wide Screening to Elucidate Metformin Action Through in vitro Assays 369
4. Studies Related to Metformin Candidate Genes 371
   4.1 Metformin Pharmacokinetics 371
   4.2 Metformin Pharmacodynamics 372
5. Genetic Studies of Other Antidiabetic Drugs 375
   5.1 Sulfonylureas 375
   5.2 Thiazolidinediones 377
   5.3 Meglitinides 378
   5.4 Acarbose 379
   5.5 SGLT2 Inhibitors (Gliflozins) 379
   5.6 Glucagon-Like Peptide-1-Based Therapies 379
   5.7 Pharmacogenetics of Adverse Reactions and Off-Target Effects of Antidiabetic Drugs 380
6. Conclusion 381
Acknowledgment 382
References 382

Abstract

Pharmacogenetic studies of antidiabetic drugs have so far focused largely on response to metformin, which is the first-line therapy for treatment of type 2 diabetes (T2D). The first studies of metformin pharmacogenetics were focused on candidate genes that were implicated in metformin pharmacokinetics and transport. Since 2011, genome-wide association studies have been conducted in large cohorts of individuals with T2D identifying genes that are associated with glycemic response to metformin. There have been fewer pharmacogenetic studies of other antidiabetic drugs, and those have

Advances in Pharmacology, Volume 83
ISSN 1054-3589
https://doi.org/10.1016/bs.apha.2018.04.005

been largely limited to candidate gene studies with small sample sizes. Understanding the pharmacogenetics of antidiabetes medications is important for the integration of genetic screening into therapeutic decision making, and to achieve the goal of "precision medicine" for patients with T2D. In this chapter, we provide a review of the pharmacogenetics investigations of metformin and other antidiabetes medications. In addition, we highlight the importance of collaborative efforts with large sample size and representation from multiple ethnic groups in pharmacogenetics studies.

1. INTRODUCTION

Pharmacogenetic studies of antidiabetic drugs have focused largely on metformin, which is now first-line therapy for type 2 diabetes. Prior to 2011, metformin pharmacogenetics studies were largely based on candidate genes, focused on genes encoding transporters that are involved in metformin pharmacokinetics. Since 2011, several genome-wide association studies (GWAS) have been published, in large multiethnic cohorts. These studies have revealed some genes which are associated with glycemic response to metformin in patients with type 2 diabetes, at genome-wide level of significance. For other antidiabetic drugs, there have been few pharmacogenetic studies, and all have been focused on candidate genes. In general, the studies have been small and largely centered on associations between drug-metabolizing enzymes and transporters with the pharmacokinetics or pharmacodynamics of the drugs. In this chapter, we begin by reviewing the pharmacogenetic studies of metformin disposition and response, mostly focused on pharmacogenetic associations in healthy volunteers and patients with diabetes on metformin. Afterward we include a brief review of pharmacogenetic studies of other classes of antidiabetic drugs including sulfonylureas, thiazolidinediones, meglitinides, acarbose, and SGLT2 inhibitors (Fig. 1). A brief conclusion is included.

2. DISCOVERY OF GENETIC LOCI RELATED TO METFORMIN RESPONSE THROUGH GENOME-WIDE APPROACHES

GWAS have revealed many loci, genes, and individual SNPs, which are critical for therapeutic and adverse drug response and drug disposition. A recent commentary reported that only 216 pharmacogenomics GWAS are available in the GWAS Catalog (MacArthur et al., 2017), and that the majority of the pharmacogenomic GWAS have focused on drugs used in the

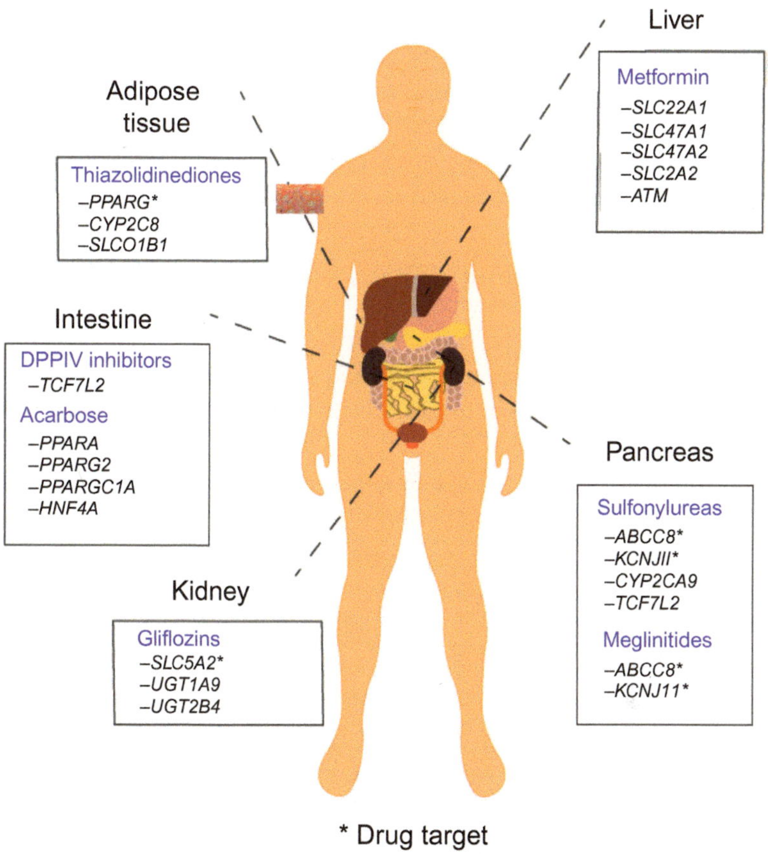

Fig. 1 Major sites of action of antidiabetic drugs and genes associated with pharmacokinetics or clinical response. *Note*: Listed drugs may have other secondary sites of action.

treatment of cancer, neuropsychiatric disorders, and cardiovascular diseases (Giacomini et al., 2017). One of the major challenges to pharmacogenomic GWAS has been sample size. In particular, pharmacogenomic phenotypes are more difficult to obtain than phenotypes for other human traits, since multiple kinds of information are needed to assess drug response. For example, drug dosage, adherence to medications, and baseline and on-drug measurements of the phenotype of interest need to be collected in each individual for a robust study. This information may be difficult to procure in large numbers of patients. Thus, to enhance sample size of primary and replication cohorts, several pharmacogenomics consortia have been established. These include the International Consortium on Lithium Genetics (Schulze et al., 2010), the International SSRI Pharmacogenomics Consortium (ISPC) (Biernacka et al., 2015), the Pharmacogenetics of

Drug-Induced Liver Injury Group (DILIGEN) (Urban et al., 2017), and the Pharmacogenomics in Childhood Asthma (PiCA) Consortium (Farzan et al., 2017). For antidiabetic drugs, two consortia largely centered on metformin genetics have been established: the metformin genetics consortium, MetGen (http://www.pgrn.org/metgen.html) and the DIRECT (DIabetes REsearCh on patient straTification) (http://www.direct-diabetes.org/). The effort of MetGen consortium is to engage researchers from around the world who have datasets for metformin and also other antidiabetic drugs to enhance the discovery of genetic biomarkers of clinical response to antidiabetic drugs. Importantly, this consortium encourages the inclusion of other ethnic populations in metformin and other antidiabetic drug pharmacogenomics studies. MetGen has already published GWAS focused on metformin, which are described later.

In terms of identification of genetic factors that associate with response to antidiabetic drugs, only two GWAS have been published. Both studies focused on metformin and one involved the MetGen consortium (Zhou et al., 2011, 2016). Given that over 100 risk alleles for type 2 diabetes have been discovered, with the inclusion of clinical data collected from diverse ethnic populations (Flannick & Florez, 2016; Florez, 2017), the fact that genome-wide association methods have only been applied to metformin response underscores the immense need for pharmacogenomics GWAS in patients on antidiabetic drugs.

In both of the metformin GWAS focused on response, retrospective observational approaches, using information in the electronic health record (EHR), were employed. For response measurements, glycated hemoglobin (HbA1c), a reliable biomarker for assessing average plasma glucose levels, was obtained from the EHR. The first metformin GWAS, published in 2011 (Zhou et al., 2011), identified genetic determinants of metformin response, where response was defined as achieving the treatment target goal of $<7\%$ HbA1c level within 18 months after starting metformin. The study identified a SNP, rs11212617, in a locus, which included ATM (Ataxia-Telangiectasia). The C-allele of rs11212617 was associated with treatment success ($n=3920$ European ancestry, $P=2.9\times10^{-9}$, odds ratio$=1.35$, 95% CI 1.22–1.49). Further replication of the SNP revealed a significant association in a meta-analysis of five cohorts of European ancestry (van Leeuwen et al., 2012), and conflicting results in other ethnic groups (Shokri et al., 2016; Zhou et al., 2014). However, in prediabetes patients, the SNP did not appear to be associated with response to metformin (Florez et al., 2012).

Since the discovery of the association of ATM with metformin response, several follow-up studies have been performed to evaluate (a) the effect of metformin in cultured cells on the activation or phosphorylation of ATM and its downstream targets (Corominas-Faja et al., 2012; Feng et al., 2015 #224; Storozhuk et al., 2013; Vazquez-Martin, Oliveras-Ferraros, Cufi, Martin-Castillo, & Menendez, 2011; Woods, Leiper, & Carling, 2012); (b) the effect of patients with ATM mutations on glucose–insulin homeostasis and indices of insulin secretion and sensitivity (Connelly et al., 2016); (c) the association of ATM variants with metformin response in prediabetic patients (Florez et al., 2012) and in patients with polycystic ovary syndrome (Pedersen, Stage, Glintborg, Andersen, & Christensen, 2018). These studies highlight the importance of follow-up studies to elucidate the mechanisms by which ATM modulates response to metformin in diabetes and other conditions. However, two independent studies showed that the ATM inhibitor, KU-55933 used to elucidate the mechanism by which ATM modulates response to metformin, reduces metformin uptake (Woods et al., 2012; Yee, Chen, & Giacomini, 2012), and in particularly, inhibits OCT1, the primary transporter for metformin in liver cells (Yee et al., 2012). Since metformin uptake via OCT1 was shown to be independent of ATM (Yee et al., 2012), the studies question the effect of ATM on modulating response to metformin via activation of AMPK and suggest that other mechanisms may be involved (Woods et al., 2012; Yee et al., 2012).

Five years after the first GWAS of clinical response to metformin in people with type 2 diabetes, a second GWAS involving MetGen was published. The study identified a minor C-allele in an intron SNP (rs8192675) of a glucose transporter, GLUT2, *SLC2A2*, which was associated with greater change in HbA1c from baseline (Table 1) as a quantitative trait in discovery and replication cohorts (Zhou et al., 2016). A meta-analysis of the SNP was performed in MetGen (http://www.pgrn.org/metgen.html), which included over 10,000 participants in 10 cohorts from Europe and the United States. Strikingly, the results reached genome-wide level significance in both models of change in HbA1c (on metformin) adjusted (beta 0.075, $P=2.0\times10^{-8}$) and nonadjusted (beta 0.17, $P=6.6\times10^{-14}$) with baseline HbA1c ($n=10{,}557$). Since *SLC2A2* is known to play a role in the development of type 2 diabetes and to have an effect on fasting glucose, genetic variation in the transporter may impact the glucose-lowering effect of antidiabetic therapy. The result showed that the SNP that associated with higher baseline HbA1c was associated with greater HbA1c reduction after initiation of metformin. This phenomenon has been observed in other

Table 1 Genes Associated with Metformin Pharmacokinetics or Response

Gene	Study Population	Metformin Dose	Variant	Phenotype
SLC22A1 (OCT1)	20 healthy volunteers	2 doses 1000 and 850 mg	R61C (rs12208357), G401S (rs34130495), 420del (rs72552763 and G4665R/rs34059508)	Impaired response to oral glucose tolerance test (Shu et al., 2007)
	20 healthy volunteers	2 doses 1000 and 850 mg	R61C (rs12208357), G401S (rs34130495), 420del (rs72552763 and G4665R/rs34059508)	Higher AUC, higher C_{max}, lower oral volume of distribution (Shu et al., 2008)
	103 healthy male Caucasian volunteers	1 dose of 500 mg	G465R	Increased renal clearance and decreased hepatic uptake (Tzvetkov et al., 2009)
	1531 GoDARTS subjects with type 2 diabetes	Average dose 1260 mg/day	R61C and M420del	No effect on HbA1c reduction (Zhou et al., 2009)
	159 Danish South Danish Diabetes Study participants with type 2 diabetes	1000 mg twice a day	R61C (rs12208357), G401S (rs34130495), 420del (rs72552763 and G4665R/rs34059508)	Decrease in trough steady-state metformin concentration and less change in HbA1c over 6 months (Christensen et al., 2011)
	1915 metformin tolerant and 251 metformin intolerant GoDARTS participants	Average dose 1000 mg/day	R61C (rs12208357), G401S (rs34130495), 420del (rs72552763 and G4665R/rs34059508)	Two reduced function alleles associated with metformin intolerance. Higher odds of intolerance in the presence of OCT1 interacting drugs (Dujic et al., 2015)
	102 subjects with type 2 diabetes from Rotterdam Study	Average dose 677 mg/day	rs622342	Less reduction in HbA1c level (Becker et al., 2009b)
	148 drug naïve Caucasian patients with type 2 diabetes	Average dose ~1400 mg/day	rs622342	No effect on HbA1c reduction (Tkac et al., 2013)
	990 multiethnic DPP participants with prediabetes	850 mg twice a day	rs622342	No evidence of interaction with metformin (Jablonski et al., 2010)

SLC22A2 (OCT2)	15 healthy Chinese participants	A single dose of 500 mg	808G > T	Reduced metformin renal tubular clearance (Wang, Yin, Tomlinson, & Chow, 2008)
	26 healthy Korean subjects	A single dose of 500 mg of metformin	596C > T, 602C > T, and 808G > T	Higher C_{max}, AUC, and lower renal clearance (Song et al., 2008)
	23 healthy Caucasian and African American volunteers	A single dose of 850 mg of metformin	808G > T	Decreased renal clearance and renal clearance by secretion of metformin (Chen et al., 2009)
	371 Danish participants with type 2 diabetes from South Danish Diabetes Study	1000 mg twice a day	rs316019	No effect on metformin concentration or HbA1c response (Christensen et al., 2011)
	990 multiethnic DPP participants with prediabetes	850 mg twice a day	rs316019	No evidence of interaction with metformin (Jablonski et al., 2010)
SLC47A1 (MATE1) and *SLC47A2* (MATE2)	57 healthy volunteers	2 doses 1000 and 850 mg	rs2252281 (MATE1) rs12943590 (MATE2)	Renal and secretory clearance of metformin higher in MATE2 carriers who were MATE1 reference. Enhanced OGTT response with MATE1, reduced response with MATE2 (Stocker et al., 2013)
	145 patients with type 2 diabetes	Average dose 938 mg/day	rs2252281 (MATE1)	Greater change in HbA1c level with MATE1 (Stocker et al., 2013)
	253 Caucasian and African American subjects with type 2 diabetes	Average dose 938 mg/day	rs12943590 (MATE2-K)	Less reduction in HbA1c (Choi et al., 2011)
	116 Caucasian subjects with type 2 diabetes	Average dose 741 mg	rs2289669 (MATE1)	Decrease in HbA1c (Becker et al., 2009a)
	148 drug naïve Caucasian patients with type 2 diabetes	Average dose ~1400 mg/day	rs2289669 (MATE1)	Greater reduction in HbA1c (Tkac et al., 2013)

Continued

Table 1 Genes Associated with Metformin Pharmacokinetics or Response—cont'd

Gene	Study Population	Metformin Dose	Variant	Phenotype
	990 multiethnic DPP participants with prediabetes	850 mg twice a day	rs8065082 (In LD r^2 0.8 with rs2289669) (MATE1)	Poorer response to metformin (Jablonski et al., 2010)
	371 Danish participants with type 2 diabetes from South Danish Diabetes Study	1000 mg twice a day	rs2252281, rs2289669 (MATE1) rs34399035 (MATE2)	No effect on metformin concentration or change in HbA1c (Christensen et al., 2011)
ATM	1024 Scottish subjects with type 2 diabetes (GWAS Discovery cohort) 2896 Caucasian subjects with type 2 diabetes (2 Replication cohorts)	The average daily dose during the 3 months prior to the minimum HbA1c was achieved	rs11212617 (intron of C11orf65), in LD with $r^2>0.8$ with SNPs in several genes including ATM, NPAT, KDELC2	Minor C-allele of rs11212617 is associated with treatment success (Zhou et al., 2011). Treatment success was defined as achieving HbA1c <7% in the first 18 months of metformin initiation ($n=3920$, $P=2.9\times10^{-9}$, odds ratio = 1.35)
SLC2A2 (GLUT2)	3103 Scottish subjects with type 2 diabetes (GWAS Discovery cohort) 7454 Caucasian subjects with type 2 diabetes (9 Replication cohorts) 2526 Non-European subjects with type 2 diabetes (3 different ethnic groups)	The average daily dose during the 3 months prior to the minimum HbA1c was achieved	rs8192675 (intron of *SLC2A2*)	Minor C-allele of rs8192675 is associated with greater response to metformin (Zhou et al., 2016). Response to metformin was defined as baseline HbA1c minus the minimum treatment HbA1c in the first 18 months of metformin initiation ($n=10{,}557$ Caucasians, $P=2.0\times10^{-8}$, beta = 0.075 (baseline-adjusted model); $P=6.6\times10^{-14}$, beta = 0.17 (baseline nonadjusted model)). Also significant in the combined non-European subjects ($n=2566$ Non-Europeans, $P=0.006$, beta = 0.077 (baseline-adjusted model); $P=0.005$, beta = 0.15 (baseline nonadjusted model)) Minor C-allele of rs8192675 is associated with lower SLC2A2 transcript levels in human liver tissue samples ($n=1226$, $P<5\times10^{-8}$) and other tissues (fibroblasts, islet, intestine) (Zhou et al., 2016)

pharmacogenetic studies, where a SNP, which has an effect on a baseline trait, also impacts drug response. For example, SNPs in PCSK9 and APOE, which are associated with baseline LDL-C levels, are also significantly associated with LDL-C reduction and fractional LDL-C reduction in response to rosuvastatin (Chasman et al., 2012). These studies suggest that pharmacogenomic studies of drug response should consider SNPs known to be associated with disease as those SNPs may also play a role in drug response. Further, the studies suggest that performing the association analyses with and without adjusting for baseline is important particularly for genes known to play a role in baseline trait measured. Other results worth mentioning from the more recent GWAS of metformin response (Zhou et al., 2016) include:

- The rs8192675 minor C-allele of SLC2A2 was associated with lower expression levels of *SLC2A2* in the human liver.
- There was a stronger HbA1c reduction induced by metformin in individuals who were obese (BMI $\geq$ 30 kg/m^2) and who harbored the C-allele of rs8192675 compared to individuals with the C-allele but who have BMI $<$ 30 kg/m^2.
- The rs8192675 minor C-allele of *SLC2A2* was associated with metformin response in non-European populations. The combined *P*-values in the non-European populations were $P=0.006$ and $P=0.005$ in baseline adjusted and nonadjusted models, respectively. Both models showed that the minor C-allele was associated with greater HbA1c reduction upon metformin treatment, similar to the results obtained in the European cohorts.

The fact that GLUT2 is the major transporter for hepatic glucose output (Seyer et al., 2013) and metformin has a primary pharmacologic effect of reducing hepatic glucose output (Foretz et al., 2010; Madiraju et al., 2014) suggests a strong mechanism by which the variant may modulate response to metformin. Further studies are warranted to replicate these findings and to elucidate whether genetic information can be used in precision medicine to guide therapy with metformin.

3. GENOME-WIDE SCREENING TO ELUCIDATE METFORMIN ACTION THROUGH IN VITRO ASSAYS

The mechanism of action of metformin is complex. In brief, the drug appears to reduce mitochondrial energy production via inhibition of complex 1. The lower levels of adenosine triphosphate (ATP) (and higher AMP to ATP ratio) lead to phosphorylation or activation of the energy sensor,

AMP-kinase, AMPK (Zhou et al., 2001). The molecular components LKB1/STK11 and ATM have been shown to play a role in the phosphorylation of AMPK in the presence of metformin, though these are not direct targets of metformin (Foretz & Viollet, 2011). Activation of AMPK results in reduced gluconeogenesis, increased insulin sensitivity, and enhanced peripheral glucose uptake. There is also evidence to suggest that metformin inhibits hepatic gluconeogenesis independent of the LKB1/AMPK pathway (Foretz et al., 2010). Another way by which gluconeogenesis is reduced is by increased AMP levels which functions as a key signaling mediator that inhibits CAMP-PKA signaling through suppression of adenylate cyclase, by allosteric inhibition of fructose-1,6-bisphosphatase and by activation of AMPK (Rena, Pearson, & Sakamoto, 2013). Metformin also likely has beneficial effects beyond the treatment of type 2 diabetes. An increasing number of observational studies suggest that treatment with metformin (relative to other glucose-lowering therapies) is associated with reduced risk of cancer (Giovannucci et al., 2010).

Different genome-wide approaches using in vitro cell-based assays have been used to identify genes associated with metformin action (Luizon et al., 2016; Niu et al., 2016). For example, RNA-seq and ChIP-seq (chromatin immunoprecipitation with massively parallel DNA sequencing) have been used to identify genes and DNA regions regulated by metformin after exposing primary human hepatocytes to metformin. These methods demonstrated that the transcript levels of ATF3, a transcription factor that plays an important role in modulating glucose homeostasis, are significantly increased by metformin (Jadhav & Zhang, 2017; Luizon et al., 2016). Further the studies also add mechanistic support to the finding that rs11212617 in the ATM gene is associated with response to metformin. That is, the SNP lies in an important enhancer region which is regulated by treatment with metformin (Luizon et al., 2016; Zhou et al., 2011). Application of GWAS to 266 human lymphoblastoid cell lines treated with metformin resulted in the identification of genetic biomarkers associated with metformin cytotoxicity (Niu et al., 2016). Some of the genes identified in the cytotoxicity assays may also influence metformin's antidiabetic actions through common pathways, such as the LKB1/AMPK pathway and PI3K/mTOR signaling pathway which are important for cellular growth as well as energy homeostasis (Niu et al., 2016; Snima, Pillai, Cherian, Nair, & Lakshmanan, 2014). For example, STUB1, a E3 ubiquitin ligase, is involved in activation of AMPK through the LKB pathway (Niu et al., 2016).

4. STUDIES RELATED TO METFORMIN CANDIDATE GENES

Prior to the onset of GWAS that offered the ability to interrogate the entire genome, research related to metformin pharmacogenetics was limited to preexisting biological knowledge of metformin through a candidate gene approach. Studies were mainly centered on the cellular transporters that regulated metformin disposition, and the majority of work focused on organic cation transporters (OCTs). In order to understand the role of candidate genes in metformin response, it is helpful to have an understanding of the pharmacokinetics and pharmacodynamics of metformin.

4.1 Metformin Pharmacokinetics

Metformin is a hydrophilic molecule that diffuses poorly across biological membranes. As such, for its disposition, metformin requires membrane transporters, and in particular, OCTs in the intestine, liver, and kidney. Metformin is excreted unchanged in the urine and has an elimination half-life of approximately 5 h in patients with normal renal function. Metformin is primarily eliminated through active tubular secretion in the kidney. The oral absorption, hepatic uptake, and renal excretion of metformin are largely mediated by OCTs (Graham et al., 2011). Though the exact transporters that contribute to the absorption, distribution, and elimination of metformin in patients are not known, in vitro studies and studies in animal models provide support for several transporters. For example, the intestinal absorption of metformin may involve the plasma membrane monoamine transporter (PMAT encoded by gene *SLC29A4*), the organic cation transporter 3 (OCT3 encoded by gene *SLC22A3*), the thiamine transporter (THTR2 encoded by *SLC19A3*) (Liang et al., 2015), and the serotonin transporter (SERT encoded by *SLC6A4*) (Han et al., 2015; Zhou, Xia, & Wang, 2007). These transporters are expressed on the luminal membrane of enterocytes. To mediate flux from the enterocyte into the portal circulation, OCT1 (gene *SLC22A1*), which is expressed on the basolateral surface, appears to be involved. For hepatic distribution of metformin to targets in the liver, evidence in OCT1 knockout mice and humans using imaging of 11C-metformin suggests that OCT1 (*SLC22A1*) is primarily involved (Jensen et al., 2016; Sundelin et al., 2017). Additionally, in OCT1-deficient mice the glucose-lowering effects of metformin are completely abolished (Shu et al., 2007). Metformin excretion into bile appears to involve multidrug and toxin extrusion 1 (MATE1 encoded by *SLC47A1*) (Otsuka et al., 2005), though in humans the bulk of metformin is excreted unchanged into the urine (Graham et al., 2011). The uptake of metformin from the circulation into renal epithelial cells is primarily facilitated by OCT2 (*SLC22A2*) located on the basolateral membrane of renal proximal tubule cells (Takane, Shikata, Otsubo, Higuchi, & Ieiri, 2008). MATE1 (*SLC47A1*) and MATE2-K (*SLC47A2*), expressed on the apical membrane, appear to be responsible for excretion of metformin into the urine (Masuda et al., 2006; Otsuka et al., 2005; Tanihara et al., 2007). OCT1 and PMAT are also expressed on the apical membrane of renal epithelial cells, and these transporters may also play a role in metformin renal disposition (Gong, Goswami, Giacomini, Altman, & Klein, 2012).

4.2 Metformin Pharmacodynamics

Metformin lowers both fasting and postprandial glucose levels primarily by reducing excessive hepatic glucose production through suppression of gluconeogenesis. Metformin may also increase peripheral glucose utilization and has downstream effects on decreasing fatty acid and triglyceride production (Hundal et al., 2000; Rena et al., 2013). As metformin does not stimulate endogenous insulin production, it does not cause hypoglycemia, which is an adverse effect that is associated with several antidiabetic medications.

The molecular mechanisms of metformin action are described earlier. Below we describe candidate gene studies that have provided information on genes, proteins, and pathways involved in the absorption, disposition, and response to metformin in healthy volunteers and in patients with type 2 diabetes (Table 1).

4.2.1 OCT1

The most studied transporter in relation to metformin genetics and disposition is OCT1, which is essential for the hepatic uptake of metformin. OCT1 is encoded by the gene *SLC22A1* which is highly polymorphic and a number of coding missense SNPs affect its activity (Kerb et al., 2002; Leabman et al., 2002; Sakata et al., 2004; Shu et al., 2003). In a study of 20 healthy volunteers, it was demonstrated that the presence of at least one of four reduced function variants (R61C/rs12208357, G401S/rs34130495, 420del/rs72552763, and/or G465R/rs34059508) attenuates the effects of a short course of metformin on glucose tolerance tests (Shu et al., 2007).

A follow-up study demonstrated that individuals carrying any of the reduced function OCT1 alleles showed a higher area under the concentration-time curve (AUC), higher peak serum concentration (C_{max}), and a lower volume of distribution compared to individuals carrying wild-type alleles (Shu et al., 2008). A subsequent study in 103 healthy volunteers found that G465R was associated with increased renal clearance and decreased hepatic uptake. However, the reduced function allele did not lead to differences in metformin AUC (Tzvetkov et al., 2009). In a large retrospective observation study of 1531 subjects with type 2 diabetes assembled by GoDARTS, the two most common reduced-function polymorphisms (R61C and M420del) were not associated with four different measures of clinical response whether defined as initial HbA1c reduction, odds of achieving a target HbA1c of less than 7%, average HbA1c or hazard of monotherapy failure. It is important to note that since the study was observational, the metformin dose, prescription of other antidiabetic agents, and timing of HbA1c measurements were at the discretion of the prescribing clinician (Zhou et al., 2009). In the South Danish Diabetes Study, which is a prospective interventional study of 159 participants, both trough and steady-state metformin concentrations and 6 months change in HbA1c were lower with increasing number of reduced-function alleles (i.e., R61C, G401S, M420del, and G465R) (Christensen et al., 2011). In terms of response, the retrospective Rotterdam study reported the association of *SLC22A1* intronic SNP rs622342 with metformin response in subjects with type 2 diabetes (Becker et al., 2009b), but this association was not observed in several later studies (Christensen et al., 2011; Jablonski et al., 2010; Tkac et al., 2013). Despite consistent data from various studies (Shu et al., 2008; Sundelin et al., 2017; Tzvetkov et al., 2009) that OCT1-reduced-function variants are associated with metformin pharmacokinetics, their role in metformin response has not been observed in some studies (Zhou et al., 2009) including the recent large observational study in diabetic patients conducted by the MetGen consortium (Dujic et al., 2017). Reasons for this discrepancy may be related to differences in analysis of the data or the fact that genes involved in the pharmacokinetics of metformin do not contribute much to variation in the pharmacodynamics of the drug.

4.2.2 OCT2

The renal transporter OCT2 appears to have less functional variation than OCT1, and the effect of variation in OCT2 with respect to metformin has been studied to a lesser extent than OCT1. A study of 15 healthy Chinese participants showed that the reduced-function 808G > T polymorphism (Ala270Ser) was associated with reduced metformin renal tubular clearance and that in the presence of cimetidine, metformin clearance was decreased in all participants, but the decrease was significantly lower in homozygous TT participants compared to GG participants (18.7% vs 48.2%, $P=0.029$) (Wang et al., 2008). Similarly, a study in Korean healthy participants showed that reduced-function genetic variants of OCT2 (596C > T, 602C > T, and 808G > T) were associated with higher peak plasma concentration and area under the curve measurements and lower renal clearance (Song et al., 2008). In contrast, in a study of 23 healthy volunteers of Caucasian and African-American ancestries, though an association between the renal clearance of metformin and 808G > T was observed, the direction of effect was the opposite and subjects who were homozygous for the reference allele 808G > G ($P<0.005$) had reduced renal clearance of metformin (Chen et al., 2009). The reasons for these differences are likely related to small sample sizes and differences in the ethnicities of the participants. Studies of association between genetic variation in OCT2 and metformin response have not shown positive results (Christensen et al., 2011; Jablonski et al., 2010).

4.2.3 MATE1 and MATE2

Studies have examined the effects of promoter variants in both MATE1 and MATE2 on variation in metformin disposition and response. In a study of 57 healthy volunteers who received metformin, the renal and secretory clearances of metformin were higher in carriers of MATE2 variants who also carried the reference alleles for MATE1. Additionally, 145 patients with type 2 diabetes carrying the MATE1 variant showed enhanced response to metformin (Stocker et al., 2013). In the Rotterdam study, the intronic SNP rs2289669 in MATE1 was associated with change in HbA1c after metformin initiation, with the minor allele enhancing the reduction in HbA1c (Becker et al., 2009a). Similar findings were observed in Tkac et al. (2013) and in the Diabetes prevention program where rs8065082 in MATE1 which is in high linkage disequilibrium with rs2289669 was associated with lower diabetes incidence in the metformin arm and not in the placebo arm in subjects who were at risk for the development of diabetes (Jablonski et al., 2010). However, this finding was not observed in the South Danish Diabetes Study (Christensen et al., 2011; Dujic et al., 2017) or in a large meta-analysis conducted by the Metformin Genetics (MetGen) Consortium.

Overall, the results of genetic associations between transporters and pharmacokinetics of metformin have led to conflicting results. Differences in data analyses, study design and in the characteristics of the participants such as their ethnicities or disease status, may have led to some of the discrepancies among studies. Most of the studies have been small and underpowered, so clearly larger well-powered studies in multiple ethnic groups are needed to understand which variants and genes may associate with the pharmacokinetics of metformin.

5. GENETIC STUDIES OF OTHER ANTIDIABETIC DRUGS

5.1 Sulfonylureas

Sulfonylureas are among the most widely used antidiabetic drugs and act by directly stimulating insulin secretion from the pancreatic beta cells. Serious side effects of these drugs are hypoglycemia and weight gain. Sulfonylureas were previously considered as a first-line treatment for type 2 diabetes, but now are mainly used as a second-line treatment in combination with metformin (Marathe, Gao, & Close, 2017; Nathan et al., 2009). Sulfonylureas stimulate insulin secretion by binding to the ATP-sensitive potassium channel (K_{ATP}) which is composed of four subunits of the sulfonylurea receptor (SUR1, *ABCC8*) and four subunits of the potassium inward rectifier channel (Kir) 6.2. Sulfonylurea binding leads to closure of the K_{ATP} channel which alters the resting potential of the cell, leading to calcium influx and stimulation of insulin secretion (Thule & Umpierrez, 2014). Sulfonylureas are metabolized in the liver primarily by the polymorphic cytochrome P450 isoenzyme 2C9 encoded by *CYP2C9*. Substitution of arginine with cysteine at amino acid position 144 (Arg144Cys) and isoleucine with leucine at position 359 (Ile359Leu) gives rise to mutant alleles CYP2C9*2 and CYP2C9*3, respectively, which have reduced catalytic activity when compared to the wild-type CYP2C9*1.

Several studies have investigated the effect of genetic variation in CYP2C9 (the rate-limiting step of metabolism) on the pharmacokinetics and pharmacodynamics of sulfonylureas. Studies in healthy subjects show that reduced-function alleles of CYP2C9 are associated with increased plasma concentrations and decreased clearance of sulfonylureas after oral administration. While small-scale studies have shown differences in sulfonylurea metabolism, studies on actual measured drug response are few. In a large retrospective study of 1073 subjects from GoDARTS, carriers of loss-of-function CYP2C9*2 or CYP2C9*3 alleles had a 3.4-fold increased likelihood of achieving therapeutic target effects on blood glucose compared to carriers of the wild-type alleles. This translated to a 0.5% greater HbA1c reduction in individuals with the variant CYP2C9 alleles (Zhou et al., 2010). In addition to CYP2C9 polymorphisms, CYP2C19 polymorphisms have been reported to be influential in gliclazide pharmacokinetics (Shao et al., 2010; Zhang, Si, et al., 2007).

The identification of SU-binding sites SUR1 and Kir6.2 (encoded by *ABCC8* and *KCNJ11*, respectively) has led to various pharmacogenetic explorations of variations in these genes. Nonsynonymous variants E23K in KCNJ11 and S1369A in ABCC8 form a haplotype, and pharmacogenetic studies of these variants show conflicting results. Association of S1369A with glycemic control has been reported in 115 Chinese patients who were on gliclazide for 8 weeks with carriers of the minor allele demonstrating a greater reduction in HbA1c than the wild-type carriers (Zhang, Liu, Kuang, Yi, & Xing, 2007). In a study that investigated the effect of the E23K variant KCNJ11 gene on gliclazide-modified release treatment in 108 newly diagnosed patients with type 2 diabetes mellitus, at baseline, patients with the KK genotype had higher blood glucose and lower serum insulin levels after oral glucose administration than patients with the EE and EK genotypes ($P < 0.05$ for all). During treatment, individuals with the KK genotype had lower fasting glucose levels and were more likely to attain the target fasting glucose level than E-allele carriers, suggesting that the KCNJ11 E23K variant is associated with a greater effect of sulfonylurea treatment in newly diagnosed Chinese patients with type 2 diabetes (Li et al., 2014). However, results from UKPDS are conflicting. In this study they evaluated 364 subjects with type 2 diabetes randomized to sulfonylurea treatment and determined that the presence of the K-allele in E23K did not predict failure to treatment with sulfonylureas at 1 year (Gloyn et al., 2001).

The *KCNQ1* gene encodes the pore-forming subunit of a voltage-gated K+ channel (KvLQT1), and studies have indicated that *KCNQ1* polymorphisms are related to impaired insulin secretion (Hu et al., 2009) and type 2 diabetes in several GWAS (see GWAS Catalog (https://www.ebi.ac.uk/gwas/home)). A study evaluated the effect *KCNQ1* genotype on sulfonylurea therapy in addition to metformin therapy on glycemic control in 87 patients with type 2 diabetes. The results showed that carriers of the T-allele achieved significantly lower fasting glucose levels in compared with patients with the GG genotype (6.95 ± 0.13 vs 7.50 ± 0.21 mmoL/L, $P = 0.033$) (Schroner et al., 2011).

The TCF7L2 gene is strongly associated with the development of type 2 diabetes with one of the highest effect sizes for common variants (Grant et al., 2006; Helgason et al., 2007). Several studies have focused on the rs7903146 variant in *TCF7L2* as a determinant of drug response. In a large GoDARTS retrospective study of subjects with type 2 diabetes, of 901 users of sulfonylureas, homozygotes for the type 2 diabetes T risk allele at *TCF7L2* rs7903146 were less likely to respond to sulfonylureas, with an odds ratio of failure of 1.73 (95% CI 1.11–2.70, $P=0.015$) (Pearson et al., 2007). This was in contrast to results from the Study to Understand the Genetics of the Acute Response of metformin and glipizide in humans (SUGAR-MGH) study where 608 participants who were healthy or at risk for type 2 diabetes were given a single dose of 5 mg of glipizide with biochemical data measured after the dose. Results from SUGAR-MGH showed that the T-allele of rs7903146 at *TCF7L2* was associated with a significantly shorter time and a steeper slope to trough glucose levels after glipizide administration (Srinivasan et al., 2018). These contrasting results suggest that it is possible that the genotype has a differential effect in subjects in whom diabetes has not yet developed compared with subjects with established type 2 diabetes, in whom some degree of beta cell failure may have already occurred.

5.2 Thiazolidinediones

The thiazolidinediones (TZDs) are a group of drugs that increase insulin sensitivity by acting on adipose tissue, muscle, and liver to increase glucose utilization and decrease glucose production. The mechanism by which the thiazolidinediones exert their effect is not fully understood but is thought to relate to activation of one or more peroxisome proliferator-activated receptors (PPARs), which regulate gene expression in response to ligand binding. Hepatic uptake of TZDs is mediated by OATP1B1, and TZDs are metabolized by CYP2C8. Homozygous carriers of the gain-of-function allele for CYP2C8, CYP2C8*3 coding for the Arg139Lys and Lys399Arg amino acid substitutions have lower rosiglitazone plasma concentrations and higher weight-adjusted clearance when compared to wild-type carriers (Aquilante et al., 2008; Kirchheiner et al., 2006). In addition to the role of OATP1B1 encoded by *SLCO1B1* and CYP2C8 in thiazolidinediones pharmacokinetics, a recent study in 833 Scottish patients showed that CYP2C8*3 and OATP1B1 nonsynonymous variant (Val174Ala, rs4149056) alter drug efficacy (Dawed et al., 2016). In particular, gain-of-function CYP2C8*3 was associated with reduced glycemic response to rosiglitazone ($P=0.01$) and less weight gain ($P=0.02$) (27271184), which is in agreement with the effect of this variant to cause increase drug clearance and lower plasma levels (Aquilante et al., 2008; Kirchheiner et al., 2006). *PPARG* is a target of TZDs and has been explored in pharmacogenetic investigations. A study in 250 Chinese patients showed that carriers of the minor allele of variant rs1801282 in *PPARG* had a higher odds of being responders to pioglitazone when compared to carriers of wild-type alleles (Hsieh et al., 2010). Studies have also looked at other adipokinins including adiponectin, leptin, resistin, and tumor necrosis factor-alpha based on the role they play in insulin resistance with variable results obtained. A study of 42 Chinese patients with type 2 diabetes treated with 12 weeks of rosiglitazone monotherapy demonstrated an attenuated effect of rosiglitazone on fasting glucose, 2 h glucose, and HOMA-IR values in subjects with adiponectin variant C-11377G (rs266729) CG and GG genotypes compared to CC genotype; however, the effects were enhanced in patients with the diplotype C-11377 (rs266729)/T45G (rs2241766) CGTT in adiponectin (Sun et al., 2008). The investigators also evaluated the impact of genetic polymorphisms of leptin and TNF-alpha on rosiglitazone response in the same group of subjects. They found an enhanced rosiglitazone effect in patients with G-2548A (rs7799039) AA genotype of leptin on fasting and 2 h insulin values compared with GG and GA genotypes. They also showed an attenuated rosiglitazone effect in patients with GA and AA genotypes of TNF-alpha G-308A (rs1800629) on fasting insulin values compared with GG genotype (Liu et al., 2008).

5.3 Meglitinides

The meglitinides, repaglinide and nateglinide, are short-acting glucose-lowering drugs that are structurally distinct from sulfonylureas and exert their effects via different pancreatic beta cell receptors, but they act similarly by regulating ATP-sensitive potassium channels (K-ATP channels) in pancreatic beta cells, thereby increasing insulin secretion. Meglitinides have a rapid onset and short duration of action. They are transported into the liver by OATP1B1 encoded by *SLCO1B1* after which metabolism occurs via CYP family isoenzymes. There have been a few pharmacogenetic studies of meglitinides. Genetic polymorphisms in CYP2C8 have been found to be associated with reduced plasma concentrations of repaglinide (Niemi et al., 2003). Repaglinide pharmacokinetics has also been shown to be modulated by genetic variants in SLCO1B1 (Kalliokoski, Backman, Neuvonen, & Niemi, 2008). Several candidate genes studies have evaluated the effect of genetic variation in genes implicated in type 2 diabetes risk on response to meglitinides (Semiz, Dujic, & Causevic, 2013). These include SNPs in *KCNQ1* (Dai et al., 2012; Yu et al., 2011), *SLC30A8* (Huang et al., 2010), *TCF7L2* and *KCNJ11* (Yu et al., 2010). However, these studies have small sample size and were performed only in Chinese patients with type 2 diabetes and therefore the results cannot be extrapolated to other populations.

5.4 Acarbose

The alpha-glucosidase inhibitor, acarbose, when taken orally, inhibits the upper gastrointestinal enzymes (alpha-glucosidases) that convert complex polysaccharide carbohydrates into monosaccharides in a dose-dependent fashion thereby slowing the absorption of glucose. Interactions between acarbose and PPAR-alpha (PPARA) with PPAR-gamma2 (PPARG2), PPAR-gamma coactivator 1alpha (PPARGC1A), and hepatic nuclear factor 4alpha (HNF4A) were evaluated in the STOP-NIDDM trial with modest associations revealed (Andrulionyte, Kuulasmaa, Chiasson, & Laakso, 2007). The clinical significance of these associations remains to be tested.

5.5 SGLT2 Inhibitors (Gliflozins)

SGLT2 inhibitors are a new class of drugs that promote the renal excretion of glucose and thereby modestly lower elevated blood glucose levels in patients with type 2 diabetes. They are mainly eliminated through O-glucuronidation by uridine diphosphate glucuronosyl transferases. A study of 134 subjects including both healthy and subjects with type 2 diabetes demonstrated that carriers of reduced-function variant, UGT1A9*3 and UGT2B4*2, had an increased plasma concentration of canagliflozin, an SGLT2 inhibitor when compared to carriers of the wild-type alleles (Francke et al., 2015). Recently, a cross-sectional study in a population at risk for type 2 diabetes in which 603 subjects received empagliflozin, an SGLT2 inhibitor, and 305 received placebo showed no association of common *SLC5A2* variants that encode SGLT2 with empagliflozin response (Zimdahl et al., 2017).

5.6 Glucagon-Like Peptide-1-Based Therapies

Glucagon-Like Peptide-1 (GLP-1)-based therapies (e.g., GLP-1 receptor agonists, dipeptidyl peptidase-4 (DPP-4) inhibitors) are a very promising group of drugs that affect glucose control through several mechanisms, including enhancement of glucose-dependent insulin secretion, slowed gastric emptying, and reduction of postprandial glucagon and of food intake. There are very few pharmacogenetic studies of GLP-1-based therapies. In a study of the association of *TCF7L2* on the response to treatment with the DPP-4 inhibitor linagliptin in 61 patients with type 2 diabetes, no significant treatment differences were seen between nonrisk variant CC carriers and heterozygous CT subjects, although HbA1c response was reduced in homozygous TT subjects when compared with CC subjects (Zimdahl et al., 2014).

5.7 Pharmacogenetics of Adverse Reactions and Off-Target Effects of Antidiabetic Drugs

In addition to studies of pharmacokinetics and response, there have been candidate gene studies of pharmacogenetics of adverse reactions to antidiabetic drugs. The most common side effect of metformin therapy is gastrointestinal distress with symptoms of taste alteration, nausea, abdominal discomfort, diarrhea, or mild anorexia. Metformin therapy can cause gastrointestinal distress in upto 40% of patients on treatment and around 5% of patients have to discontinue metformin because of side effects (Bailey, 2015). A study of adverse effects by GoDARTS investigators was undertaken in 1915 participants with type 2 diabetes who had evidence of metformin intolerance including gastrointestinal side effects and the need to discontinue the drug and 251 subjects who were metformin tolerant. Their results showed that the presence of two or more reduced-function alleles of OCT1 (at R61C, C88R/rs55918055, G401S, M420del, or G465R) increased the odds of metformin intolerance by more than twofold. Further, concomitant use of OCT1-inhibiting medications such as verapamil, citalopram, or proton pump inhibitors increased the odds by fourfold, presumably by increasing metformin concentrations in the intestine (Dujic et al., 2015). Hypoglycemia is the most common side effect of sulfonylureas. Loss-of-function CYP2C9 variants have been associated with increased drugs levels of gliclazide with significantly increased risk of hypoglycemia (Gokalp et al., 2011). The DREAM (Diabetes REduction Assessment with Ramipril and rosiglitazone Medication) trial evaluated adverse effects of rosiglitazone on edema in 4197 participants. A single SNP rs6123045 in *NFATC2* was significantly associated with edema, and the interaction between the SNP and rosiglitazone for edema was significant (Bailey et al., 2010). Studies are required to evaluate the pharmacogenetics of adverse effects of other newer drugs such as SGLT2 inhibitors and incretin-based therapies.

Few studies have evaluated the pharmacogenetics factors involved in off-target effects of antidiabetic drugs. In addition to its beneficial effect on glycemic control, metformin has been shown to have cardiovascular benefit in patients with type 2 diabetes (Lamanna, Monami, Marchionni, & Mannucci, 2011). A small Russian study of 52 subjects evaluated the type 2 diabetes associated PPRA-gamma2 pro12Ala polymorphism in relation to metformin therapy in patients with coronary heart disease and metabolic syndrome or type 2 diabetes. They found that patients with coronary artery disease who carried the Pro allele showed a significant metformin-induced reduction in weight, waist circumference, body mass index, and plasma levels of cardiovascular markers including total cholesterol, C-peptide, and cytokines, such IL-1beta, IL-6, IL-8, and TNF-alpha. Further studies are clearly needed to evaluate the pharmacogenetics of off-target effects of metformin and other antidiabetic drugs (Lavrenko, Shlykova, Kutsenko, Mamontova, & Kaidashev, 2012).

6. CONCLUSION

In summary, there are few pharmacogenomics studies of antidiabetic drugs other than metformin. For metformin, two GWAS have been conducted and have revealed that genetic variants in ATM and *SLC2A2* are associated with response to the drug in large populations of patients with type 2 diabetes treated with metformin. Though these results need replication in additional cohorts, they pave the way for precision medicine in guiding selection and dosing of metformin in diabetic patient populations. Candidate gene studies focused on metformin pharmacokinetics have been small, and there is a clear need for larger studies to identify the genes that play a role in variation in pharmacokinetics of the drug. Pharmacogenomic studies are clearly needed for other antidiabetic drugs beyond metformin, as to date, most pharmacogenomic studies of other antidiabetic drugs are small and focused on candidate genes. The goal of precision medicine is to tailor medical therapy according to patient characteristics to achieve optimal therapeutic response while minimizing adverse effects. For precision medicine to be used in guiding selection of antidiabetic drugs for individual patients based on genetic (and other) factors, there is a clear need for larger studies focused on efficacy of both metformin and other antidiabetic drugs. In addition, because many antidiabetic drugs are associated with dose-limiting toxicities, further studies are needed to identify the genetic factors that underlie adverse drug reactions in order to enhance the optimal selection of drug and dose in the treatment of type 2 diabetes.

ACKNOWLEDGMENT

S.S., S.W.Y. and K.M.G would like to acknowledge funding from National Institute of Health (grant number GM117163).

CONFLICT OF INTEREST

S.S. does not have any conflict of interest. K.M.G. and S.W.Y. are cofounders of Apricity Therapeutics, Inc., which focuses on transporters in drug discovery and development.

REFERENCES

Andrulionyte, L., Kuulasmaa, T., Chiasson, J. L., & Laakso, M. (2007). Single nucleotide polymorphisms of the peroxisome proliferator-activated receptor-alpha gene (PPARA) influence the conversion from impaired glucose tolerance to type 2 diabetes: The STOP-NIDDM trial. *Diabetes*, *56*(4), 1181–1186. https://doi.org/10.2337/db06-1110.

Aquilante, C. L., Bushman, L. R., Knutsen, S. D., Burt, L. E., Rome, L. C., & Kosmiski, L. A. (2008). Influence of SLCO1B1 and CYP2C8 gene polymorphisms on rosiglitazone pharmacokinetics in healthy volunteers. *Human Genomics*, *3*(1), 7–16.

Bailey, C. J. (2015). Safety of antidiabetes medications: An update. *Clinical Pharmacology and Therapeutics*, *98*(2), 185–195. https://doi.org/10.1002/cpt.125.

Bailey, S. D., Xie, C., Do, R., Montpetit, A., Diaz, R., Mohan, V., et al. (2010). Variation at the NFATC2 locus increases the risk of thiazolidinedione-induced edema in the Diabetes REduction Assessment with ramipril and rosiglitazone Medication (DREAM) study. *Diabetes Care*, *33*(10), 2250–2253. https://doi.org/10.2337/dc10-0452.

Becker, M. L., Visser, L. E., van Schaik, R. H., Hofman, A., Uitterlinden, A. G., & Stricker, B. H. (2009a). Genetic variation in the multidrug and toxin extrusion 1 transporter protein influences the glucose-lowering effect of metformin in patients with diabetes: A preliminary study. *Diabetes*, *58*(3), 745–749. https://doi.org/10.2337/db08-1028.

Becker, M. L., Visser, L. E., van Schaik, R. H., Hofman, A., Uitterlinden, A. G., & Stricker, B. H. (2009b). Genetic variation in the organic cation transporter 1 is associated with metformin response in patients with diabetes mellitus. *The Pharmacogenomics Journal*, *9*(4), 242–247. https://doi.org/10.1038/tpj.2009.15.

Biernacka, J. M., Sangkuhl, K., Jenkins, G., Whaley, R. M., Barman, P., Batzler, A., et al. (2015). The International SSRI Pharmacogenomics Consortium (ISPC): A genome-wide association study of antidepressant treatment response. *Translational Psychiatry*, *5*, e553. https://doi.org/10.1038/tp.2015.47.

Chasman, D. I., Giulianini, F., MacFadyen, J., Barratt, B. J., Nyberg, F., & Ridker, P. M. (2012). Genetic determinants of statin-induced low-density lipoprotein cholesterol reduction: The Justification for the Use of Statins in Prevention: An Intervention Trial Evaluating Rosuvastatin (JUPITER) trial. *Circulation. Cardiovascular Genetics*, *5*(2), 257–264. https://doi.org/10.1161/circgenetics.111.961144.

Chen, Y., Li, S., Brown, C., Cheatham, S., Castro, R. A., Leabman, M. K., et al. (2009). Effect of genetic variation in the organic cation transporter 2 on the renal elimination of metformin. *Pharmacogenetics and Genomics*, *19*(7), 497–504. https://doi.org/10.1097/FPC.0b013e32832cc7e9.

Choi, J. H., Yee, S. W., Ramirez, A. H., Morrissey, K. M., Jang, G. H., Joski, P. J., et al. (2011). A common 5'-UTR variant in MATE2-K is associated with poor response to metformin. *Clinical Pharmacology and Therapeutics*, *90*(5), 674–684. https://doi.org/10.1038/clpt.2011.165.

Christensen, M. M., Brasch-Andersen, C., Green, H., Nielsen, F., Damkier, P., Beck-Nielsen, H., et al. (2011). The pharmacogenetics of metformin and its impact on plasma metformin steady-state levels and glycosylated hemoglobin A1c. *Pharmacogenetics and Genomics*, *21*(12), 837–850. https://doi.org/10.1097/FPC.0b013e32834c0010.

Connelly, P. J., Smith, N., Chadwick, R., Exley, A. R., Shneerson, J. M., & Pearson, E. R. (2016). Recessive mutations in the cancer gene ataxia telangiectasia mutated (ATM), at a locus previously associated with metformin response, cause dysglycaemia and insulin resistance. *Diabetic Medicine*, *33*(3), 371–375. https://doi.org/10.1111/dme.13037.

Corominas-Faja, B., Quirantes-Pine, R., Oliveras-Ferraros, C., Vazquez-Martin, A., Cufi, S., Martin-Castillo, B., et al. (2012). Metabolomic fingerprint reveals that metformin impairs one-carbon metabolism in a manner similar to the antifolate class of chemotherapy drugs. *Aging (Albany NY)*, *4*(7), 480–498. https://doi.org/10.18632/aging.100472.

Dai, X. P., Huang, Q., Yin, J. Y., Guo, Y., Gong, Z. C., Lei, M. X., et al. (2012). KCNQ1 gene polymorphisms are associated with the therapeutic efficacy of repaglinide in Chinese type 2 diabetic patients. *Clinical and Experimental Pharmacology & Physiology*, *39*(5), 462–468. https://doi.org/10.1111/j.1440-1681.2012.05701.x.

Dawed, A. Y., Donnelly, L., Tavendale, R., Carr, F., Leese, G., Palmer, C. N., et al. (2016). CYP2C8 and SLCO1B1 variants and therapeutic response to thiazolidinediones in patients with type 2 diabetes. *Diabetes Care*, *39*(11), 1902–1908. https://doi.org/10.2337/dc15-2464.

Dujic, T., Zhou, K., Donnelly, L. A., Tavendale, R., Palmer, C. N., & Pearson, E. R. (2015). Association of organic cation transporter 1 with intolerance to metformin in type 2 diabetes: A GoDARTS study. *Diabetes*, *64*(5), 1786–1793. https://doi.org/10.2337/db14-1388.

Dujic, T., Zhou, K., Yee, S. W., van Leeuwen, N., de Keyser, C. E., Javorsky, M., et al. (2017). Variants in pharmacokinetic transporters and glycemic response to metformin: A Metgen meta-analysis. *Clinical Pharmacology and Therapeutics*, *101*(6), 763–772. https://doi.org/10.1002/cpt.567.

Farzan, N., Vijverberg, S. J., Andiappan, A. K., Arianto, L., Berce, V., Blanca-Lopez, N., et al. (2017). Rationale and design of the multiethnic pharmacogenomics in childhood asthma consortium. *Pharmacogenomics*, *18*(10), 931–943. https://doi.org/10.2217/pgs-2017-0035.

Feng, T., Li, L., Ling, S., Fan, N., Fang, M., Zhang, H., et al. (2015). Metformin enhances radiation response of ECa109 cells through activation of ATM and AMPK. *Biomedicine and Pharmacotherapy*, *69*, 260–266. https://doi.org/10.1016/j.biopha.2014.11.021.

Flannick, J., & Florez, J. C. (2016). Type 2 diabetes: Genetic data sharing to advance complex disease research. *Nature Reviews Genetics*, *17*(9), 535–549. https://doi.org/10.1038/nrg.2016.56.

Florez, J. C. (2017). Mining the genome for therapeutic targets. *Diabetes*, *66*(7), 1770–1778. https://doi.org/10.2337/dbi16-0069.

Florez, J. C., Jablonski, K. A., Taylor, A., Mather, K., Horton, E., White, N. H., et al. (2012). The C allele of ATM rs11212617 does not associate with metformin response in the diabetes prevention program. *Diabetes Care*, *35*(9), 1864–1867. https://doi.org/10.2337/dc11-2301.

Foretz, M., Hebrard, S., Leclerc, J., Zarrinpashneh, E., Soty, M., Mithieux, G., et al. (2010). Metformin inhibits hepatic gluconeogenesis in mice independently of the LKB1/AMPK pathway via a decrease in hepatic energy state. *The Journal of Clinical Investigation*, *120*(7), 2355–2369. https://doi.org/10.1172/jci40671.

Foretz, M., & Viollet, B. (2011). Regulation of hepatic metabolism by AMPK. *Journal of Hepatology*, *54*(4), 827–829. https://doi.org/10.1016/j.jhep.2010.09.014.

Francke, S., Mamidi, R. N., Solanki, B., Scheers, E., Jadwin, A., Favis, R., et al. (2015). In vitro metabolism of canagliflozin in human liver, kidney, intestine microsomes, and recombinant uridine diphosphate glucuronosyltransferases (UGT) and the effect of genetic variability of UGT enzymes on the pharmacokinetics of canagliflozin in humans. *Journal of Clinical Pharmacology*, *55*(9), 1061–1072. https://doi.org/10.1002/jcph.506.

Giacomini, K. M., Yee, S. W., Mushiroda, T., Weinshilboum, R. M., Ratain, M. J., & Kubo, M. (2017). Genome-wide association studies of drug response and toxicity: An opportunity for genome medicine. *Nature Reviews Drug Discovery*, *16*(1), 1. https://doi.org/10.1038/nrd.2016.234.

Giovannucci, E., Harlan, D. M., Archer, M. C., Bergenstal, R. M., Gapstur, S. M., Habel, L. A., et al. (2010). Diabetes and cancer: A consensus report. *Diabetes Care*, *33*(7), 1674–1685. https://doi.org/10.2337/dc10-0666.

Gloyn, A. L., Hashim, Y., Ashcroft, S. J., Ashfield, R., Wiltshire, S., & Turner, R. C. (2001). Association studies of variants in promoter and coding regions of beta-cell ATP-sensitive K-channel genes SUR1 and Kir6.2 with type 2 diabetes mellitus (UKPDS 53). *Diabetic Medicine*, *18*(3), 206–212.

Gokalp, O., Gunes, A., Cam, H., Cure, E., Aydin, O., Tamer, M. N., et al. (2011). Mild hypoglycaemic attacks induced by sulphonylureas related to CYP2C9, CYP2C19 and CYP2C8 polymorphisms in routine clinical setting. *European Journal of Clinical Pharmacology*, *67*(12), 1223–1229. https://doi.org/10.1007/s00228-011-1078-4.

Gong, L., Goswami, S., Giacomini, K. M., Altman, R. B., & Klein, T. E. (2012). Metformin pathways: Pharmacokinetics and pharmacodynamics. *Pharmacogenetics and Genomics*, *22*(11), 820–827. https://doi.org/10.1097/FPC.0b013e3283559b22.

Graham, G. G., Punt, J., Arora, M., Day, R. O., Doogue, M. P., Duong, J. K., et al. (2011). Clinical pharmacokinetics of metformin. *Clinical Pharmacokinetics*, *50*(2), 81–98. https://doi.org/10.2165/11534750-000000000-00000.

Grant, S. F., Thorleifsson, G., Reynisdottir, I., Benediktsson, R., Manolescu, A., Sainz, J., et al. (2006). Variant of transcription factor 7-like 2 (TCF7L2) gene confers risk of type 2 diabetes. *Nature Genetics*, *38*(3), 320–323. https://doi.org/10.1038/ng1732.

Han, T. K., Proctor, W. R., Costales, C. L., Cai, H., Everett, R. S., & Thakker, D. R. (2015). Four cation-selective transporters contribute to apical uptake and accumulation of metformin in Caco-2 cell monolayers. *The Journal of Pharmacology and Experimental Therapeutics*, *352*(3), 519–528. https://doi.org/10.1124/jpet.114.220350.

Helgason, A., Palsson, S., Thorleifsson, G., Grant, S. F., Emilsson, V., Gunnarsdottir, S., et al. (2007). Refining the impact of TCF7L2 gene variants on type 2 diabetes and adaptive evolution. *Nature Genetics*, *39*(2), 218–225. https://doi.org/10.1038/ng1960.

Hsieh, M. C., Lin, K. D., Tien, K. J., Tu, S. T., Hsiao, J. Y., Chang, S. J., et al. (2010). Common polymorphisms of the peroxisome proliferator-activated receptor-gamma (Pro12Ala) and peroxisome proliferator-activated receptor-gamma coactivator-1 (Gly482Ser) and the response to pioglitazone in Chinese patients with type 2 diabetes mellitus. *Metabolism*, *59*(8), 1139–1144. https://doi.org/10.1016/j.metabol.2009.10.030.

Hu, C., Wang, C., Zhang, R., Ma, X., Wang, J., Lu, J., et al. (2009). Variations in KCNQ1 are associated with type 2 diabetes and beta cell function in a Chinese population. *Diabetologia*, *52*(7), 1322–1325. https://doi.org/10.1007/s00125-009-1335-6.

Huang, Q., Yin, J. Y., Dai, X. P., Wu, J., Chen, X., Deng, C. S., et al. (2010). Association analysis of SLC30A8 rs13266634 and rs16889462 polymorphisms with type 2 diabetes mellitus and repaglinide response in Chinese patients. *European Journal of Clinical Pharmacology*, *66*(12), 1207–1215. https://doi.org/10.1007/s00228-010-0882-6.

Hundal, R. S., Krssak, M., Dufour, S., Laurent, D., Lebon, V., Chandramouli, V., et al. (2000). Mechanism by which metformin reduces glucose production in type 2 diabetes. *Diabetes*, *49*(12), 2063–2069.

Jablonski, K. A., McAteer, J. B., de Bakker, P. I., Franks, P. W., Pollin, T. I., Hanson, R. L., et al. (2010). Common variants in 40 genes assessed for diabetes incidence and response to metformin and lifestyle intervention in the diabetes prevention program. *Diabetes*, *59*(10), 2672–2681. https://doi.org/10.2337/db10-0543.

Jadhav, K., & Zhang, Y. (2017). Activating transcription factor 3 in immune response and metabolic regulation. *Liver Research*, *1*(2), 96–102. https://doi.org/10.1016/j.livres.2017.08.001.

Jensen, J. B., Sundelin, E. I., Jakobsen, S., Gormsen, L. C., Munk, O. L., Frokiaer, J., et al. (2016). [11C]-Labeled metformin distribution in the liver and small intestine using dynamic positron emission tomography in mice demonstrates tissue-specific transporter dependency. *Diabetes*, *65*(6), 1724–1730. https://doi.org/10.2337/db16-0032.

Kalliokoski, A., Backman, J. T., Neuvonen, P. J., & Niemi, M. (2008). Effects of the SLCO1B1*1B haplotype on the pharmacokinetics and pharmacodynamics of repaglinide and nateglinide. *Pharmacogenetics and Genomics*, *18*(11), 937–942. https://doi.org/10.1097/FPC.0b013e32830d733e.

Kerb, R., Brinkmann, U., Chatskaia, N., Gorbunov, D., Gorboulev, V., Mornhinweg, E., et al. (2002). Identification of genetic variations of the human organic cation transporter hOCT1 and their functional consequences. *Pharmacogenetics*, *12*(8), 591–595.

Kirchheiner, J., Thomas, S., Bauer, S., Tomalik-Scharte, D., Hering, U., Doroshyenko, O., et al. (2006). Pharmacokinetics and pharmacodynamics of rosiglitazone in relation to CYP2C8 genotype. *Clinical Pharmacology and Therapeutics*, *80*(6), 657–667. https://doi.org/10.1016/j.clpt.2006.09.008.

Lamanna, C., Monami, M., Marchionni, N., & Mannucci, E. (2011). Effect of metformin on cardiovascular events and mortality: A meta-analysis of randomized clinical trials. *Diabetes, Obesity & Metabolism*, *13*(3), 221–228. https://doi.org/10.1111/j.1463-1326.2010.01349.x.

Lavrenko, A. V., Shlykova, O. A., Kutsenko, L. A., Mamontova, T. V., & Kaidashev, I. P. (2012). Pharmacogenetic features of the effect of metformin in patients with coronary heart disease in the presence of metabolic syndrome and type 2 diabetes mellitus in terms of PPAR-gamma2 gene polymorphism. *Terapevticheskiĭ Arkhiv*, *84*(9), 35–40.

Leabman, M. K., Huang, C. C., Kawamoto, M., Johns, S. J., Stryke, D., Ferrin, T. E., et al. (2002). Polymorphisms in a human kidney xenobiotic transporter, OCT2, exhibit altered function. *Pharmacogenetics*, *12*(5), 395–405.

Li, Q., Chen, M., Zhang, R., Jiang, F., Wang, J., Zhou, J., et al. (2014). KCNJ11 E23K variant is associated with the therapeutic effect of sulphonylureas in Chinese type 2 diabetic patients. *Clinical and Experimental Pharmacology & Physiology*, *41*(10), 748–754. https://doi.org/10.1111/1440-1681.12280.

Liang, X., Chien, H. C., Yee, S. W., Giacomini, M. M., Chen, E. C., Piao, M., et al. (2015). Metformin is a substrate and inhibitor of the human thiamine transporter, THTR-2 (SLC19A3). *Molecular Pharmaceutics*, *12*(12), 4301–4310. https://doi.org/10.1021/acs.molpharmaceut.5b00501.

Liu, H. L., Lin, Y. G., Wu, J., Sun, H., Gong, Z. C., Hu, P. C., et al. (2008). Impact of genetic polymorphisms of leptin and TNF-alpha on rosiglitazone response in Chinese patients with type 2 diabetes. *European Journal of Clinical Pharmacology*, *64*(7), 663–671. https://doi.org/10.1007/s00228-008-0483-9.

Luizon, M. R., Eckalbar, W. L., Wang, Y., Jones, S. L., Smith, R. P., Laurance, M., et al. (2016). Genomic characterization of metformin hepatic response. *PLoS Genetics*, *12*(11), e1006449. https://doi.org/10.1371/journal.pgen.1006449.

MacArthur, J., Bowler, E., Cerezo, M., Gil, L., Hall, P., Hastings, E., et al. (2017). The new NHGRI-EBI Catalog of published genome-wide association studies (GWAS Catalog). *Nucleic Acids Research*, *45*(D1), D896–D901. https://doi.org/10.1093/nar/gkw1133.

Madiraju, A. K., Erion, D. M., Rahimi, Y., Zhang, X. M., Braddock, D. T., Albright, R. A., et al. (2014). Metformin suppresses gluconeogenesis by inhibiting mitochondrial glycerophosphate dehydrogenase. *Nature*, *510*(7506), 542–546. https://doi.org/10.1038/nature13270.

Marathe, P. H., Gao, H. X., & Close, K. L. (2017). American Diabetes Association standards of medical care in diabetes 2017. *Journal of Diabetes*, *9*(4), 320–324. https://doi.org/10.1111/1753-0407.12524.

Masuda, S., Terada, T., Yonezawa, A., Tanihara, Y., Kishimoto, K., Katsura, T., et al. (2006). Identification and functional characterization of a new human kidney-specific H+/organic cation antiporter, kidney-specific multidrug and toxin extrusion 2. *Journal of the American Society of Nephrology*, *17*(8), 2127–2135. https://doi.org/10.1681/asn.2006030205.

Nathan, D. M., Buse, J. B., Davidson, M. B., Ferrannini, E., Holman, R. R., Sherwin, R., et al. (2009). Medical Management of Hyperglycemia in type 2 diabetes: A consensus algorithm for the initiation and adjustment of therapy: A consensus statement of the American diabetes association and the European association for the study of diabetes. *Diabetes Care*, *32*(1), 193–203. https://doi.org/10.2337/dc08-9025.

Niemi, M., Leathart, J. B., Neuvonen, M., Backman, J. T., Daly, A. K., & Neuvonen, P. J. (2003). Polymorphism in CYP2C8 is associated with reduced plasma concentrations of repaglinide. *Clinical Pharmacology and Therapeutics*, *74*(4), 380–387. https://doi.org/10.1016/s0009-9236(03)00228-5.

Niu, N., Liu, T., Cairns, J., Ly, R. C., Tan, X., Deng, M., et al. (2016). Metformin pharmacogenomics: A genome-wide association study to identify genetic and epigenetic biomarkers involved in metformin anticancer response using human lymphoblastoid cell lines. *Human Molecular Genetics*, *25*(21), 4819–4834. https://doi.org/10.1093/hmg/ddw301.

Otsuka, M., Matsumoto, T., Morimoto, R., Arioka, S., Omote, H., & Moriyama, Y. (2005). A human transporter protein that mediates the final excretion step for toxic organic cations. *Proceedings of the National Academy of Sciences of the United States of America*, *102*(50), 17923–17928. https://doi.org/10.1073/pnas.0506483102.

Pearson, E. R., Donnelly, L. A., Kimber, C., Whitley, A., Doney, A. S., McCarthy, M. I., et al. (2007). Variation in TCF7L2 influences therapeutic response to sulfonylureas: A GoDARTs study. *Diabetes*, *56*(8), 2178–2182. https://doi.org/10.2337/db07-0440.

Pedersen, A. J. T., Stage, T. B., Glintborg, D., Andersen, M., & Christensen, M. M. H. (2018). The pharmacogenetics of metformin in women with polycystic ovary syndrome: A randomized trial. *Basic & Clinical Pharmacology & Toxicology*, *122*(2), 239–244. https://doi.org/10.1111/bcpt.12874.

Rena, G., Pearson, E. R., & Sakamoto, K. (2013). Molecular mechanism of action of metformin: Old or new insights? *Diabetologia*, *56*(9), 1898–1906. https://doi.org/10.1007/s00125-013-2991-0.

Sakata, T., Anzai, N., Shin, H. J., Noshiro, R., Hirata, T., Yokoyama, H., et al. (2004). Novel single nucleotide polymorphisms of organic cation transporter 1 (SLC22A1) affecting transport functions. *Biochemical and Biophysical Research Communications*, *313*(3), 789–793.

Schroner, Z., Dobrikova, M., Klimcakova, L., Javorsky, M., Zidzik, J., Kozarova, M., et al. (2011). Variation in KCNQ1 is associated with therapeutic response to sulphonylureas. *Medical Science Monitor*, *17*(7), Cr392–Cr396.

Schulze, T. G., Alda, M., Adli, M., Akula, N., Ardau, R., Bui, E. T., et al. (2010). The international consortium on lithium genetics (ConLiGen): An initiative by the NIMH and IGSLI to study the genetic basis of response to lithium treatment. *Neuropsychobiology*, *62*(1), 72–78. https://doi.org/10.1159/000314708.

Semiz, S., Dujic, T., & Causevic, A. (2013). Pharmacogenetics and personalized treatment of type 2 diabetes. *Biochemia Medica (Zagreb)*, *23*(2), 154–171.

Seyer, P., Vallois, D., Poitry-Yamate, C., Schutz, F., Metref, S., Tarussio, D., et al. (2013). Hepatic glucose sensing is required to preserve beta cell glucose competence. *The Journal of Clinical Investigation*, *123*(4), 1662–1676. https://doi.org/10.1172/jci65538.

Shao, H., Ren, X. M., Liu, N. F., Chen, G. M., Li, W. L., Zhai, Z. H., et al. (2010). Influence of CYP2C9 and CYP2C19 genetic polymorphisms on pharmacokinetics and pharmacodynamics of gliclazide in healthy Chinese Han volunteers. *Journal of Clinical Pharmacy and Therapeutics*, *35*(3), 351–360. https://doi.org/10.1111/j.1365-2710.2009.01134.x.

Shokri, F., Ghaedi, H., Ghafouri Fard, S., Movafagh, A., Abediankenari, S., Mahrooz, A., et al. (2016). Impact of ATM and SLC22A1 polymorphisms on therapeutic response to metformin in Iranian diabetic patients. *International Journal of Molecular and Cellular Medicine*, *5*(1), 1–7.

Shu, Y., Brown, C., Castro, R. A., Shi, R. J., Lin, E. T., Owen, R. P., et al. (2008). Effect of genetic variation in the organic cation transporter 1, OCT1, on metformin pharmacokinetics. *Clinical Pharmacology and Therapeutics*, *83*(2), 273–280. https://doi.org/10.1038/sj.clpt.6100275.

Shu, Y., Leabman, M. K., Feng, B., Mangravite, L. M., Huang, C. C., Stryke, D., et al. (2003). Evolutionary conservation predicts function of variants of the human organic cation transporter, OCT1. *Proceedings of the National Academy of Sciences of the United States of America*, *100*(10), 5902–5907. https://doi.org/10.1073/pnas.0730858100.

Shu, Y., Sheardown, S. A., Brown, C., Owen, R. P., Zhang, S., Castro, R. A., et al. (2007). Effect of genetic variation in the organic cation transporter 1 (OCT1) on metformin action. *The Journal of Clinical Investigation*, *117*(5), 1422–1431. https://doi.org/10.1172/jci30558.

Snima, K. S., Pillai, P., Cherian, A. M., Nair, S. V., & Lakshmanan, V. K. (2014). Antidiabetic drug metformin: Challenges and perspectives for cancer therapy. *Current Cancer Drug Targets*, *14*(8), 727–736.

Song, I. S., Shin, H. J., Shim, E. J., Jung, I. S., Kim, W. Y., Shon, J. H., et al. (2008). Genetic variants of the organic cation transporter 2 influence the disposition of metformin. *Clinical Pharmacology and Therapeutics*, *84*(5), 559–562. https://doi.org/10.1038/clpt.2008.61.

Srinivasan, S., Kaur, V., Chamarthi, B., Littleton, K. R., Chen, L., Manning, A. K., et al. (2018). TCF7L2 genetic variation augments incretin resistance and influences response to a sulfonylurea and metformin: The study to understand the genetics of the acute response to metformin and glipizide in humans (SUGAR-MGH). *Diabetes Care*, *41*(3), 554–561. https://doi.org/10.2337/dc17-1386.

Stocker, S. L., Morrissey, K. M., Yee, S. W., Castro, R. A., Xu, L., Dahlin, A., et al. (2013). The effect of novel promoter variants in MATE1 and MATE2 on the pharmacokinetics and pharmacodynamics of metformin. *Clinical Pharmacology and Therapeutics*, *93*(2), 186–194. https://doi.org/10.1038/clpt.2012.210.

Storozhuk, Y., Hopmans, S. N., Sanli, T., Barron, C., Tsiani, E., Cutz, J. C., et al. (2013). Metformin inhibits growth and enhances radiation response of non-small cell lung cancer (NSCLC) through ATM and AMPK. *British Journal of Cancer*, *108*(10), 2021–2032. https://doi.org/10.1038/bjc.2013.187.

Sun, H., Gong, Z. C., Yin, J. Y., Liu, H. L., Liu, Y. Z., Guo, Z. W., et al. (2008). The association of adiponectin allele 45T/G and -11377C/G polymorphisms with type 2 diabetes and rosiglitazone response in Chinese patients. *British Journal of Clinical Pharmacology*, *65*(6), 917–926. https://doi.org/10.1111/j.1365-2125.2008.03145.x.

Sundelin, E., Gormsen, L. C., Jensen, J. B., Vendelbo, M. H., Jakobsen, S., Munk, O. L., et al. (2017). Genetic polymorphisms in organic cation transporter 1 attenuates hepatic metformin exposure in humans. *Clinical Pharmacology and Therapeutics*, *102*(5), 841–848. https://doi.org/10.1002/cpt.701.

Takane, H., Shikata, E., Otsubo, K., Higuchi, S., & Ieiri, I. (2008). Polymorphism in human organic cation transporters and metformin action. *Pharmacogenomics*, *9*(4), 415–422. https://doi.org/10.2217/14622416.9.4.415.

Tanihara, Y., Masuda, S., Sato, T., Katsura, T., Ogawa, O., & Inui, K. (2007). Substrate specificity of MATE1 and MATE2-K, human multidrug and toxin extrusions/H(+)-organic cation antiporters. *Biochemical Pharmacology*, *74*(2), 359–371. https://doi.org/10.1016/j.bcp.2007.04.010.

Thule, P. M., & Umpierrez, G. (2014). Sulfonylureas: A new look at old therapy. *Current Diabetes Reports*, *14*(4), 473. https://doi.org/10.1007/s11892-014-0473-5.

Tkac, I., Klimcakova, L., Javorsky, M., Fabianova, M., Schroner, Z., Hermanova, H., et al. (2013). Pharmacogenomic association between a variant in SLC47A1 gene and therapeutic response to metformin in type 2 diabetes. *Diabetes, Obesity & Metabolism*, *15*(2), 189–191. https://doi.org/10.1111/j.1463-1326.2012.01691.x.

Tzvetkov, M. V., Vormfelde, S. V., Balen, D., Meineke, I., Schmidt, T., Sehrt, D., et al. (2009). The effects of genetic polymorphisms in the organic cation transporters OCT1, OCT2, and OCT3 on the renal clearance of metformin. *Clinical Pharmacology and Therapeutics*, *86*(3), 299–306. https://doi.org/10.1038/clpt.2009.92.

Urban, T. J., Nicoletti, P., Chalasani, N., Serrano, J., Stolz, A., Daly, A. K., et al. (2017). Minocycline hepatotoxicity: Clinical characterization and identification of HLA-B *35:02 as a risk factor. *Journal of Hepatology*, *67*(1), 137–144. https://doi.org/10.1016/j.jhep.2017.03.010.

van Leeuwen, N., Nijpels, G., Becker, M. L., Deshmukh, H., Zhou, K., Stricker, B. H., et al. (2012). A gene variant near ATM is significantly associated with metformin treatment response in type 2 diabetes: A replication and meta-analysis of five cohorts. *Diabetologia*, *55*(7), 1971–1977. https://doi.org/10.1007/s00125-012-2537-x.

Vazquez-Martin, A., Oliveras-Ferraros, C., Cufi, S., Martin-Castillo, B., & Menendez, J. A. (2011). Metformin activates an ataxia telangiectasia mutated (ATM)/Chk2-regulated DNA damage-like response. *Cell Cycle*, *10*(9), 1499–1501. https://doi.org/10.4161/cc.10.9.15423.

Wang, Z. J., Yin, O. Q., Tomlinson, B., & Chow, M. S. (2008). OCT2 polymorphisms and in-vivo renal functional consequence: Studies with metformin and cimetidine. *Pharmacogenetics and Genomics*, *18*(7), 637–645. https://doi.org/10.1097/FPC.0b013e328302cd41.

Woods, A., Leiper, J. M., & Carling, D. (2012). The role of ATM in response to metformin treatment and activation of AMPK. *Nature Genetics*, *44*(4), 360–361. https://doi.org/10.1038/ng.2235.

Yee, S. W., Chen, L., & Giacomini, K. M. (2012). The role of ATM in response to metformin treatment and activation of AMPK. *Nature Genetics*, *44*(4), 359–360. https://doi.org/10.1038/ng.2236.

Yu, W., Hu, C., Zhang, R., Wang, C., Qin, W., Lu, J., et al. (2011). Effects of KCNQ1 polymorphisms on the therapeutic efficacy of oral antidiabetic drugs in Chinese patients with type 2 diabetes. *Clinical Pharmacology and Therapeutics*, *89*(3), 437–442. https://doi.org/10.1038/clpt.2010.351.

Yu, M., Xu, X. J., Yin, J. Y., Wu, J., Chen, X., Gong, Z. C., et al. (2010). KCNJ11 Lys23Glu and TCF7L2 rs290487(C/T) polymorphisms affect therapeutic efficacy of repaglinide in Chinese patients with type 2 diabetes. *Clinical Pharmacology and Therapeutics*, *87*(3), 330–335. https://doi.org/10.1038/clpt.2009.242.

Zhang, H., Liu, X., Kuang, H., Yi, R., & Xing, H. (2007). Association of sulfonylurea receptor 1 genotype with therapeutic response to gliclazide in type 2 diabetes. *Diabetes Research and Clinical Practice*, 77(1), 58–61. https://doi.org/10.1016/j.diabres.2006.10.021.

Zhang, Y., Si, D., Chen, X., Lin, N., Guo, Y., Zhou, H., et al. (2007). Influence of CYP2C9 and CYP2C19 genetic polymorphisms on pharmacokinetics of gliclazide MR in Chinese subjects. *British Journal of Clinical Pharmacology*, *64*(1), 67–74. https://doi.org/10.1111/j.1365-2125.2007.02846.x.

Zhou, K., Bellenguez, C., Spencer, C. C., Bennett, A. J., Coleman, R. L., Tavendale, R., et al. (2011). Common variants near ATM are associated with glycemic response to metformin in type 2 diabetes. *Nature Genetics*, *43*(2), 117–120. https://doi.org/10.1038/ng.735.

Zhou, K., Donnelly, L., Burch, L., Tavendale, R., Doney, A. S., Leese, G., et al. (2010). Loss-of-function CYP2C9 variants improve therapeutic response to sulfonylureas in type 2 diabetes: A go-DARTS study. *Clinical Pharmacology and Therapeutics*, *87*(1), 52–56. https://doi.org/10.1038/clpt.2009.176.

Zhou, K., Donnelly, L. A., Kimber, C. H., Donnan, P. T., Doney, A. S., Leese, G., et al. (2009). Reduced-function SLC22A1 polymorphisms encoding organic cation transporter 1 and glycemic response to metformin: A GoDARTS study. *Diabetes*, *58*(6), 1434–1439. https://doi.org/10.2337/db08-0896.

Zhou, Y., Guo, Y., Ye, W., Wang, Y., Li, X., Tian, Y., et al. (2014). RS11212617 is associated with metformin treatment response in type 2 diabetes in Shanghai local Chinese population. *International Journal of Clinical Practice*, *68*(12), 1462–1466. https://doi.org/10.1111/ijcp.12534.

Zhou, G., Myers, R., Li, Y., Chen, Y., Shen, X., Fenyk-Melody, J., et al. (2001). Role of AMP-activated protein kinase in mechanism of metformin action. *The Journal of Clinical Investigation*, *108*(8), 1167–1174. https://doi.org/10.1172/jci13505.

Zhou, M., Xia, L., & Wang, J. (2007). Metformin transport by a newly cloned proton-stimulated organic cation transporter (plasma membrane monoamine transporter) expressed in human intestine. *Drug Metabolism and Disposition*, *35*(10), 1956–1962. https://doi.org/10.1124/dmd.107.015495.

Zhou, K., Yee, S. W., Seiser, E. L., van Leeuwen, N., Tavendale, R., Bennett, A. J., et al. (2016). Variation in the glucose transporter gene SLC2A2 is associated with glycemic response to metformin. *Nature Genetics*, *48*(9), 1055–1059. https://doi.org/10.1038/ng.3632.

Zimdahl, H., Haupt, A., Brendel, M., Bour, L., Machicao, F., Salsali, A., et al. (2017). Influence of common polymorphisms in the SLC5A2 gene on metabolic traits in subjects at increased risk of diabetes and on response to empagliflozin treatment in patients with diabetes. *Pharmacogenetics and Genomics*, *27*(4), 135–142. https://doi.org/10.1097/fpc.0000000000000268.

Zimdahl, H., Ittrich, C., Graefe-Mody, U., Boehm, B. O., Mark, M., Woerle, H. J., et al. (2014). Influence of TCF7L2 gene variants on the therapeutic response to the dipeptidylpeptidase-4 inhibitor linagliptin. *Diabetologia*, *57*(9), 1869–1875. https://doi.org/10.1007/s00125-014-3276-y.

Kolibri 360 GmbH
Ferdinand-Jühlke-Straße 7
99095 Erfurt, Deutschland
produktsicherheit@kolibri360.de